Dietary Supplements and Functional Foods

T0369681

Dietary Supplements and Functional Foods

Second Edition

Geoffrey P. Webb
Senior Lecturer in Nutrition and Physiology
University of East London
School of Health and Bioscience

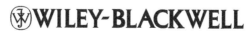

A John Wiley & Sons, Ltd., Publication

This edition first published 2011
© 2011 and 2006 Blackwell Publishing Ltd

Blackwell Publishing was acquired by John Wiley & Sons in February 2007. Blackwell's publishing program has been merged with Wiley's global Scientific, Technical and Medical business to form Wiley-Blackwell.

Registered Office
John Wiley & Sons Ltd, The Atrium, Southern Gate, Chichester, West Sussex, PO19 8SQ, UK

Editorial Offices
9600 Garsington Road, Oxford, OX4 2DQ, UK
The Atrium, Southern Gate, Chichester, West Sussex, PO19 8SQ, UK
2121 State Avenue, Ames, Iowa 50014-8300, USA

For details of our global editorial offices, for customer services and for information about how to apply for permission to reuse the copyright material in this book please see our website at www.wiley.com/wiley-blackwell.

Library of Congress Cataloging-in-Publication Data

Webb, Geoffrey P.
  Dietary supplements and functional foods / Geoffrey P. Webb. – 2nd ed.
      p. ; cm.
  Includes bibliographical references and index.
  ISBN 978-1-4443-3240-7 (pbk. : alk. paper)
1. Dietary supplements. 2. Functional foods. I. Title.
  [DNLM: 1. Dietary Supplements. 2. Functional Food. QU 145.5]
  RM258.5.W43 2011
  615′.1–dc22
                                                    2010040968

A catalogue record for this book is available from the British Library.

This book is published in the following electronic formats: ePDF 9781444340068; ePub 9781444340075

Set in 10/12pt Sabon by SPi Publisher Services, Pondicherry, India

1 2011

Contents

Preface

In the preface to the first edition of this book, I stated that one of my major objectives was to give order and structure to the topic of dietary supplements and functional foods. Hundreds of substances are marketed as dietary supplements and so one approach would have been to select a number of the most popular substances, arrange them alphabetically and then discuss each of them separately, perhaps using a series of common subheadings. Mason (2007) had already used this approach in the first edition of her very useful reference book on supplements, so rather than produce a similar competing book, I tried to structure this book in the way one might organise the syllabus and teaching for an undergraduate module: emphasising common themes, logical groupings and general principles and concepts.

As with an undergraduate module, I have started with an overview of the topic: the types and uses of supplements, the extent of usage, potential hazards of taking supplements, the legal regulation of supplements and a thorough review of the sources of information and the scientific methods used to determine their effectiveness and safety. An understanding of the methodology used in their assessment is essential not only for those considering a research project in this area, but also to anyone who wants to read and evaluate the scientific literature.

The traditional motivation for using supplements was to ensure adequacy of essential micronutrients. In Chapter 2 there is an assessment of the extent to which one can assume adequacy in industrialised countries and the numbers and types of people for whom this assumption of adequacy would be misplaced. For non-nutritionists this chapter also includes an overview of how the adequacy of micronutrient intakes is defined and measured and how micronutrient status can be assessed.

Chapters 3, 4 and 6 deal with individual micronutrients, the vitamins and minerals, and also with natural oils that are sources of essential fatty acids. Since 2004, there has been a lot of published research relating to vitamin D. This research relates not only to its importance in maintaining bone health, but also to its effects outside of bone and emerging evidence linking low vitamin D status to conditions like diabetes, multiple sclerosis and hypertension; the expanded section on vitamin D reflects this new focus. When I wrote the first edition, I was confident that mandatory fortification of flour in the UK with folic acid was imminent; this has not happened and in Chapter 3, I discuss at length why the authorities have delayed introducing this measure. In the section on fish oils in Chapter 6, I include a new section dealing with claims that these supplements might affect mood, attention and behaviour, especially in children. Much media attention has been given to studies that claim to show benefits for fish oil supplements in schoolchildren, but my literature search suggests that there is almost no proper scientific research into this claim.

As in the first edition, Chapter 5 deals with antioxidants and the oxidant theory of disease. Although substances with antioxidant activity are in all categories of supplements, I took the decision in 2004 to deal with them together as a separate grouping. A large proportion of the news reports about the benefits of 'superfoods' and supplements relate to their antioxidant effects and there is a general assumption that antioxidants are good for us and that large intakes will help in preventing and treating disease; observational evidence also tends to support this view. However, I noted in the first edition that the evidence that large supplemental intakes actually confer long-term health benefits is not supported by the results of clinical trials, and that most of the supposed long-term benefits are extrapolated from short-term, reductionist studies. In 2004, I considered this scepticism to be a minority view, but in its consideration of 'health claims' for particular foods or ingredients, the European Food Standards Agency has recently given a negative opinion about antioxidant claims, because there is a lack of evidence of real physiological benefit associated with improvements in measures of oxidant stress or antioxidant status.

As in the first edition, Chapter 7 deals with a number of organic substances that are mostly natural metabolites with vitamin-like functions. These are not considered essential nutrients, because endogenous synthesis is thought to be sufficient to meet our physiological needs for them. The rationale for taking these substances as supplements is the belief that in some people or in some circumstances (for example disease) endogenous synthesis is not sufficient for optimal functioning, or that supplemental intakes may prevent or ameliorate disease.

Chapter 8 deals mainly with plant extracts that have been sold as food supplements. Although some of these substances are derived from accepted foods, others would be from plants that would not be recognised as mainstream foods in the UK. One major difficulty I have had in writing this new edition has been to decide if and how the EU Traditional Herbal Medicinal Products Directive might (in April 2011) affect the availability of these substances when sold over the counter as food supplements. My understanding from discussions with the FSA and the MHRA is that four of the substances singled out for discussion in this chapter (Agnus castus, Echinacea, milk thistle and St John's wort) need to be sold as registered traditional medicines rather than as food supplements. It seems probable that extracts of these herbs will continue to be available for sale over the counter, but only those produced by authorised manufacturers will be available from sources within the EU. It is the bio-activity of secondary metabolites in these plant extracts that is the basis for believing that they might have beneficial effects when taken as supplements. There are many tens of thousands of these secondary metabolites but, in line with my objective of trying to give order and structure, I have made the point that they can be divided into a small number of categories of substances with common structural features, characteristics and synthetic origins within plants.

The final chapter deals with functional foods. The sales growth of functional foods is outstripping growth in the total food market and probably taking some market share from the food supplement market, which has been growing only slowly in recent years. The list of substances sold as supplements has grown and is expanding, so I considered adding extra substances to my list of extracts in Chapter 8. Many of these new supplements are extracts of ordinary or exotic foods that are claimed to have particularly high levels of particular nutrients or other substances like antioxidants, and these have been termed 'superfoods'. All of the substances that I considered adding to my list of natural extracts are extracts of one of these superfoods and so, rather than discuss them individually, I have added a short section on superfoods to Chapter 9.

1 An Overview of Dietary Supplements and Functional Foods

The evolving rationale for supplement use

Adequacy and the prevention of deficiency diseases

Traditionally, dietary supplements like cod liver oil, iron tablets and multivitamins were taken to ensure the adequacy of our diet: that it contained enough essential nutrients to prevent overt deficiency disease and that we did not suffer other, more subtle adverse effects of marginal nutrient inadequacy. While this remains an important motivation for many people, others now also take supplements in the hope that they will have additional health benefits, for example:

- To reduce the risk of developing a chronic age-related disease such as cancer, heart disease, osteoporosis or type 2 diabetes.
- To compensate for some (perceived) individual idiosyncrasy that may increase the requirement for an accepted nutrient or make another substance an essential nutrient for that person.
- To 'boost the immune system'.
- To treat or lessen the symptoms of a non-deficiency disease such as clinical depression or arthritis.
- To boost intake during periods of (perceived) increase in requirement, such as in pregnancy, illness or old age.
- To boost athletic performance.

One ironic consequence of these new circumstances is that the high levels of vitamin A and D in cod liver oil, the traditional reason for taking it, may actually be seen as a disadvantage. These vitamins are toxic in excess and may prevent us from safely taking large doses of the essential polyunsaturated fats that are now regarded as the most important active ingredients of fish and fish liver oils (see Chapter 6).

During the first half of the twentieth century it was found that certain foods and essential nutrients extracted from these foods could prevent or cure several common, serious and frequently fatal diseases, such as those listed below:

Dietary Supplements and Functional Foods, 2nd Edition. Geoffrey P. Webb.
© 2011 Blackwell Publishing Ltd.

- Vitamin C cures scurvy, a frequently fatal disease experienced by those undertaking long voyages by sail or expeditions where they were required to live for long periods without access to fruit or vegetables. It is characterised by bleeding gums, excessive bruising and a tendency to haemorrhage internally.
- Niacin (vitamin B$_3$) cures pellagra, a fatal disease that is associated with a subsistence diet composed largely of maize. It is characterised by the '4 Ds': diarrhoea, dermatitis, dementia and ultimately death.
- Thiamin (vitamin B$_1$) cures beriberi, another potentially fatal disease that is associated with a diet heavily dependent on polished (white) rice. It is characterised by degeneration of sensory and motor nerves, loss of peripheral sensation, paralysis, brain damage, oedema and heart failure.
- Iodine supplements cure goitre and the iodine deficiency diseases, which are still endemic in many areas where the soil iodine content is low. They are characterised by low metabolic rate and mental deterioration in adults (myxoedema), severe and irreversible impairment of mental and physical development in children (cretinism), as well as high risk of miscarriage, stillbirth and birth defects.
- Vitamin D cures rickets, a disease once prevalent among children in the northern industrialised cities of Europe due to a combination of poor diet and low exposure of the skin to summer sunlight. Rickets leads to characteristic abnormalities in the skeleton like bow legs (which may not be entirely reversible), as well as poor growth, muscle weakness and high susceptibility to infection.
- Vitamin A prevents and 'cures' xerophthalmia, in which there is progressive deterioration of the eyes leading ultimately to permanent and irreversible blindness. Vitamin A deficiency also increases susceptibility to, and death from, infectious diseases. Deficiency occurs in populations subsisting largely on starchy foods who eat practically no animal fats and few green or brightly coloured fruits or vegetables.

Some of these diseases are still very prevalent in some parts of the world. Vitamin A deficiency causes hundreds of thousands of children in the Third World to go blind each year and is a major contributory factor in the high child and infant mortality seen in some countries. Iodine deficiency and goitre still affect hundreds of millions of people globally and iodine deficiency is the world's most common preventable cause of mental deficiency in children.

Most us who now live in one of the wealthy industrialised countries will probably have had no direct experience of any of the classic dietary deficiency diseases, with the exception of iron-deficiency anaemia. This was not true in the nineteenth century and the first half of the twentieth century, when these diseases were not merely confined to developing countries but some, like the examples below, were prevalent even in countries that are now part of the industrialised world.

- Pellagra (niacin deficiency) caused tens of thousands of deaths in the southern states of the USA in the early twentieth century and epidemics also occurred in parts of southern Europe where maize was adopted as a staple food.

- In the first decades of the twentieth century, beriberi (thiamin deficiency) exacted a heavy toll in the countries of the Far East like Japan and the Philippines where white rice was the dietary staple.
- Also in the early decades of the twentieth century, the majority of children from poor families living in the northern industrialised cities of Britain would have been affected by rickets (vitamin D deficiency).
- Goitre (iodine deficiency) was once common in the states bordering the Great Lakes in the USA and in the Cotswolds and Peak District in England.

As their dietary origins were unravelled, so it became common knowledge that simple dietary changes could prevent and cure these serious and frequently fatal diseases. As the active components of the diet were identified and purified, they were found to be equally effective when taken as supplements in the form of pills or potions. The major impact of these studies is illustrated by the observation that between 1929 and 1943, eleven people shared seven Nobel prizes (Physiology/Medicine/Chemistry) for vitamin-related work. Clear evidence that dietary changes or supplements of substances found in food could dramatically cure several very common serious and often fatal diseases has probably left a 'legacy of expectation' that perhaps dietary cures might work for other serious diseases. The dramatic and demonstrable benefits of taking small amounts of these nutrient supplements would surely have encouraged the use of larger supplements to 'optimise' intakes and perhaps prevent other, more subtle adverse effects of deficiency. Dietary supplements were thus proven to have major benefits for some people and might be a useful safety net for anyone concerned about the adequacy of their own or their family's diet.

The notion of widespread use of dietary supplements was born. It was reinforced by scientific advisers who persuaded governments to fortify common foods with extra vitamins and minerals, which seemingly gave official confirmation that ordinary food could not guarantee nutrient adequacy. For example, the British government made it mandatory to fortify white bread and flour with iron, calcium and some B vitamins and to fortify margarine with added vitamins A and D.

Diet as a means to prevent chronic, age and wealth-related diseases

In the latter decades of the twentieth century, the nutritional focus, and the health focus generally, changed in industrialised countries. As affluence increased, so the focus shifted away from the problems associated with poverty and deprivation, such as infectious and deficiency diseases, towards the chronic diseases that afflict middle-aged and elderly people in affluent populations: diseases like cancer, heart disease, diabetes and osteoporosis. These chronic diseases now cause most of the deaths and chronic ill-health in these long-lived populations. The reasons for this change of emphasis are illustrated by the British mortality statistics listed below.

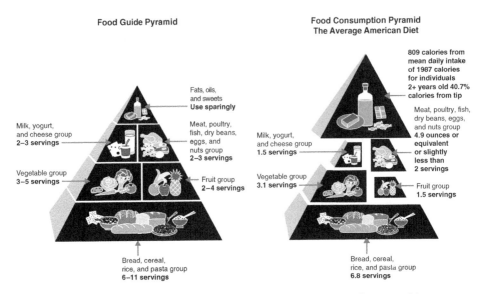

Figure 1.1   The American food guide pyramid and the food consumption pyramid (what Americans really eat).

In Britain in 1901:

- Average life expectancy was only around 47 years.
- Less than half of people lived to see their 65th birthday.
- A fifth of all deaths were due to infectious diseases.
- Less than a quarter of deaths were due to cancer and heart disease combined.

A hundred years later:

- Average life expectancy had increased by about 30 years.
- Most people lived beyond their 65th year.
- Only around 1 in 200 of all deaths was due to infection.
- Three-quarters of all deaths were due to cancer and cardiovascular diseases.

Dietary advice and guidelines are today aimed not only at ensuring adequacy and preventing deficiency, but also at preventing or delaying the onset of these 'diseases of industrialisation' or 'diseases of longevity'. Most nutritionists and dieticians would agree that such a 'prudent' diet should be built around starchy staples such as potatoes, bread and other cereals. It should have substantial amounts of fruit and vegetables (at least five portions a day), moderate amounts of lean meat, fish and low-fat dairy produce (or vegetarian alternatives), with only sparing use of sugary and fatty foods. This diet is visually represented in the USA by a 'food guide pyramid' (Figure 1.1) and in Britain by a 'food guide plate' (Figure 1.2).

This is not the diet that most affluent people choose to eat when guided merely by preference and convenience. Fats and sugars improve the palatability of foods,

Fruit and vegetables
Choose a wide variety

Bread, other cereals and potatoes
Eat all types and choose high fibre
kinds whenever you can

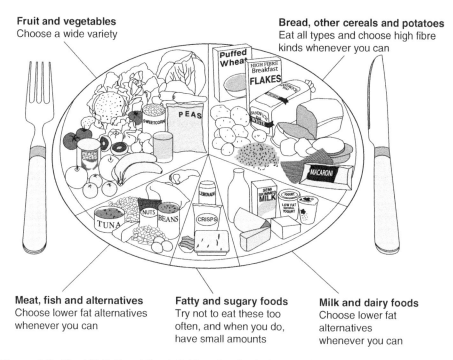

Meat, fish and alternatives
Choose lower fat alternatives
whenever you can

Fatty and sugary foods
Try not to eat these too
often, and when you do,
have small amounts

Milk and dairy foods
Choose lower fat
alternatives
whenever you can

Figure 1.2   The UK National Food Guide – the tilted plate model.
Source: Redrawn with permission from the Food Standards Agency, London.

whereas starchy foods are essentially bland, so as populations become more affluent and the economic and supply constraints on food selection are loosened, people
tend to replace much of the starchy food in their diet with more expensive and
more palatable foods. They tend to choose diets that are rich in fat and sugar but
low in starch. In a poor population in a Third World country, starch may provide
three-quarters of the daily calories, whereas in Britain and the USA it provides only
around a quarter of calories. Increasing affluence and industrialisation generally
lead to a sharp decline in the consumption of cereals and potatoes but increased
consumption of meat, dairy foods, sugar and sugary products, as well as fats and
oils. Figure 1.1 also shows in 'food guide pyramid' form what the diet that
Americans (and Britons) actually choose to eat is like.

Supplements versus dietary change for the prevention
of chronic disease

It is sometimes argued that health promotion and dietary guidelines are pointless,
because people ignore advice about diet and healthy eating. This does not seem to
be consistent with the health-driven changes in the British diet that have occurred
in the last few decades. Despite their preferences, many people have been prepared to make major changes in their diet in order to try to improve their weight

Table 1.1 Health driven changes in the British diet in the last quarter of the twentieth century

- Butter has decreased from around 70% of the 'yellow fat' market to around 25%
- Low-fat spreads have risen from zero to capture over half the yellow fat market
- Vegetable oil has increased from less than a quarter of the cooking fat market to more than three-quarters
- Animal fats have reduced from over three-quarters of the cooking fat market to under a quarter
- Low-fat milk (skimmed and semi-skimmed) has risen from almost zero to around two-thirds of milk sales
- Low-calorie soft drinks have risen from very little to capture over 20% of the soft drink market
- Sales of sugar per se have decreased by around two-thirds
- Sales of wholemeal bread have risen from very small to almost a fifth of bread sales
- Around a third of men and half of women take some dietary supplements

control and long-term health prospects. Some aspects of the typical British and American diet have been totally transformed by health promotion. Table 1.1 charts some of these health-driven dietary changes in Britain in the last 25 years of the twentieth century.

Most people are nowadays aware that deficiency diseases can be cured, and adequate intakes of essential nutrients assured, by taking purified nutrients either as supplements or in fortified foods. By analogy, perhaps some of the benefits of the modern recommended diet could be obtained by taking supplements that contain the active ingredients of foods that may help to prevent diseases like cancer, heart disease and osteoporosis. This would allow us to eat our preferred 'unhealthy', fat- and sugar-rich diet, but still enjoy at least some of the health benefits of eating a more prudent diet. Most of the dietary changes listed in Table 1.1 involve simple substitution of a traditional and perhaps preferred product for a similar product that is perceived to be healthier or less fattening. Many people are prepared to make these relatively simple and 'painless' substitutions for health reasons, but may be less willing to make more complex and far-reaching structural changes to their diet.

'Popping a pill' or buying a modified functional food could be seen as the ultimate example of this willingness to make changes that are easy, convenient and 'painless'. For example:

- Instead of eating five daily portions of antioxidant-rich fruit and vegetables, we could take the substances that have antioxidant properties in pill form.
- Rather than eating one or two portions of oily fish each week, we could swallow capsules containing fish oil.
- Rather than eating foods naturally rich in dietary fibre, we could sprinkle wheat bran on to our preferred low-fibre foods or buy a fibre-enriched breakfast cereal.
- Rather than eating a diet that is low in saturated fat and cholesterol to lower our blood cholesterol, we could spread on to our bread margarine containing a plant sterol that reduces blood cholesterol concentration by interfering with cholesterol absorption.

Dietary supplements and natural remedies as a safer alternative to modern medicine?

In recent decades, major scientific and engineering advances have led to the increasing development of expensive, high-technology medical and surgical procedures and drug therapies. Paradoxically, recent decades have also seen increased numbers of people turning to alternative medical therapies, which often have little or no formal scientific basis and may be based on traditional folk medicine or on theories put forward before the explosive growth of scientific knowledge in the twentieth century. Many alternative therapies stress the importance of a 'good diet' in maintaining and restoring health. The perceived 'naturalness' of many of these therapies contrasts sharply with the high-technology image of modern medicine. The media provide us with an endless stream of stories about iatrogenic (physician-induced) problems that may undermine confidence in the safety of modern medicine. Stories abound about medical accidents, untoward side-effects of common treatments, hospital-acquired infections and patients being infected by infected health workers, surgical instruments or contaminated therapeutic products.

In these circumstances, people may see diet therapy, dietary supplements and non-invasive alternative therapies as a safer, less technological and more natural way of maintaining health and treating illness. If something is naturally present in the diet and is perhaps even an essential nutrient, then surely it must be safer to take than an artificially manufactured or genetically engineered drug? Self-selected supplements or alternative therapies also allow people to play a more active role in their own health management, rather than always having to be purely passive recipients of whatever treatment the health 'expert' decides to administer. These alternatives may be seen as empowering the individual patient/consumer and shifting the locus of control away from the medical establishment.

People may also turn to these alternatives when orthodox medicines or surgery 'fails'. Despite the undoubted advances in conventional medical and surgical therapy, it still has limits; many of the fatal or chronic disabling conditions that are responsible for most deaths and disability are, by definition, still incurable.

It would be unwise to assume that high doses of purified nutrients, food extracts or herbal products are always harmless. Overdoses of several nutrients, for example vitamins A and D and iron, have well-known toxic and potentially fatal effects. Indeed, iron poisoning is the most common cause of accidental poisoning in children. It is also believed that there may be adverse long-term consequences associated with other supplements. For example, large β-carotene supplements taken to prevent cancer and heart disease may actually accelerate the development of these conditions in some groups (see Chapter 5). Many common foods contain natural toxicants and these may become hazardous if unusually large amounts or concentrated extracts of a food are consumed regularly. Many conventional medicines are derived from substances present in plants that may be harmful in excess, and some potent poisons are also of plant origin (for a list of examples, see the section on alkaloids in Chapter 8).

In this book, I will look at the suggested effects of particular supplements and any scientific rationale for these effects, and offer an overview of the evidence of their effectiveness. I will also deal with safety issues and any evidence of harmful effects. If supplements really do have the potential to improve health and alleviate illness, then it would be illogical not to consider that they also have the potential to do harm.

Defining dietary supplements

Almost anything that is swallowed in pill or potion form that is not a licensed medicine has by default been legally classified as a dietary or food supplement in the UK and the USA. Many substances that have origins in herbal or traditional medicine are currently (2010) sold as food supplements in order to avoid the expense of getting approval as a licensed medicine. Before a medicinal licence is granted by the Medicines and Healthcare Products Regulatory Authority (MHRA) in the UK, the Authority must receive satisfactory evidence of the product's safety and efficacy. There is the real possibility that despite huge financial investment by the applicant, the application will be rejected.

The definitions of dietary supplements and functional foods in this section will determine the scope of the book. If one took the broadest definitions of dietary supplements and functional foods, then the scope of this book would be impossibly large. For example, dietary supplements could include food preparations designed to meet all or part of the nutritional and energy needs of invalids, sports drinks, slimming foods and hundreds of herbal medicines that have been sold as dietary supplements. The term 'functional foods' could include every fortified food and every food for which some sort of health claim has been made, such as most breakfast cereals (see Chapter 9 for a working definition of functional foods).

There are many formal definitions of dietary supplements that attempt to delineate what is and is not covered by the term. Some of the important elements of these definitions are listed below and in general only substances that satisfy these criteria have been included. I have not attempted to produce a contrived definition, but rather to delineate what is and is not covered in the book, and also to try to produce a logical classification of the types of supplements in common use. Note that legal definitions of food/dietary supplements in the UK, EU and USA are discussed later in this chapter.

- Dietary supplements are taken orally and in specified doses in the form of pills, capsules, powders or liquid preparations.
- They are intended to be additional to the normal diet.
- They are not the sole source of energy or fluid or a major contributor to energy or fluid intake.
- They usually carry some health claims, either on the label or in other promotional material (e.g. in sales brochures or press advertisements).

In a review, Webb (2007) identified five broad categories into which most dietary supplements fall and these are listed below:

- Single or combined products containing vitamins and minerals or occasionally other essential nutrients like amino acids. The general issue of micronutrient adequacy and the part supplements might play in ensuring adequacy is dealt with in Chapter 2. The individual vitamins and minerals are then discussed in Chapters 3 and 4.
- Organic substances that are natural body metabolites but are not normally considered to be essential nutrients because of endogenous synthesis, e.g. glucosamine, s-adenosylmethionine, co-enzyme Q_{10} and L-carnitine. It is suggested that in some circumstances endogenous synthesis may not be enough for optimal functioning and thus that supplemental intakes of these substances may have health benefits or even the potential to alleviate disease (these are dealt with in Chapter 7).
- Natural fats and oils such as fish oil, evening primrose oil or flaxseed oil (these are dealt with in Chapter 6).
- Plant or occasionally animal extracts that contain essential nutrients, natural metabolites or other bioactive substances claimed to have health-enhancing properties, e.g. garlic, ginseng, Ginkgo biloba and royal jelly. A select list of some of the most commonly used of these substances and some of those with the most valid claims to be derived from potential foods are dealt with in Chapter 8. Note that from May 2011 some of these will be sold as traditional herbal medicines rather than food supplements within the UK and the EU.
- Substances with antioxidant activity. This category will include essential nutrients and other substances listed in the other categories above. However, the oxidant theory of disease and the putative role of antioxidants in preventing or treating disease is now such a major element in claims made for foods and supplements that these have been separated out and dealt with together in Chapter 5.

Legal regulation of dietary supplements (the UK and EU perspective)

Medicines

A medicine is a substance that is used to cure, treat or prevent a disease. As a result of an EU Directive, the definition of a medicinal product has been widened to cover anything that meets either of the following criteria (MHRA, 2007):

> *Any substance or combination of substances presented as having properties for treating or preventing disease in human beings.*

> *Any substance or combination of substances which may be used in or administered to human beings either with a view to restoring, correcting or modifying physiological function by exerting a pharmacological, immunological or metabolic action, or to making a medical diagnosis.*

In the UK, only substances licensed as medicines have historically been permitted to make medicinal claims; that is, claims that they can cure, prevent or treat a disease. Given this wider definition, only licensed medicines are permitted to claim that they restore or correct physiological functions; these sorts of claims are not permitted for food or dietary supplements. These restrictions apply not only to the packaging of the product but also to advertising material for the product and to company websites. In the UK, control and licensing of medicines is the responsibility of the Medicines and Healthcare Products Regulatory Authority (MHRA). In order to obtain a product licence, medicines must satisfy this authority as to their safety and effectiveness. Some medicines can be sold over the counter at a variety of retail outlets (GSL, general sales list medicines), some can only be sold in pharmacies (P) and some are prescription-only medicines (POM) that can only be provided if prescribed by a doctor or sometimes another medical professional.

A few of the substances used as dietary supplements are also licensed medicines, including some generic vitamins (vitamins A and D, folic acid and cyanocobalamin, vitamin B_{12}); a multivitamin preparation designed to meet the needs of children (Abidec); a fish oil preparation (Maxepa); and an iron and folic acid supplement intended for pregnant women (Pregaday). It is permissible to make medicinal claims for these products, for example that Maxepa lowers raised plasma triacylglycerols and so helps to prevent heart attacks and pancreatitis.

In 2002, medicinal licences for two preparations of evening primrose oil, Epogam and Efamast, were withdrawn. These had been widely used and prescribed to treat eczema and mastalgia (breast pain). However, a re-evaluation of the evidence persuaded the licensing authority that the evidence for their efficacy did not meet the standard required for licensing for the treatment of these conditions. Evening primrose oil was freely available as a dietary supplement and continues to be available, but claims that it is effective in treating these conditions are no longer legal for any evening primrose preparations.

Some herbal remedies are exempt from licensing if they consist solely of a dried or crushed part of the plant that is sold under its botanical name with no written recommendations for use on the packaging, and provided they are made by someone who holds a special manufacturing licence. This 'section 12(1) exemption' (from the Medicines Act) was intended to be used by herbalists who produce their own remedies for supply to their patients. It is has also been possible for bulk manufacturers to sell products under this exemption (section 12(2)). The Traditional Herbal Medicinal Products Directive means that from April 2011, herbal products will no longer be permitted to be sold under the section 12(2) exemption, although individual herbalists will still be permitted to supply herbal products under the section 12(1) exemption. Since April 2004 this Directive has also prevented the marketing of any new traditional herbal medicine under exemption 12(2) unless it was already being legally sold before 30 April 2004. The impact of the Directive on herbal preparations currently sold as food supplements is discussed later in this chapter.

When the Traditional Herbal Medicinal Products Directive was first passed it proposed a system for fast-tracking the pharmaceutical registration of a number of traditional herbs where there is a substantial history of safe use. The European

Commission proposed that products should be eligible for 'simplified pharmaceutical registration' if they have been in use for 30 years or more, with at least 15 years of use within an EU member state. All of the herbal products discussed in Chapter 8 would be eligible for fast-tracking for pharmaceutical registration by these criteria. Note that the registration process applies to a single product and registration for one product is not a blanket registration for all products containing that ingredient. Manufacturers may choose to supply their registered product to other suppliers to market it under their own label. While this process is much less onerous than that for a new pharmaceutical drug, it still requires considerable time and resources, especially for small or medium-sized producers of herbal products.

Non-medicinal supplements

To get a medicine licensed can take up to a decade and cost many millions of pounds and so many manufacturers of nutrients, 'natural substances' and herbal preparations have chosen to market them as food supplements instead. This means that they are subject to legal regulations relating to food rather than to medicines. Anything that is taken orally and not classified as a medicine is, by default, classified as food.

This has major commercial advantages for the manufacturer, who not only bypasses the expensive and slow process of getting the product licensed, but is also subject to the much less stringent legal regulations relating to food. It is illegal to sell food that is harmful to health and it is illegal to dishonestly describe or advertise a food. This means that it is theoretically illegal to make false health claims for a dietary supplement, but it has historically been necessary for a prosecution to 'prove' a claim to be false, whereas a medicine must be shown to be safe and effective before it is licensed.

In the UK there has been no agency like the MHRA to oversee the regulation of dietary supplements; enforcement of food safety laws and advertising claims has been the responsibility of Environmental Health Officers and Trading Standards Officers employed by local authorities. The Food Standards Agency is now taking a more active role in overseeing the regulation of supplements and the new EU regulations relating to permitted health claims (see later) will have an increasing impact on this situation.

Borderline products

There are many substances currently (2010) sold as food supplements that are on the 'borderline' between medicines and food supplements, including many herbal products. Some of the products discussed in Chapter 8 have well-established food uses, whereas others have less wide food uses and are more likely to be considered by many people to be or to have origins as herbal medicines. The definition of a food supplement within the EU is:

> foodstuffs the purpose of which is to supplement the normal diet and which are concentrated sources of nutrients or other substances with a nutritional or physiological effect, alone or in combination, marketed in dose form.

On the MHRA website (www.mhra.gov.uk) there is a 50-page downloadable document published in 2007 entitled 'Guidance note 8. A guide to what is a medicinal product'. This sets out in some detail how the MHRA decides whether a substance should be classified as a medicine and thus subject to its regulation. Other substances that are taken orally will be classified as food or food supplements. There is no definitive list of substances that are classified as medicines or as foods and the MHRA document suggests that products need to be considered on a case-by-case basis using a number of criteria, including the way the product is marketed and claims made about it; the extent to which it has been used as a food; and its perception by consumers. The MHRA website also contains an extensive list of herbal ingredients along with details of their recorded uses as foods and for medicinal purposes. This can be accessed at the following web address by clicking on the term herbal ingredients: www.mhra.gov.uk/Howweregulate/Medicines/Doesmyproduct-needalicence/Borderlineproducts/index.htm.

My discussions with representatives of the MHRA and FSA indicate that several of the herbal products discussed in Chapter 8 will from May 2011 no longer be permitted to be sold as food supplements in the UK and the EU, namely Agnus castus, Echinacea, milk thistle and St John's wort. These substances, together with a number of other herbal extracts currently sold as food supplements (e.g. black cohosh), will need to be registered as traditional herbal medicines. It will only be legal to sell registered products in the UK (excluding those dispensed by herbal practitioners under section 12(1) of the Medicines Act). Each registration will cover a single formulation produced by a single manufacturer, although retailers may then market these under different labels. While registered products must satisfy quality and safety criteria and demonstrate their past safe use within the EU, efficacy will not be a specific consideration. This means that for those covered by registration, products should actually contain the amounts of 'bioactive' ingredients listed on the label, which as will be seen later is not always the case with substances sold as food or dietary supplements.

Note that retailers will be permitted to sell existing stocks of supplements that have been reclassified. These supplements will gradually disappear and be replaced by registered products, which should still be freely available for over-the-counter sales. It will also remain legal for individuals to import 'supplements' from areas outside EU jurisdiction, provided they are solely for their own use. This means, for example, that it will be legal to make internet purchases of dietary supplements of St John's wort or Echinacea from the USA.

Health claims

Even though medicinal claims for foods and supplements (as outlined earlier) are not permitted, more general health claims that do not imply that a supplement prevents or treats a specific disease are permitted in the UK. Some examples of unacceptable claims for supplements are listed below:

- helps to prevent osteoporosis'
- 'prevents heart disease'

- 'helps to prevent cancer'
- 'helps to prevent or treat arthritis'
- 'prevents colds and flu'
- 'treats eczema'

Appendix 1 of 'Guidance note 8. A guide to what is a medicinal product', referred to earlier, contains a list of about 40 words or phrases that have contributed to a determination by the MHRA that they were associated with a medicinal product, along with an indication of what in some contexts the term may suggest or imply about a product, including the terms listed below:

- alleviates (may imply a claim to treat a disease)
- avoids (may imply prevention of a disease)
- boosts the immune system
- calms, calm or calming (to imply sedates)
- can benefit those who suffer from (implies treatment)
- can lower cholesterol
- clinically proven/clinical trials evidence (implies that efficacy in treating a disease has been demonstrated)
- combats, cure/cures, fights or heals (all can imply efficacy in treating or preventing a disease)
- helps maintain a normal mood balance (implies helpful in treating depression)
- prevents/preventing
- remedies
- traditionally used for (can imply a claim to treat or prevent an adverse condition)
- treats/treatment/treating

In 2000, the Joint Health Claims Initiative (JHCI) began operating in the UK as a joint venture between consumer organisations, enforcement authorities and industry trade associations to try to establish a code of practice for health claims relating to foods. It was set up in response to the growth in the market for functional foods. Its stated aim was to ensure that health claims on foods were:

- scientifically true
- legally acceptable in the UK
- meaningful to consumers and not confusing

However, this group ceased operations at the end of March 2007 because EU regulations aimed at harmonising rules about nutrition and health claims made on food started to be applied in 2007 and effectively superseded this attempt at a voluntary code of practice. The EU regulation means that the European Commission and member states will act together to authorise a positive list of health claims that will be allowed to be used on food. The European Food Standards Agency (EFSA) became responsible for assessing health claims based on dossiers submitted to it by the UK Food Standards Agency and equivalent bodies in other member states.

In 2006, the UK Food Standards Agency began asking businesses to submit health claims for consideration for inclusion on this European list of permitted health claims. The decisions about whether claims were justified and thus permitted would be based on evaluation of published scientific data in academic journals. The lists from member states had to be submitted during 2007 and towards the end of 2009 opinions on the first batch of over 500 health claims were published by the EFSA. Only about a third of these first batch of claims were given favourable evaluations; that is, that there was sufficient scientific evidence to support the claims. These favourable outcomes related mainly to the functions of vitamins and minerals. Other favourable outcomes covered, for example, the effects of dietary fibre, the role of fatty acid on blood cholesterol levels and the benefits of sugar-free chewing gum for dental health. The second batch of over 400 health claims released in February 2010 resulted in just nine favourable outcomes, including:

- 'Vitamin D contributes to the normal function of the immune system and healthy inflammatory response', 'Vitamin D contributes to the maintenance of normal muscle function'.
- 'Regular consumption of guar gum' (a source of soluble fibre) 'contributes to the maintenance of normal blood cholesterol levels'.
- 'Potassium contributes to normal muscular and neurological function' and 'Potassium helps maintain normal blood pressure'.

Some high-profile claims were not given approval. For example, some claims relating to antioxidants were rejected because there was insufficient evidence that any effects in reducing oxidative damage to cellular components constituted a beneficial physiological effect. Claims relating to probiotics and to some herbal products did not achieve positive decisions either, largely because of lack of information to identify the substance for which the benefit is claimed. It is expected that during 2011 the assessment of the initial group of health claims submitted in 2007 will be completed and the first positive list of permitted health claims established. Once this process is completed and fully implemented, only listed claims or those under consideration by the EFSA will be permitted to be made.

Despite any legal restrictions on claims, it is not difficult to make the public aware of claims that substances sold as food or supplements may help in the treatment or prevention of disease. Newspaper and other media articles frequently extol the virtues of particular foods, food components or supplements; these articles are often written by people with little or no academic or clinical training in nutrition. Companies or organisations wishing to promote a particular food or supplement may sponsor academic research and the resulting academic papers may be used to generate highly positive headlines about the substance that could not be used in advertising material. For instance, none of the following headline claims could legally be made for a substance sold as a food or supplement, even without recent legal changes (all from a search of the BBC news website, http://news.bbc.co.uk):

- Curry spice can 'help for arthritis'.
- Olive oil 'can cut cancer risk'.
- Spice 'may fight cystic fibrosis'.
- Watercress 'may cut cancer'.
- Pomegranates 'slow tumour growth'.
- Berries 'help prevent dementia'.
- 'Green tea compound Alzheimer's hope'.
- Vitamin D 'slashes cancer risk'.
- 'High vitamin D levels cut MS risk'.

Much more sensational headlines could easily be found in a trawl through back issues of newspapers. The full BBC articles usually give a fairly balanced account of recent published research data and provide sufficient information to allow the original scientific article to be traced easily; this is not the case with all media outlets. However, whether the full article is balanced or not, the public has been made aware of a medicinal claim for a food and that claim is often based on very limited or highly reductionist evidence.

Consider the watercress example above. This headlines refers to some research (sponsored by the Watercress Alliance) indicating that eating 85 g of watercress (more than most people eat in total over eight weeks) every day for eight weeks increases blood antioxidant levels, reduces acute measures of oxidant stress and increases resistance of blood to the effect of an oxidising agent. Dark green leafy vegetables are well known to be rich sources of substances with antioxidant activity, so wouldn't it actually be more surprising if very large supplements of watercress did not have such effects? I do not question the veracity of the scientific data, but I do question whether this really provides significant positive evidence that eating normal amounts of watercress reduces cancer risk, and whether any number of other similar vegetables taken in this way might not produce similar effects (see Webb, 2009).

Commercial sponsors can commission research that tests the effects of a large supplement of, say, a plant extract, an exotic fruit juice or some other food product on short-term measures of antioxidant activity or other putative disease risk indicators. One might argue that the purpose of such a study is not primarily to advance scientific knowledge. It may be to satisfy the requirements of the EFSA about food claims, provide marketing ammunition for the sponsor or to enhance the profile of the researchers; good publicity can be fostered by a carefully written press release. The study may be technically well designed and executed and so its results may be technically accurate, but does this alone make it scientifically worthwhile?

Vitamin and mineral supplements

There have been a number of steps taken towards harmonisation of the legislation relating to food supplements within the EU. The first stage in this process was the Food Supplements Directive that was passed into EU law in 2002 and has been integrated into the national laws of the member states. These regulations came into force on 1 August 2005 and they contain two positive lists relating to vitamins and minerals, which may be seen in the Food Supplements (England) Regulations 2003 (HMSO, 2003). These two positive lists are:

- A list of vitamins and minerals that may be used in the manufacture of food supplements.
- A list of the forms in which these vitamins and minerals may be used in the manufacture of food supplements.

Any substance that is not included in these positive lists cannot be used in food supplements. The first list did not contain, for example, boron, nickel, silicon, tin or vanadium, which had all previously been included in some dietary supplements. Several forms of vitamins and minerals that had been widely used were also not in the second list and the only permitted form of folate was folic acid, which is not actually present in ordinary food. Since 2003, there have been some significant additions to both lists, including the following:

- Silicon and boron have been added to the list of permitted minerals (although this does mean that they are now considered to be essential; see Chapter 4).
- Menaquinone has been added to the permitted forms of vitamin K.
- Calcium-L-methylfolate has been added as a permitted form of folate.
- Chromium picolinate has been added as a permitted organic form of chromium.

Prior to European harmonisation there have been very diverse regulations regarding the maximum permitted doses of vitamins and minerals that may be legally included in products available for over-the-counter sale as dietary supplements. The intention is that over the coming years, the European Commission will set maximum permitted levels of vitamins and minerals that can be present in products marketed as food supplements for general sale. The Commission will be guided in this process by an expert committee, the Scientific Committee for Food.

In some countries, such as the UK, there has been a very liberal framework with few restrictions on the levels of most vitamins and minerals available for general sale. Those few generic vitamins that are known to be harmful in high doses are licensed medicines; there are maximum levels set for these when available for general sale (GSL), that is:

- 2250 µg of vitamin A
- 10 µg of vitamin D
- 10 µg of cyanocobalamin (vitamin B_{12})
- 200 µg of folic acid

Doses in excess of these amounts are restricted either to pharmacy-only (P) or prescription-only sale (POM). Of course, general food law still applies to all dietary supplements, thus they must not be injurious to health and they cannot carry medicinal claims. This means that it is possible to buy 'megadoses' of many essential nutrients in the UK with a view to achieving some benefit beyond simply ensuring dietary adequacy and prevention of deficiency. It is, for example, legal to buy and sell vitamin C preparations containing 20 or more times the EU recommended daily allowance (RDA) (60 mg).

In contrast to this liberal position in countries like the UK and Sweden, in other countries, such as France, the general philosophy is that doses up to the RDA or a low multiple of it are regarded as foods, but anything in excess of this is regarded as a medicine. In these countries the vitamins and minerals in food supplements are seen as being there almost exclusively to ensure nutritional adequacy and prevent deficiency. Between these two extremes there has been a whole spectrum of regulations within the countries of the EU. Clearly, it is going to be extremely contentious to set common regulations when individual countries have evolved such diverse regulatory frameworks and philosophies, and where manufacturers, suppliers, consumer groups and individual consumers may be keen to preserve their existing practices and rights.

My understanding from discussions with representatives of the FSA is that European legislation regulating the maximum permitted doses of vitamins and minerals is not imminent. In the UK, there were discussions between the FSA and representatives of the food supplements industry, which established a voluntary code in 2004. According to this code manufacturers and suppliers of supplements were encouraged to include advisory notes on labels for products containing more than specified amounts of some vitamins and minerals, and in a few cases encouraged to reformulate their product. The main recommendations of this voluntary agreement are listed below:

- Preparations containing more than 1000 mg/day of vitamin C, 20 mg iron, 1500 mg calcium, 400 mg magnesium and 250 mg phosphorus should carry a warning that they might cause mild stomach upsets.
- Preparations containing >7 mg/day of β-carotene should carry a warning that they should not be taken by heavy smokers and suppliers were encouraged to reformulate to below 7 mg/day.
- Products containing >20 mg/day of nicotinic acid should warn of the possibility of causing skin flushing and suppliers were encouraged to reformulate using nicotinamide.
- Preparations containing more than 4 mg/day of manganese should carry a warning that long-term consumption of this amount might lead to muscle pain and fatigue.
- Preparations with more than 100 mg/day of vitamin B_6 should carry a warning that long-term consumption of this amount might lead to tingling and numbness and suppliers were encouraged to reformulate to a lower amount.

A 2006 Mintel survey commissioned by the FSA suggested that higher-dose products accounted for 12–15% of the vitamin and mineral market. Most of the companies supplying these products said, when contacted, that they had either already added these advisory statements to their labels or were in the process of doing so. Products showing these advisory statements started appearing on retailers' shelves in 2006.

Regulation in the USA

This topic has been concisely reviewed by Hathcock (2001) and Forbes and McNamara (2006). The regulation of dietary supplements in the USA is in many ways similar to that existing in the UK prior to the influence of EU directives. As in the UK, dietary supplements are regulated as foods rather than drugs by the Food and Drug Administration (FDA). Manufacturers have a legal duty to ensure that the product is safe and that the labelling accurately reflects what the product contains. Unlike with drugs, there is no requirement for manufacturers to demonstrate the efficacy of their product unless they make a specific health claim.

Provided that a food meets certain compositional criteria, then some relationships between nutrients and disease are regarded as sufficiently well established for them to be used as health claims on food labels. These include the relationships between:

- calcium and osteoporosis
- sodium and hypertension
- saturated fat and cholesterol and heart disease
- fat and cancer
- folic acid and neural tube defects

This means that supplements containing calcium or folic acid may be able to make use of these established and permitted health claims. Full details of permitted health claims in the USA may be found in Forbes and McNamara (2006).

The Dietary Supplement Health Education Act (DSHEA) of 1994 further said that certain nutrition support claims could be made for a dietary supplement without the need for it to be regulated as a drug. These nutritional support claims cover areas such as:

- claims about classic nutritional deficiencies
- structure or function effects
- mechanisms for structure or function effects
- general health and well-being

This Act also gives a very broad definition of *dietary supplements* that seems to offer a legal basis for selling many substances as dietary supplements in a medicinal presentation (pills or potions) that would not ordinarily be regarded as food:

> *product... intended to supplement the diet that bears or contains... a vita-min;... a mineral; an herb or other botanical;... an amino acid;... a dietary substance for use by man to supplement the diet by increasing the total dietary intake; or... a concentrate, metabolite, constituent, extract, or com-bination [of any ingredient described above]. (taken from Forbes and McNamara, 2006)*

This very broad definition would encompass every substance discussed specifically in this book and would give suppliers a clear legal justification for selling their product as a dietary supplement. In effect, it provides a legal umbrella that protects suppliers from interference in the sale of products covered by the very broad definition.

The DSHEA requires that manufacturers have evidence to support claims for nutritional support and the manufacturer may be required to include a disclaimer stating that the claim has not been evaluated by the FDA. However, this appears to have been lightly enforced. For example, up to 2001 several warnings had been issued to companies in the USA about their making claims for products that would require them to be approved as drugs to be legal, but according to Hathcock (2001) very few warnings had questioned the level of substantiation for claims. As an example of one of these warnings, it is noted in Chapter 7 that a company making claims that methylsulphonylmethane (MSM) could be beneficial in the treatment of a large number of medical conditions was warned that such a claim could not be legally made for substances other than approved drugs.

Supplement quality

Medicines are subject to strict quality controls, but there are few such controls over dietary supplements. There are a number of quality control concerns about dietary supplements, as summarised below:

- Do they actually contain the ingredients that are listed on the packaging and that the consumer is entitled to expect? In the case of natural extracts, it may be unclear what the active ingredients are; even where the active agents are known, different preparations may contain variable amounts of these. In Chapter 8, for example, it is noted that not only do many St John's wort preparations contain less than the advertised amount of hypericin and hyperforin rather than hypericin is also probably the active constituent.
- In the case of herbal extracts, there needs to be authentication of the plant used for the extract to ensure that it is actually the correct species. It is also important to ensure that the correct part of the plant has been used to make the extract.
- Do they contain the advertised amount of the ingredients?
- Do they contain acceptable levels of potentially harmful contaminants? Some supplements may be contaminated with harmful amounts of heavy metals and there have been cases of synthetic and sometimes unlicensed drugs being added to some ethnic medicines sold under the umbrella of dietary supplements.
- Does the product disintegrate after ingestion so that it can be absorbed and utilised?

There is an independent testing organisation in the USA called ConsumerLab, which has carried out a very large number of product tests of dietary supplements. It tests various brands of supplements for identity, strength, purity and bio-availability. Further details of this testing, and sample results, can be found on the ConsumerLab website (www.consumerlab.com), although a subscription is required for full access to test results. Some sample findings of these product tests are given below:

- Seven out of eight milk thistle products contained less than the stated amount of silymarin (47–67%).
- A small minority of fish oil supplements contained only small amounts of EPA or DHA, with sometimes misleading labels.
- Of ten St John's wort products tested, four contained unacceptable levels of cadmium and three contained only 36% or less of the stated content of hyperforin or hypericin.
- One tested phytosterol preparation would not break apart to release its contents and so was likely to be ineffective.
- Some probiotic preparations contained as little as 7–58% of the number of cells listed on the labels.
- Several gluosamine products were contaminated with lead and two chondroitin preparations contained 6% or less of the stated chondroitin content.
- One saw palmetto preparation contained no saw palmetto.
- One vitamin C supplement provided less than half the stated vitamin C content.
- 30% of multivitamin preparations tested had defects, for example:
  - Three of four children's multivitamins were too high in vitamin A.
  - One 'vitamin water' had 15 times the stated level of folic acid.

In reviews that were current at the time of the first edition of this book, ConsumerLab had found one coenzyme Q_{10} preparation contained no coenzyme Q_{10} and one brand of s-adenosylmethionine that contained only about 30% of the amount claimed.

These deficiencies are of great practical importance for people buying supplements, particularly those containing extracts of plants or other natural products. Even if high-quality clinical trials using a high-quality defined extract indicate that it may have beneficial effects, there is still no guarantee that an over-the-counter preparation will also have the same effects.

Note that herbal products that obtain registration as traditional herbal medicines will be required to meet standards of quality as to their composition and bioavailability. This should ultimately mean that in the future such products should be of consistent quality and be reliable in their compositional claims in the UK.

The market for supplements

According to the marketing intelligence organisation Mintel, in the year 2000 just over a third of UK men and nearly half of women said that they took dietary supplements and around three-quarters of these users said that they took them daily (Mintel 2001). In all age groups, use of supplements was greater in women than men and there was a pronounced trend for usage to increase with age. In the 55–64-year age group, 44% of men and 55% of women said that they used supplements. At that time (2001) Mintel estimated that the total UK market for supplements was worth around £355 million per annum, which was about 8% less in real terms than the value of the market in 1996.

In its latest report on the UK vitamins and supplements market (2009), Mintel estimated that the market had reached an estimated £396 million. In the five-year period 2004–2009 the sales of vitamins and other supplements grew by less than 9% in the UK; Mintel projects that sales will only increase by a further 10% in the period 2009–2014. This means that there is very slow growth in the UK supplement market, particularly when compared to the growth of functional food products discussed in Chapter 9. A number of factors are inhibiting the growth in the supplement market, such as the following:

- The increasing availability of cheaper own-brand products and discounting by suppliers, which reduces overall market value (Mintel suggests that over 6 million adults perceive supplements to be too expensive and they are often seen as non-essential items that can be cut back on during a recession).
- Competition from products like functional foods.
- A shift in consumer preference towards more natural sources of nutrients.
- A decrease in the proportion of people using supplements.

The latest Mintel report also gives a breakdown of this market for supplements into supplement categories and individual supplements. Some highlights from the report are listed below and further quantitative details are given in Table 1.2:

Table 1.2 Approximate breakdown by value of the market for dietary supplements in the UK

Supplement category	Value	% of total	Change 2007–9 (%)
All vitamins & supplements	396	100	+6.4
All vitamin products	114	29	–5.8
Cod liver oil	62	22	+3.3
Evening primrose/ starflower oil	21	7	–16.0
Omega-3 (fish oil)	47	17	+46.9
Glucosamine	48	17	+60.0
Minerals	15	5	–
Garlic	12	4	–14.3
Ginseng	10	4	–
St John's wort	7	2	–
Ginkgo biloba	9	3	–
All others (including tonics)	51	18	+4.1

Source: Mintel (2009).

- The natural oils cod liver oil, evening primrose oil (EPO)/starflower oil and omega-3 fish oils accounted for 33% of the total supplement market in 2009. Sales of EPO/starflower oil fell by 16% between 2007 and 2009, whereas sales of omega-3 oils grew by 47%.
- Sales of single and multivitamin preparations made up 29% of the supplement market in 2009 and this represented a drop of about 6% since 2007.
- Sales of glucosamine grew by 60% between 2007 and 2009.
- Sales of garlic fell by over 14% in the period 2007–2009.

These numbers look small in comparison to sales of supplements in the USA, where the market was estimated to be worth $18.5 billion in 2002 and growing at a similar rate to that in the UK. In 2009 around 65% of adult US consumers reported that they took dietary supplements and no less than 54% take a multivitamin preparation. In the EU sales of supplements in 2005 were estimated to value around €5 billion.

Reasons for taking supplements

As suggested at the beginning of this chapter, people take supplements for a variety of reasons. These have been grouped into the four major categories discussed below.

To compensate for a perceived or potential inadequacy in the diet

Although overt deficiency diseases are rarely seen among the general population in industrialised countries, avoiding these is still an important motivation for many of those who take vitamin and/or mineral supplements. There are some groups within the populations of these countries for whom the general assumption of even basic dietary adequacy may not always be secure. As noted earlier, some overt deficiency diseases are still very prevalent in many developing countries.

As a general rule, nutrient deficiencies are unlikely if people eat enough food to satisfy their energy needs and consume a variety of foods from each of the four major food groups, listed below:

- The bread and cereals group, including rice, pasta, breakfast cereals.
- The milk group, including other dairy foods such as cheese, yoghurt and also vegetarian milk substitutes.
- The fruit and vegetable group.
- The meat group, including fish, eggs, poultry, pulses and vegetarian meat substitutes.

Different foods have different profiles of essential nutrients. For example, milk is rich in calcium and B vitamins but low in vitamin C and iron. Muscle meat is rich in iron and protein but essentially devoid of vitamins A and C. Many fruits and vegetables provide plenty of vitamins C and A (as carotene) but little zinc or vitamin E. For this reason, nutritionists have always encouraged people to eat a varied diet. The original idea of food groups was to ensure dietary adequacy by encouraging people to eat a minimum number of portions from each food group each day to ensure that they got enough vitamins, minerals and protein. A varied diet also makes it less likely that any of the natural toxins or potentially toxic contaminants in some foods will be consumed in hazardous amounts.

A specific nutrient deficiency becomes increasingly more likely the lower the total amount of food eaten and/or the narrower the range of foods selected.

Unless there are major differences in dietary composition, one would expect that intakes of essential vitamins and minerals should rise with increasing calorie consumption; that is, those who eat the most food would tend to have the highest intakes of nutrients. For example, on average men eat more than women and men thus tend to have higher intakes of essential nutrients than women.

Affluent populations usually have an abundant quantity and variety of foods to select from and so should be at very low risk of nutrient deficiency. Despite this, any circumstance that reduces total food intake, narrows the range of foods eaten or increases the requirement for a nutrient will increase the likelihood of deficiency (see Chapter 2). Average adult intakes of almost all the major vitamins and minerals in the UK comfortably exceed estimated average requirements, with the clear exception of the iron intake of women. However, as we will see in Chapter 2, many individuals do have intakes of some nutrients that are clearly unsatisfactory and/or show biochemical evidence of unsatisfactory status. Similar findings have also been reported for children and elderly people.

Intakes of essential nutrients tend to be lower in the lower social classes and supplement use is also less frequent in the lower socio-economic groups; thus those in the social groups most likely to need supplements are the least likely to take them. Growing children, the elderly, pregnant or lactating women and those with illnesses or serious injuries have traditionally been seen as at higher risk of nutrient deficiency. Whether this perception of increased deficiency risk in these groups is justified or not is discussed more fully in Chapter 2.

When the aim of supplementation is to ensure adequacy or prevent deficiency, then the dose is likely to be relatively modest and will be based on estimates of normal requirements. This also makes it unlikely that any supplements will be taken in amounts that are likely to be acutely toxic and less likely that they will have any long-term adverse consequences. Long-term doses that do not go above 2–3 times normal requirements can usually be regarded as safe. There are occasions when even relatively modest overdoses of a nutrient can be harmful, however. For example, it is recommended by the UK panel on dietary standards (COMA, 1991) that infants and young children should not take in more than 2–3 times their normal requirements of vitamin A (retinol). Excess retinol, but not carotene, is also known to cause birth defects when consumed by pregnant animals or women, so pregnant women are advised not to take non-prescribed vitamin A supplements and to avoid liver products, because they can contain very high levels of vitamin A.

To compensate for some perceived increase in need or defective handling of a nutrient

Certain medical conditions or other circumstances may, or may be seen to, increase the need for a particular nutrient, such as those listed below:

- *Pernicious anaemia.* This is an auto-immune disease that results in a failure to produce a gastric 'intrinsic factor' that is necessary for the absorption of vitamin B_{12}. This leads to vitamin B_{12} deficiency, which in turn leads to a severe and potentially fatal anaemia, as well as damage to the spinal cord and brain that can cause progressive paralysis. These symptoms can be alleviated by regular injections of vitamin B_{12} (or by very high oral intakes).
- *Blood loss.* A normal healthy man loses less than 1 mg of iron per day, but 1 ml of blood contains around 0.5 mg of iron and so chronic blood loss or substantial acute losses greatly increase iron losses and the risk of iron deficiency anaemia. A bleeding stomach ulcer, gut cancer, intestinal parasites, and heavy menstruation or repeated pregnancies in young women can all substantially increase iron losses and so increase iron requirements (see Chapter 4).
- *Pregnancy and folic acid.* Since the early 1990s, women in Britain and the USA have been advised to take folic acid supplements when they first become or plan to become pregnant. It has been shown that these folic acid supplements reduce the risk of the baby having a neural tube defect (NTD) such as anencephaly or spina bifida. Expert committees in both the UK and the USA have recommended that a common food (flour and bread) should be fortified with extra folic acid to minimise the occurrence of NTD and this recommendation has been implemented in the USA (see Chapter 3).
- *Vitamin D supplements for the elderly.* For most people, the major source of vitamin D is by its production in their skin when exposed to the ultraviolet rays in summer sunshine. Anyone who is not regularly exposed to the sun during the summer months is at risk of vitamin D deficiency unless they take supplements. It now seems probable that lack of vitamin D is an important contributory factor in the development of osteoporosis in elderly, largely housebound people. In the UK it is recommended that all elderly people take vitamin D supplements unless they are regularly exposed to summer sunlight (COMA, 1991).

In Chapter 7, several examples are given of substances that are not normally regarded as essential nutrients being essential for some individuals or under some circumstances (conditionally essential). For example, L-carnitine is not normally an essential nutrient, but it may be essential for some individuals who have genetic defects in their synthetic pathway for carnitine. Premature babies may require long-chain omega-3 and omega-6 fatty acids to be provided in their diet because the elongation and desaturation enzymes needed to make them from the parent compounds linoleic and linolenic acids may not be developed.

To treat or prevent non-deficiency diseases

This category of usage can be split into two overlapping divisions: first, where the expected benefit is fairly acute; and second, where the aim is the long-term prevention of chronic diseases such as cancer, heart disease or osteoporosis. Note that it is not legal to make claims that a substance sold as a food or food supplement has such effects, although as we have seen earlier it is not difficult to make sure that the public is aware of such claims.

Some examples follow where the effect of the supplement or functional food is expected to become apparent within days, weeks or months:

- Evening primrose oil is widely taken by women in the belief that it will reduce the symptoms of pre-menstrual syndrome or reduce the breast tenderness (mastalgia) that many women experience at certain times during their menstrual cycle (Chapter 6).
- Fish oil preparations have been claimed to give symptomatic relief from the pain of arthritis (Chapter 6).
- Certain fermented foods containing living cultures of bacteria (probiotics) are claimed to reduce the incidence of gut or vaginal infections (Chapter 9).

As the results of treatment are expected to manifest fairly quickly – that is, within weeks or months – then these would seem relatively amenable to proper controlled testing, as described later in the chapter.

Listed below are some examples of supplement or functional food usage where the tangible benefit to the consumer is expected to be long term; that is, measured in years or even decades. In these cases, proper controlled testing is much more difficult. As an alternative, one can try to assess the likely long-term impact by monitoring the impact of the product on some short-term marker of disease likelihood, but such changes can only be classed as a benefit if they really do herald a later reduction in disease risk.

- It is suggested that taking calcium supplements or eating foods with enhanced calcium levels when women are young may reduce the risk of their suffering osteoporosis fractures in old age. Changes in bone density measured after weeks or months may be used as an early indication of 'success' (Chapter 4).
- Supplements of plant pigments with antioxidant activity, like beta-carotene or lycopene, may reduce the risk of developing cancer or heart disease or any other disease in which it has been suggested that oxidative damage by free radicals may play an aetiological role. It may be argued that the laboratory demonstration of the antioxidant potential of these substances or an 'improvement' in acute measures of a person's antioxidant status is an indication that they will prevent chronic disease (Chapter 5).
- Margarine and other foods with high levels of certain plant sterols are justifiably claimed to lower the blood cholesterol concentration. Although high blood cholesterol concentration is asymptomatic, it is associated with a high risk of coronary disease and so these products are promoted and used in the belief that they will, in the long term, reduce the risk of death from coronary heart disease.

This category of use is perhaps the one that that causes the most controversy and is the one with the greatest potential to do harm. Often when supplements are used for this purpose the doses involved will be pharmacological and will bear no relationship to the amounts consumed in a normal diet or required to prevent deficiency. Other substances that would not normally be consumed or only consumed occasionally may be taken regularly, over extended periods and in high doses as supplements, such as many of the substances covered in Chapter 8. It has been claimed, for example, that large doses of vitamin C can prevent or treat colds and other conditions, with doses of 10 to 100 times 'normal requirements' advocated by some enthusiasts for this vitamin. When taken in doses that may exceed the usual maximum by an order of magnitude, then the possibility of harmful side-effects is clearly much greater than if doses are around that normally consumed or that recommended to ensure adequacy.

All substances are poisonous; there is none which is not a poison. The right dose differentiates a poison and a remedy. (Paracelsus 1493–1541)

When used with the aim of long-term disease prevention, relatively large doses of supplements (or functional foods) may be taken over several decades with no immediate apparent benefit for the consumer. The theoretical risks of some net adverse effects are probably greatest when supplements are used for this purpose. As the benefits of 'treatment' are expected to take some years to manifest, this is also the most difficult category to test for effectiveness and safety.

To improve athletic performance

There is a large and rapidly expanding literature on the effects of dietary manipulation and supplementation on athletic performance, so this aspect of dietary supplements could be the subject of a large book in its own right. Some of the individual substances favoured by athletes, such as creatine, ginseng and glucosamine, will be dealt with in the appropriate chapters, but some other supplements taken primarily by athletes will not be covered.

Heavy training may increase to a limited extent the requirement for some vitamins, minerals and protein, therefore supplements – sometimes large supplements – of these essential nutrients are frequently taken by athletes. However, if athletes are meeting their increased energy requirements while training, they should also be taking in more nutrients than the average inactive person. The nutrient supplements taken by most athletes are probably unnecessary and may even be detrimental; excesses of some essential nutrients are toxic and some may reduce performance. Problems may arise in those sports where leanness is perceived to be advantageous (e.g. gymnastics) and so athletes (often female athletes) train heavily and also restrict their energy intake. Any deficiencies in athletes are likely to be the result of a restricted food intake rather than increased requirements due to the effects of training (Maughan, 1994).

Do supplements and functional foods work? Testing their effectiveness and safety

In many cases it is very difficult to give a definitive answer or even a fairly confident answer to the question of whether supplements or functional foods are actually effective (or even safe). In this section, I will briefly review the ways in which evidence on effectiveness and safety is gathered and try to explain why it is still difficult to give an authoritative assessment of a supplement's safety and effectiveness, even when it has been used for many years and sometimes despite the publication of hundreds of research studies. I will concentrate on broad principles rather than trying to assess the effectiveness or safety of any particular supplement or functional food. The effectiveness of individual products is assessed in later chapters where particular supplements and functional foods are covered.

Scientific papers about dietary supplements, or indeed about any other scientific or medical topic, can be found using an appropriate and specific search engine. Abstracts of papers can usually be accessed free from any web-connected computer and in some cases there are links to (free) full-text versions. Abstracts of most of the journal articles listed in the references at the end of this book can be obtained in this way. PubMed is a service of the National Library of Medicine in the USA and this has been used for electronic searches in the preparation of this book (www. ncbi.nlm.nih.gov/entrez).

Measures of outcome

When trying to assess the effectiveness of a dietary supplement or functional food, one must decide what measure or measures are going to be used as indicators of success or failure. If one is interested in the use of a supplement to ensure adequacy of one or more essential nutrients, then one could use biochemical measures of nutrient status to assess whether this outcome had been achieved. In some other cases, one can monitor the effect of a supplement on the signs and/or symptoms of a disease. Thus when dietary deficiency diseases were first being identified, one could confirm the beneficial effects of a vitamin or mineral by testing the effect on symptoms and the disease progression of purified supplements or foods rich in the nutrient. For example, one could show that vitamin C alleviates the symptoms of scurvy and iodine cures goitre. As a more recent example, if a fish oil supplement is claimed to be beneficial in treating arthritis, then one can monitor patients' assessment of the effect on joint pain levels; or one can use more objective radiological measures of disease progression such as narrowing of the joint space. Note that the more subjective the outcome measure, the higher is the likely 'placebo effect'; that is, benefits that are due to the psychological response to treatment and that are also obtained with a sham treatment (placebo) if the subject believes it to be real. It will be seen later in the chapter that on occasion up to half of subjects may report beneficial effects from an inactive placebo 'treatment'.

When testing whether taking a supplement or functional food reduces the risk of developing and/or dying from a particular disease, these 'outcomes' may take a long time to materialise in currently healthy subjects. If these outcome measures are used it may be necessary to monitor very large samples of people for many years in prospective studies (looking forward to see how current behaviour affects future disease risk), or else to use a retrospective approach (comparing past behaviour in those with and without the disease).

There are alternative outcome measures that give more immediate results. For example, one could measure the effect of a supplement or functional food on some asymptomatic disease risk factor like plasma cholesterol concentration, blood pressure or some biochemical measure of antioxidant status. If it can be shown to lower plasma cholesterol concentration, then this may indicate that it will also lower the risk of heart disease. If a supplement can be shown to lower blood pressure, this may indicate that it will reduce the risk of a stroke or some other consequence of hypertension. If it can be shown to improve some measure of antioxidant status, this may indicate that it will protect against cancer, heart disease or other diseases purported to be linked to oxidative damage by free radicals. However, it must be remembered that in these cases all that has actually been demonstrated is that the supplement or functional food affects an asymptomatic risk indicator. Any claims about its net benefit are projections based on the assumption that lowering of the risk factor will indeed ultimately result in a reduced incidence of the disease, and also that the supplement or functional food will not have some other detrimental effect that will cancel out or even exceed any benefits.

The two main investigative approaches

There are two broad approaches that can be used to try to assess the effectiveness of any particular substance: the observational approach and the experimental approach.

The observational approach

The observational approach uses information from previously published sources (e.g. national statistics, survey results or perhaps sales data for foods or supplements) or from surveys conducted by the study team. This information is then assessed and variables correlated to see whether it supports a particular hypothesis or not; the approach may also be used to generate hypotheses that can then be tested using an experimental approach. The investigators do not set out to change the behaviour or the 'treatment' of the study subjects.

The observational approach may be used to identify dietary and lifestyle characteristics of populations, groups or individuals that are associated with high or low mortality or high or low risk of particular conditions. However, its use becomes much more problematical when the aim is to show a specific cause-and-effect relationship between, say, the intake of a particular dietary component and a particular disease. For example, many observational studies indicate that people who consume large amounts of fruits and vegetables have a reduced risk of developing cancer compared to those who eat few fruits and vegetables. The cumulative weight of such studies is so persuasive that dietary guidelines in many countries have recommended increased fruit and vegetable consumption, with a target of five portions per day being a widely promoted in the UK and USA. These data are also consistent with the proposition that high levels of certain nutrients (e.g. vitamin C) or antioxidants (e.g. β-carotene) that are predominantly derived from fruit and vegetables have cancer-protective properties. This in turn is used to support the case for taking these substances (or plant extracts rich in these substances) in supplement form. However, as will be seen in Chapter 5, these fruit and vegetable data are a long way short of providing a convincing demonstration that consuming purified antioxidants in pill form will always prove beneficial or even safe.

Observational studies fall into a number of categories, as detailed below.

Cross-cultural comparisons

Cross-cultural studies look at age-standardised disease frequencies in different cultural groups to see if they can be correlated with dietary or other lifestyle differences between the groups. Below are some examples from later chapters:

- Observations that Greenland Eskimos eating a traditional diet rich in marine oils had low rates of coronary heart disease and arthritis were an important stimulus for research on the benefits of eating oily fish and taking fish oil supplements (Chapter 6).
- Observations that women living in countries where there is a high intake of soy products have relatively low rates of breast cancer have led to suggestions that the phyto-oestrogens in soy foods might have a protective effect against breast cancer (Chapter 9).

Migration studies

Migration studies are an important way of differentiating between genetics and environment as causes of differences in disease rates between populations. In general, when people migrate they tend gradually to adopt aspects of the diet and lifestyle of the native population in their new home (so-called acculturation). As migrant populations acculturate with the native population, so they also start to acquire a profile of disease risk that moves towards that in their adopted country; that is, they start to suffer from and die of the same illnesses as the rest of the population in their new homeland. This suggests that most of the differences between disease frequencies seen in different populations are due to environmental rather than genetic factors. The general principle that diet and lifestyle differences are major factors in determining disease rates is essential for the credibility of supplement use and indeed for the whole field of health promotion. For example:

- In Chapter 9 it is noted that when women migrate from high soy areas like China and Japan to western countries where soy intakes are low, breast cancer rates remain low in the migrants themselves but rise in subsequent generations. This has led to suggestions that exposure to phyto-oestrogens in early life or even *in utero* may afford protection against breast cancer.

Time trend studies

In time trend studies correlations are sought between temporal changes in behaviour and disease frequency. One might, for example, correlate changes in salt consumption in a population with changes in average blood pressure or death rates from stroke.

- In Chapter 4 it is noted that the fall in rates of decayed, missing and filled teeth seen in children in many countries over recent decades is largely attributable to the growth in the use of fluoridated toothpaste.

Case-control studies

In case-control studies one attempts to compare the past behaviour of those with a disease (cases) and those free from it (controls). For example, one might try to test the notion that high intake of a dietary component protects against cancer by comparing the past intakes of matched groups of cancer sufferers (cases) and non-sufferers (controls). It may be very difficult to get reliable estimates of past diet; if one takes current diet as an indicator of past diet of the 'cases', then there is always the real possibility that their current diet is a reflection of their disease or their awareness of it. It may thus be an 'effect' of their cancer rather than a contribution to its 'cause'. Sometimes people have tried to overcome this problem by using 'markers' of past intake in samples of blood taken and stored several years before the selection of cases and controls, for instance as part of a screening programme. For example, levels of carotenoids in stored blood samples have been used as a marker for past fruit and vegetable intake.

The case-control approach has been extremely useful in assessing the impact on health of factors where clear and reliable information on past behaviour can be obtained, such as the link between cigarette smoking and lung cancer. Case-control studies have also been useful in helping to identify the causes of some relatively uncommon conditions, such as the link between the prone sleeping position of babies and the risk of cot death, and the link between occupational exposure to asbestos and a normally rare form of lung cancer (mesothelioma).

- Case-control studies have suggested that past ginseng consumption was lower in Korean people who have developed a cancer than in matched control subjects who are free from cancer (Chapter 8).
- Many case-control studies have found that people with cancer had lower fruit and vegetable intakes and lower blood β-carotene intakes than matched controls who do not have cancer (Chapter 5).

Cohort studies

In cohort studies, the behaviour of a large sample of people (the cohort) is assessed and related to their risk of developing a disease over subsequent years. For example, the fruit and vegetable intake of a large cohort of people could be assessed, the group monitored for a number of years and cases of cancer recorded. The hypothesis is that those people in the cohort with the lowest fruit and vegetable intake at the start of the study will be most likely to develop cancer, while those with the highest intake are the least likely. Cancer rates can be compared in fifths (quintiles) of the population divided according to their fruit and vegetable intake; that is, the quintile with the lowest consumption, next lowest and so on, up to the highest-consuming quintile.

Although cohort studies are regarded as the most powerful and persuasive of the observational studies, they are also very expensive and time-consuming to conduct. To get enough new cases of disease in a cohort to allow meaningful statistical analysis requires very large cohorts (sometimes tens or hundreds of thousands are monitored) and they have to be followed for long periods. For example, it would require a cohort of 100 000 middle-aged northern Europeans to be followed for five years to get 150 newly diagnosed cases of colon cancer. Note that cancers diagnosed in the first two years of the study may be excluded, because these may have already been present but undiagnosed when the study started.

Listed below are examples of cohort studies that are directly relevant to the use of dietary supplements and discussed in later chapters of the book:

- A cohort study with 120 000 Dutch people over a period of 40 months found no association between consumption of garlic supplements or any other foods of the Allium family and the risk of developing cancer. This has been interpreted as suggesting that garlic has no protective effect against bowel cancer (Chapter 8).
- A five-year cohort study of ginseng intake in 4600 Koreans found that cancer rates in those regularly consuming ginseng were around half of those in the no-ginseng group (Chapter 8).
- Two large cohort studies have shown that a high intake of vitamin E from supplements was associated with a reduced rate of coronary heart disease in men and women (see Chapter 5). Note that these subjects were not given supplements in a controlled trial but were using them of their own accord and thus these supplement users may be, for example, more health conscious than the rest of the population.

Although relatively few cohort studies dealing directly with the use of dietary supplements are referred to in this book, several large and sometimes ongoing cohort studies have done much to shape our current views of how diet and lifestyle influence health and disease risk. Some examples are listed below:

- The Framingham study was started in 1948, when a cohort of just over 5000 men and women resident in the town of Framingham, Massachusetts were recruited. A detailed physical examination and lifestyle questionnaire were completed on each of these subjects, with the aim of identifying common factors and character-istics that related to cardiovascular disease risk. Detailed medical histories and physical examinations were carried out at two-yearly intervals. In 1971 a second, similar-sized cohort was recruited composed of the adult children of the original cohort along with their spouses. (See the Framingham website for details of this study: www.nhlbi.nih.gov/about/framingham/.)

- The Nurses' Health Study was started in 1976, when around 120 000 married American nurses were recruited and asked to fill in health-related question-naires. The primary motivation with this first cohort of participants (aged 30–55 years in 1976) was to assess the long-term consequences of oral contra-ceptive use. The participants were sent follow-up questionnaires at two-year intervals and in 1980 food frequency and diet questionnaires were first included. In 1989, a second, slightly younger cohort was recruited, with the aim of looking not only at the effects of oral contraceptive use but also at diet and lifestyle as risk factors for subsequent disease. (Further details of this study can be found at the study website: www.channing.harvard.edu/nhs/index.php/history.)

- The Whitehall II study used as its target cohort all civil servants working in the London offices of 20 Whitehall departments in 1985–88. The total sample size was just over 10 000, with a 2:1 male-to-female ratio. The initial questionnaire and screening were carried out between 1985 and 1988 with regular and ongo-ing follow-ups. The overall aim of this study was to investigate the biological mechanisms that might account for the social inequalities in cardiovascular disease and diabetes, including the role of traditional and established risk fac-tors like smoking, physical activity, blood pressure and cholesterol; dietary factors were subsequently included in the study. (Further details of this study can be found at www.ucl.ac.uk/whitehallII.)

Cross-sectional studies

If one is using a risk marker or a symptom as the measure of outcome, then it is possible to get 'immediate' results using a survey of a cross-section of the popula-tion. If one assessed diet and supplement usage in a large sample of people and then measured a disease risk marker or symptom, then one could look for correlations between consumption of a particular substance and the measured outcome. Thus in a dietary context one could look at the relationship between measured saturated fat intake and blood cholesterol concentration, or between habitual salt intake and blood pressure.

- In Chapter 9 it is suggested that cross-sectional studies in populations with high average soy intakes (but not in low soy populations), women with the highest intakes of soy have the highest bone mineral density. This has been used to sup-port the case that phyto-oestrogens in soy products or supplements may protect against osteoporosis.

Limitations of observational studies

Observational studies can never 'prove' a hypothesis, although in some cases the cumulative weight of evidence from such studies may well be accepted as such. The problem of 'confounding variables' affects the validity of all such observational studies. For example, a negative correlation between fruit and vegetable intake and age-specific cancer rates in different countries does not necessarily mean that fruit and vegetables protect against cancer. There may be numerous important differences between the populations in the study and these other differences may well account for the apparent protective effect of fruit and vegetables. Time trends may show that changes in fruit and vegetable consumption have been associated with changes in age-specific cancer rates, but other dietary, lifestyle and environmental changes will also almost certainly have occurred over the same time period – so is this association really an indication of cause and effect? While a large cohort study may show that those with a high fruit and vegetable intake have a lower risk of developing cancer, this does not prove a protective effect of fruit and vegetables. High fruit and vegetable consumers are likely to be different from low consumers in other respects.

A confounding variable is one that is 'independently linked to both the suspected cause and the disease or other outcome'. Take the proposition that high alcohol consumption causes lung cancer. If it was found in a case-control or cohort study that high alcohol consumption predicted high risk of lung cancer, this would not necessarily mean that alcohol is a direct cause of lung cancer. Smoking is a well-established cause of lung cancer and it is not unreasonable to suggest that heavy drinkers might be more likely to smoke (or passively smoke in smoky bars) than moderate drinkers or non-drinkers. So the association between drinking and lung cancer could be due to the confounding effects of smoking, which is independently linked to lung cancer and in this hypothetical example to alcohol consumption.

In our fruit and vegetable example, it can be convincingly demonstrated that there is a strong association between high fruit and vegetable consumption and lower cancer risk using several different observational approaches. There are, however, many potential confounding variables, as listed below, that one would need to consider before concluding that the association is likely to be cause and effect; that is, that substances in fruit and vegetables directly protect against cancer.

- High fruit and vegetable intake may displace other 'cancer-promoting' components of the diet. For example, do high fruit and vegetable consumers have lower fat and/or meat protein intakes than low fruit and vegetable eaters?
- In Britain, fruit and vegetable consumption is affected by wealth and social class – people who are more affluent tend to consume more fruit and vegetables. Poverty is known to be a strong predictor of poor health and early mortality. Is the association between low fruit and vegetable intake and high cancer risk merely another indication that poorer people have a higher risk of developing cancer?

- Is high fruit and vegetable consumption a marker for a tendency to be more health aware? Are high fruit and vegetable consumers less likely to smoke or drink heavily, and more likely to exercise regularly, control their weight and make health a factor in their food choices?

As another example, if one found a strong link between supplement or functional food use and a low or high risk of a particular disease (e.g. vitamin E supplements and heart disease, as noted earlier), this would be an interesting observation that could generate a potentially testable hypothesis, but one would need to be cautious before assuming a 'cause-and-effect' relationship (see below):

- Users are unlikely to be typical of the whole population in terms of their socio-economic and educational status, their gender, age profile etc.
- Supplement use might well indicate a higher than typical health awareness and thus a greater tendency to adopt other 'healthy diet and lifestyle' practices.
- Conversely, vague symptoms or other early indications of disease might encourage people to try a supplement and thus lead to high supplement use among new diagnoses, which might be falsely interpreted as suggesting that the supplement has played a role in triggering the disease.

Modern observational studies are designed to minimise the influence of confounding variables and use various statistical procedures to correct for the effect of confounders. However, these processes are by no means perfect and they are applied with varying degrees of rigour by different research groups. To correct properly for confounding variables, one needs detailed quantitative information about the potential confounder that may not always be obtainable. If one wanted to correct for the effects of smoking as a confounder, then it should be possible to get reliable quantitative information from subjects about their tobacco usage. However, if one wanted to correct for differences in level of physical activity, this would be extremely difficult and error prone.

The experimental approach

Human experiments

Experiments are designed to test a particular hypothesis, for instance that a supplement alleviates the symptoms of a particular disease. In such an example, matched experimental and control groups would be selected and the experimental group given the supplement while the control group given a placebo. At the end of the experiment, pre-determined measures of outcome are compared in the control and experimental groups. In a double-blind trial, those who are carrying out the study and collecting the data should not know which subjects are receiving real and placebo treatments until after the data collection has been completed. If the two groups were well matched at the start of the trial and all other factors in the handling of the two groups are equal, then any statistically significant differences between the two groups can be confidently attributed to the effect of the 'treatment'.

A placebo is a dummy treatment that is itself inactive but should be indistinguishable from the real treatment. Any treatment may produce beneficial effects that are purely psychological rather than due to an active physiological effect of the treatment; placebos should control for this effect. The more subjective the measure of outcome, the more important it is to use a placebo to account for any psychological effects of being treated. For example, in trials of therapies for depression, it is common for a placebo to result in positive benefits in 25% or more of patients (see the section on St John's wort in Chapter 8); and in studies of treatments for menopausal hot flushes, placebos may produce benefits in up to 50% of patients (see Chapter 9, the section on phyto-oestrogens). It is also very important that those conducting the trial and assessing the participants should not know which participants are receiving which treatments until all of the data has been collected. Researchers can bias the responses of participants if they believe that the treatment will or will not work, and it can bias the way in which they collect and record results.

Experiments are generally regarded as the main way in which the advancement of scientific knowledge and understanding occurs. An hypothesis is put forward to explain observations and then an experiment or experiments designed to test the hypothesis. The hypothesis is then accepted, rejected or modified in the light of the results of the experiment(s). Many hypotheses about the potential benefits of using supplements and functional foods have arisen from observational studies like those listed above and these must then be tested in controlled experiments, ultimately where feasible in high-quality controlled clinical trials.

Consider the hypothesis that a dietary supplement reduces high blood pressure. To test this hypothesis, one could select matched groups of subjects with mild hypertension (at least matched for age, sex, use of antihypertensive drugs and initial blood pressure). One group would receive the supplement (test group) and the other would be given an identical but inert placebo (control group). In order to eliminate the possibility of bias from the experimenters, one could code the real and placebo treatments so that none of those involved know which patient is in which group until the data collection is complete. At the end of the designated period the blood pressure changes in the control and experimental groups would be compared. Several test groups taking different doses of the supplement could be used to see if any effect was dose dependent. This is a double-blind, placebo-controlled trial: the gold standard for trials of drugs, supplements and indeed any clinical treatment.

In this particular case, because the effect of the treatment is fairly acute, one might design the experiment so that all subjects spend a period on the real treatment and another period on the dummy treatment. The subjects would be randomly assigned to receive either real or placebo treatment first. The blood pressures at the end of the placebo and real treatment periods would be compared and in effect each subject would act as their own control. This is termed a double-blind, placebo-controlled, random crossover trial (see Figure 1.3 for a plan of such a study). Note that some clinical trials, especially of new drugs, compare the effectiveness of the new treatment to the current treatment rather than a placebo to see

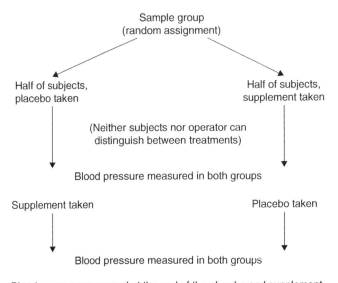

Sample group
(random assignment)

Half of subjects,
placebo taken

Half of subjects,
supplement taken

(Neither subjects nor operator can
distinguish between treatments)

Blood pressure measured in both groups

Supplement taken

Placebo taken

Blood pressure measured in both groups

Blood pressure compared at the end of the placebo and supplement
periods using a paired statistical test (e.g. 'paired' t test)

Figure 1.3   Theoretical plan of a double-blind, random, cross-over trial of a putative blood
pressure-lowering supplement.

if the new treatment is more effective. It is argued that where established effective
treatments are already available, it may be unethical to deprive the control group
of any treatment.

Clinical trials vary widely in their quality and this clearly affects confidence in
the outcome. A good trial should ideally:

- Be well-blinded so that neither subject nor researcher should know or be able to
work out which treatment a patient is receiving.
- Have an unbiased and random allocation of subjects to control and placebo
groups.
- Should describe in detail people who withdraw or drop out of the study, as high
drop-out rates can skew the results (e.g. if many treated patients fail to complete
the study because they feel that the treatment offered is ineffective).

One of the most widely used methods to grade the quality of clinical trials is the
Jadad scale (derived from the work of Jadad *et al.*, 1996). On this scale, trials are
given a score of 0 to 5 based on three criteria:

- If the study is described as randomised, it receives one point; if the method of
randomisation is described and is appropriate then an extra point is given,
although a point is subtracted if the method described is inappropriate.

- Likewise, if the study is described as double blind then a point is given and a further point if the method is described and appropriate, but a point is removed if the described method is inappropriate.
- An additional point is given if the number of withdrawals and drop-outs from each group is given along with the underlying reasons.

While this is clearly a crude and imperfect method of assessing trial quality, it can be done quickly and is widely used.

An additional problem with clinical trials involving dietary supplements is the variable or indeterminate quality of supplements, as mentioned earlier. In some countries in continental Europe such as Germany, there is a long history of substances like herbal extracts and natural metabolites being prescribed by orthodox health practitioners and being subject to pharmaceutical-level control of their quality and potency. In the UK and the USA, many of these same substances are sold over the counter as dietary/food supplements without any such regulation of their quality. Low quality and potency could affect the outcome of a clinical trial and variability in quality could also perhaps be a factor in the variability of the results of clinical trials. In addition, if good clinical trials have been conducted on high-quality, pharmaceutical-grade compounds, will similar results be obtained with each of the assortment of supplements of the same name sold over the counter in the UK and the USA?

There are many potential short-term outcome measures that can be used in these experimental trials:

- A risk marker measurement such as blood pressure or cholesterol concentration.
- An objective measure of a disease symptom or progression.
- The subject's own perception of the effects, like their perceived pain level.
- The physician's assessment of the patient's improvement.

These experiments become much more expensive and difficult if the outcome measure takes a long time to materialise, for example if the benefits of the treatment are not expected for many months or even years. If one is testing a preventive effect, such as whether a supplement or functional food prevents a chronic disease like cancer or heart disease, then one is in a similar situation as with a cohort study. One must persuade many thousands of people to remain in the study and continue taking the supplement (or placebo) for a number of years and pay people to monitor them until sufficient numbers of cases of cancer or heart disease occur to allow statistical analysis.

- In Chapter 6, two trials of fish oils in men who had previously had a heart attack (secondary intervention trials) are discussed. Both of these studies suggest that taking fish oil supplements significantly reduces total mortality in the years immediately after a first heart attack.
- In Chapter 3 there is discussion of two trials of the effects of periconceptual folic acid supplements in reducing the risk of babies being born with a neural

tube defect (NTD). These show that these supplements can reduce both the recurrence of NTDs in women with a previously affected pregnancy and also the first occurrence in women not previously affected.

- In Chapter 5 several long-term trials of β-carotene supplements in the prevention of cancer are reviewed. These suggest that, despite all the epidemiological evidence suggesting a protective effect of a β-carotene-rich diet, supplements of β-carotene may actually increase deaths from cancer in some groups, such as smokers, and perhaps also increase deaths from cardiovascular causes.

Experimental treatments may sometimes take the form of education or promotion programmes rather than actual provision of supplements, for instance an intensive programme to promote the use of a supplement. Let us say that one region was subject to a very active campaign to persuade women to take iron supplements to reduce the prevalence of anaemia, and another matched region was used as a control. One could compare changes in average blood haemoglobin concentration or rates of anaemia in the two areas over the course of the intervention.

There is currently a very active campaign in the UK to persuade women to take folic acid supplements when they are planning a pregnancy and in the early stages of pregnancy. This campaign should ultimately reduce the prevalence of NTDs in the UK, although it is hindered by the fact that maybe half of all pregnancies are unplanned, and also that those people with the lowest nutrient intakes from food are also the least likely to take a supplement. In order to overcome these obstacles, fortification of a common food(s) with folic acid has been recommended; this would ensure that all women of child-bearing age as well as the rest of the population receive extra folic acid (see discussion in Chapter 3).

Systematic reviews and meta-analyses

The costs and complexity of a controlled trial increase with the size and duration of the study. For this reason, many clinical trials of dietary supplements have used relatively small numbers of subjects. This means that even if they have been well designed and executed, they may not have the statistical power to provide a definitive judgement of the value or otherwise of the supplement unless the effect is large. The net result of this is a literature concerning supplements that often contains many individual studies addressing a particular question and giving inconclusive or even conflicting answers. These studies will vary in size and quality and in the details of their design, so simply counting how many studies are for, against or inconclusive for a particular question is not a helpful or valid procedure.

A systematic review aims to identify, using pre-set and objective search methodology, as many as possible of the studies that have addressed a particular topic. One or more electronic databases of published papers will be used to identify all published papers that use the key search words. Additional pre-set and systematic search methods may be used to find additional studies, for example the reference lists of papers from the primary search, and perhaps some method may be used for trying to get data from studies that have not been formally published, for instance clinical trials registered with the American Food and Drugs Administration (FDA).

A meta-analysis of studies identified from a systematic review involves a statistical pooling of all studies that meet pre-determined quality and eligibility criteria. The reviewers may set general eligibility criteria, for example relating to dosage, diagnostic criteria and characteristics of subjects, such as age and sex and outcome measures. The Jadad score, as described in the previous section, is widely used to select trials according to quality, for instance a minimum Jadad score may be required for eligibility for the meta-analysis. In this way a number of small studies of limited statistical power can be combined as if they were a single study of much greater statistical power. Individual component studies in the meta-analysis are weighted according to the sample size used. In theory, a well-conducted systematic review and meta-analysis should give a much better indication of the true answer to a question than a simple for-and-against count or a qualitative and subjective interpretation by the reviewer.

When studies are combined in a meta-analysis, it is assumed that they are all essentially homogeneous and that any differences between them in terms of outcome are due to chance. This is often not the case, for example differences in outcome may be due to 'real' differences in the nature of the subjects; that is, a treatment may have different effects in different categories of subject. Some of the other pitfalls of this approach are summarised below (after Naylor, 1997).

- *Publication bias*. There is much evidence that studies with a positive outcome are more likely to be published than those with a negative or inconclusive outcome. This may occur at the submission level: a high proportion of trials of supplements are funded by the manufacturers who have a vested interest in the publication of trials with a positive outcome, but are less keen to see the publication of trials with a negative outcome. Journal editors and reviewers may also favour the publication of studies with positive outcomes, as these may be seen as more interesting to readers and more likely to have a positive effect on a journal's impact. This is seen as a major problem in the area of dietary supplements, partly because of the high level of involvement of manufacturing companies in the funding of trials; it may also be a problem with drug trials for similar reasons. For example, Turner *et al.* (2008) identified 74 trials of antidepressant drugs registered with the US FDA. Only 1 of 38 trials with a positive outcome was not published, whereas 22 of the 36 studies with negative or questionable results were not published and 11 were published in a way that, in the opinion of Turner *et al.*, conveyed a positive outcome.

  In many meta-analyses authors try to detect whether substantial publication bias has occurred. One of the simplest and most widely used of these methods is the funnel plot. The assumption is made that small trials will give more variable results than larger trials of the same quality. In a funnel plot the effect estimate of each trial is plotted against the sample size. In the absence of bias, one would expect to see a symmetrical (funnel-shaped) scattering of trials around the true effect estimate. The larger and more consistent trials should be

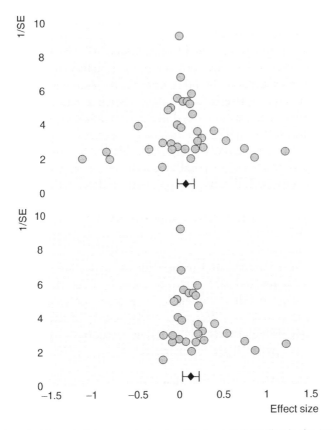

Figure 1.4 A typical funnel plot generated using 35 simulated studies in the top graph and the same plot at the bottom after removing 5 smaller trials with negative outcomes to illustrate the typical manifestation of publication bias.
Source: Reproduced from Sutton, A.J. *et al.* (2000) *British Medical Journal*, **320**, 1574.

closely grouped at the top of the funnel; as the trial size gets smaller and more inconsistent in its results, the scattering around the true result should get larger but remain broadly symmetrical. If there is a lack of symmetry (usually a lack of small trials showing a negative effect), this would suggest publication bias; that is, that some of the small negative trials have not been published. This illustrated in Figure 1.4, where a funnel plot of 35 simulated studies is shown and the plot is then redrawn as if five small trials with negative outcomes had not been published (see Sutton *et al.*, 2000 and Egger *et al.*, 1997 for further details and discussion.

- *Multiple publishing*. Some trials may be published more than once; if these are all included in a meta-analysis, this can bias its outcome. Naylor quotes the example of a single study being the source for seven different publications. These different publications of the same trial had different authorship, which would make it more difficult to identify that they all related to the same study.

- *Selection bias*. Unless the selection of papers for inclusion in the meta-analysis is done strictly using pre-set objective criteria, this may be a further source of bias. This may result in meta-analyses looking at the same question coming to different conclusions. It may also mean that authors find that when they analyse their results using different inclusion criteria, the results change. For example, in trials of a supplement the initial analysis of all trials meeting the minimum criteria may be more positive about the supplement than when the analysis is repeated using increased-quality selection criteria (e.g. McAlindon *et al.*, 2000 and Bjelakovic *et al.*, 2007). These anecdotal examples seem to be part of a general trend in which trials of low methodological quality produce a higher estimate of benefit from an intervention compared to high-quality studies. Moher *et al.* (1998) randomly selected 11 meta-analyses of various medical interventions for treatment of a variety of conditions. They conducted these meta-analyses again and divided up the studies according to quality. They found that at that time many of the trials were of low quality and that lower-quality trials were associated with a 34% increase in estimated treatment benefit compared to the better-conducted trials. This finding was consistent when two different methods were used for quality classification. This needs to be borne in mind when interpreting meta-analyses, especially where the reviewers are critical of the quality of many of the trials. Note that a simple reduction in the level of statistical significance would be expected if reviewers reduce the number of studies in a meta-analysis when setting higher-quality criteria (because sample size has been reduced), but if there is also a substantial drop in the size of the treatment effect measure, this would indicate that the lower-quality trials were biasing results in favour of the treatment.

Figure 1.5 illustrates a typical 'forest plot' presentation of results from a meta-analysis (taken from Linde *et al.*, 2008). Each of the 16 horizontal lines represents one clinical trial of St John's wort versus a placebo in the treatment of major depression. The bullet in the middle of the line represents the mean treatment effect and the limits of the lines represent the 95% confidence limits. The size of the bullet gives an indication of the weighting applied to that study. Any bullet to the left of the vertical zero line favours the placebo and any to the right favours St John's wort. The trials have been divided by precision (i.e. size) and the more precise trial results favour the effect of St John's wort over the placebo more than the lower, higher-precision trials, as is generally the case.

Numerous examples of systematic reviews and meta-analyses are referred to in the rest of this book. Just three examples are given below:

- Chapter 8 describes how a systematic review and meta-analysis of the benefits of Ginkgo biloba supplements for cognitive impairment and dementia did indicate statistically significant improvements in the physicians' assessments of the patients' improvement and other outcome measures in those taking the supplements.
- In Chapter 7, meta-analyses of trials of glucosamine for treatment of osteoarthritis of the hip and knee up to 1999 indicate that when used for at least four weeks it does produce a moderate to large beneficial effect. This study indicated

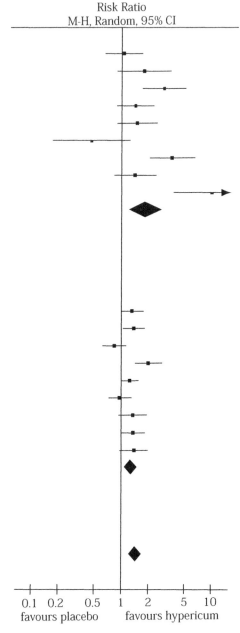

Figure 1.5   A typical forest plot presentation of the data from a meta-analysis. The plot shows results (risk ratio with 95% confidence intervals) from 18 clinical trials of St John's wort (Hypericum) against a placebo for the treatment of depression. The top 9 trials were the least precise, while the bottom 9 were the most precise. The three dark diamonds represent (from top to bottom) the combined weighted result of the 8 least precise trials; the 8 most precise trials; all 16 trials.
Source: Reproduced from Linde *et al*. (2008) *Cochrane Database of Systematic Reviews*) Oct 8;(4): CD000448.

a high probability of publication bias and the magnitude of the beneficial effects was reduced when only the larger and higher-quality studies were used for the analysis.

- Also in Chapter 8, the meta-analysis of trials of St John's wort from which Figure 1.5 is taken is discussed.

The Cochrane Library contains a very large database of high-quality systematic reviews that are widely regarded as the gold standard for assessing the efficacy of a particular healthcare intervention. Most readers of this book will have free access to the full text of these reviews online via the home page for the Cochrane library (www3.interscience.wiley.com/cgi-bin/mrwhome/106568753/HOME). The Cochrane library is published by Wiley-Blackwell for the Cochrane Collaboration, a non-profit organisation that aims to improve healthcare decision making by increasing the availability of systematic reviews of healthcare interventions.

It is usually assumed by reviewers and other readers of respected scientific journals that the researchers will have been honest, honourable and unbiased in the conduct and reporting of their research. There have, however, been several well-publicised examples of research fraud, where authors have knowingly published false research findings in order to further their careers or to gain a commercial advantage. Such proven or confessed examples of scientific fraud are thankfully rare, but presumably other examples exist in the literature that it is almost impossible for the non-specialist to spot (these papers have been peer reviewed by experts in the field who have not detected the 'fraud').

In 2005 the important American journal *Nutrition* retracted a paper published in the journal by the Canadian researcher R. K. Chandra in 2001. This paper reported a placebo-controlled trial that seemed to show that moderate doses of vitamins and minerals taken as supplements improved cognitive function in elderly people. The same author has published more than 200 articles, several of which have been widely cited; four of these papers were cited in the first edition of this book as evidence that vitamin and mineral supplements might have beneficial effects on immune function in elderly people. Only one of the author's papers had been retracted by 2005, although there must be a question mark over many of the others, especially as he made a considerable amount of money from sales of his multivitamin mixture, sold as an 'evidence-based' (his own published trials) nutrition supplement for the elderly (see Smith, 2005 and Hamblin, 2006 for fuller accounts).

In 2002, UK regulators withdrew the product licences for two evening primrose oil preparations for the treatment of atopic eczema and mastalgia (breast pain), on the basis of lack of evidence for their efficacy. Some of the circumstances leading up to this are discussed by Williams (2003) in an editorial in the *British Medical Journal*. In 1989, Morse *et al.* published a meta-analysis of nine trials of evening primrose oil for the treatment of atopic eczema. The authors of this study were from an organisation involved in the marketing of several evening primrose preparations, including those whose product licences were withdrawn. This trial found that evening primrose oil was more effective than a placebo in controlling this condition. Seven of the nine trials included in the meta-analysis were small trials sponsored by the company and, according to Williams, one relatively large independent study with negative findings was excluded from the analysis on grounds that he considered to be dubious. A more recent meta-analysis by Van Gool *et al.* (2004) found no significant benefit for evening primrose oil over a placebo. The protocol for a Cochrane review of the effect of evening primrose oil for the treatment of atopic eczema was published in 2003, but unfortunately at the time of writing no data has been published.

Statistical significance and clinical significance

Statistical analysis is used to estimate the probability that, say, a difference between two sample means or an association between two variables could have occurred simply by chance. If one tested the effects of a substance and a placebo on plasma cholesterol concentration in two matched groups of subjects, then it is unlikely that the mean change in the parameter would be identical in the two groups, even if the test compound was as inert as the placebo or even if both groups had been given identical treatments. In this instance, statistical analysis should indicate a high probability that this difference between the two treatments is due to chance.

By convention in science, if the probability of a result being due to chance is less than 5% (1 in 20), it is regarded as 'statistically significant'. This is a purely mathematical significance and does not indicate whether say the effect of a dietary supplement has a clinically meaningful value to the people taking it (see examples below).

- There is substantial evidence, reviewed in Chapter 8, that some garlic supplements produce a statistically significant reduction in plasma cholesterol concentration when compared to a placebo. However, this evidence also suggests that the effect of garlic supplements is small and probably transitory. This means that despite their statistically significant effect, garlic supplements are regarded as an ineffective means of producing clinically useful reductions in plasma cholesterol.
- In Chapter 7, substantial evidence is presented that glucosamine supplements have a statistically significant effect both in reducing the symptoms of mild osteoarthritis of the knee and in preventing the narrowing of the joint space that occurred in the placebo group. However, about half of the rheumatologists taking part in a debate on the use of glucosamine supplements were against its routine use. They argued that the symptomatic benefits were small and confined to those with mild symptoms, and that the effect on joint space was of unproven clinical usefulness.
- In Chapter 8, a sizeable controlled study is described in which large daily chitosan supplements are compared to a placebo. After six months the chitosan group had lost an average of half a kilogram more than the control group. Despite this effect being statistically significant, the authors regarded it as not

clinically significant and it did not warrant the use of chitosan for weight loss. Likewise, the chitosan group registered a statistically significant but clinically unimportant fall in their circulating LDL cholesterol.

Of course, statistical significance may also be the product of bias in the design or conduct of the experiment, from for example inadequate blinding, unsatisfactory randomisation in the allocation of subjects or a failure to take account of high drop-out rates caused by patient perception of a treatment being ineffective.

Animal experiments

Experiments with human volunteers are always fraught with difficulties and uncertainties, such as:

- Ensuring that control and experimental groups are adequately matched.
- The withdrawal of subjects before the trial is complete.
- Variable and often uncertain compliance with the treatment regimen.
- Placebo effects.
- Other influences on outcome measures during the experimental period, e.g. illnesses, injuries, pregnancy, use of prescribed drugs, major life stresses etc.

Animal experiments have fewer such problems and they afford the competent researcher the opportunity to do highly reliable and repeatable experiments at relatively low cost. Some of the advantages of animal experiments compared to those using human subjects are listed here:

- One can get extremely well-matched control and experimental groups, e.g. by using inbred strains one can get large numbers of genetically identical animals.
- One can control all aspects of diet and environment so that the only difference between the groups is the treatment under test.
- The duration of the experiment can, if necessary, be as long as the animals live.
- One can ensure 100% compliance with treatment throughout the experiment.
- One can use invasive measures of outcome.
- One can take risks that would be ethically unacceptable with human subjects, e.g. using high and possibly harmful doses.

The problem with animal experiments is their validity – are the responses of laboratory animals always a valid guide to the likely responses of people? Even if animals and people appear to respond similarly, animal experiments may be of little use in deciding on appropriate doses for humans, partly because of species differences *per se* and also because of the problem of scaling from small laboratory animals to people.

Animal experiments do have a role in the testing of supplements and functional foods. They certainly played a part in demonstrating the effects of vitamin and mineral deficiencies and in confirming that these deficiency diseases could be cured by the appropriate vitamin or mineral. Perhaps the proper role of animals should be to generate hypotheses about human responses and/or to show that these have enough credibility to be worthwhile for testing in people (the benefits and limitations of such animal experiments are discussed at length in Webb, 1992). Some examples from later chapters of this book are listed below:

- Green tea polyphenols consistently reduce the development of chemically induced cancers in animal models. When matched groups of animals are exposed to a carcinogenic chemical, those animals receiving green tea polyphenols develop fewer cancers than those not receiving them. Human epidemiological studies have not as yet, however, consistently supported a protective effect of green tea in humans (see Chapter 8).
- There is a substantial amount of data from laboratory experiments with small animals suggesting that ginsenosides extracted from ginseng improve exercise performance in controlled trials. These animal studies have often used very high doses and in some cases the ginsenosides have been injected. The data from human trials is much less consistent and, so far, much less convincing (see Chapter 8).
- In animal studies soybean feeding generally leads to increased bone density in ovariectomised female rats, suggesting that the phyto-oestrogens in soybeans improve bone health in these animals. There is some limited epidemiological data to suggest that high doses of soy products may also produce a measurable effect on bone density in the lumbar spine in women (Chapter 9).

In vitro *experiments*

In vitro experiments are literally those done 'in glass'. These would include:

- Experiments with isolated (human) cells including tumour cell lines.
- Experiments using micro-organisms.
- Experiments using cell-free systems.

Thus one could test with such systems, for example:

- Whether a substance inhibited a particular enzyme or bound to a particular receptor.
- Whether a substance had any bacteriocidal effects.
- Whether a compound was mutagenic or antimutagenic in bacteria. Mutagenicity in bacteria is used as an indicator of carcinogenicity: a compound that is mutagenic might be a potential carcinogen and one that is antimutagenic might have cancer-preventing potential.
- How a substance affected the growth or metabolism of cancer cells.

There are numerous examples of such studies throughout the book and three examples are briefly mentioned below. Note that the results of such studies must be treated with great caution until the benefits predicted from these reductionist experiments are supported by evidence from more holistic trials with human subjects.

- In Chapter 8, it is noted that lipophilic extracts of Agnus castus berries bind to dopamine receptors on isolated pituitary cells and inhibit the release of the hormone prolactin. This may explain its proposed effect in reducing the symptoms of pre-menstrual syndrome.
- Allicin from garlic has bacteriocidal effects *in vitro*. It can even kill many isolates of methacillin-resistant Staphylococcus aureus (MRSA) (see Chapter 8). This work has largely focused on the potential use of garlic as a topical antibacterial agent, but there are also claims that it has anti-infective properties when taken orally.
- Glucosamine can increase the rate of proteoglycan production in cultured chondrocytes. Chondrocytes are cartilage-forming cells and proteoglycans are key components of cartilage. Glucosamine also inhibits the production of some inflammatory mediators in these isolated cells. Even though there are doubts about whether the *in vitro* doses are a realistic indication of the amounts reaching the chondrocytes *in vivo*, this may nevertheless suggest mechanisms by which it could reduce the symptoms of osteoarthritis.

What about safety?

It should never be assumed that just because something is a 'natural' component of the diet, it is therefore inherently safe. It is not reasonable to assume that even if taking a supplement does no good, it is unlikely to do harm, so that the balance of advantage always lies with taking the supplement 'just in case'. Some supplements are expensive and so cost is a factor that should be taken in to account when weighing up the balance of advantage. It is almost a cliché to say that every substance is toxic, it is merely the dose needed for toxic effects that varies. The higher the dose used, the more likely it is that there will be harmful effects.

Many common foods contain toxins that can pose a serious threat to health under some circumstances, such as the following:

- Red kidney beans contain a substance (a haemagglutinin) that causes acute nausea, diarrhoea and vomiting if the beans are not subjected to vigorous boiling before being eaten.
- Cassava contains substances that release cyanide, which can cause poisoning if it is not properly prepared.
- Broad beans (Vicia fava) contain a substance that causes red cell breakdown. Many Mediterranean people and black Americans are very susceptible to this toxin, with acute symptoms of vomiting, abdominal pain, fever, dark urine and, in the longer term, anaemia. This condition, called favism, is associated with an

X-linked deficiency of the enzyme glucose-6-phosphate dehydrogenase and so is much more common in men; these individuals also develop these symptoms when given a widely used antimalarial drug, primaquine.

Several of the essential nutrients also have well-documented toxic, perhaps even fatal, effects when taken in excessive amounts:

- Iron is an essential nutrient, but iron poisoning from dietary supplements intended for their parents is also the most common cause of accidental poisoning in children.
- Vitamin A (retinol) is known to be acutely toxic in very high doses. It may also cause an increased risk of fracture in elderly people at doses around twice the usual recommended intake, and it is thought to cause malformations in unborn children if consumed in excess during pregnancy.
- β-carotene has a very low acute toxicity, but there is evidence that chronic high consumption may promote tumour growth in smokers and others at high risk of lung cancer.
- Large folic acid supplements may interfere with the actions of a number of drugs that work because they antagonise the effects of folic acid. It may also mask the anaemia caused by vitamin B_{12} deficiency (including pernicious anaemia) and this means that the irreversible neuropathy of B_{12} deficiency is left untreated. There have even been recent claims that it may promote the growth of bowel tumours (see Chapter 3 for a detailed discussion).

An Expert Group on Vitamins and Minerals produced a 350-page report for the Food Standards Agency (FSA, 2003) that tried to establish Tolerable Upper Intake Levels (UL) for all vitamins, essential minerals and other trace elements using previously published data. The UL is the total chronic daily intake of the substance that is judged to be unlikely to pose a risk to health. It is ideally based on the No Observed Adverse Effect Level (NOAEL), the highest intake at which no adverse effects are observed. In several cases the committee had less than ideal data to work with, for example they may have:

- had to infer doses that were chronically acceptable from relatively short-term studies;
- had to rely to some extent on animal data;
- had to use data from studies where the substance was not administered via the normal oral route.

Essentially the same types of observational and experimental methods that are used to assess efficacy are also used to assess safety. In this case the outcome measure is some 'adverse effect'; that is, a physiological, developmental or other effect that in expert opinion is either directly damaging to the individual's functioning or makes him or her more vulnerable to other stresses or environmental influences.

The quality of supplement research

Several of the substances discussed in this book, even though they are not essential nutrients, have a long history of use as supplements or traditional remedies and some have been the subject of hundreds or even thousands of research studies. For example, when St John's wort was entered into the PubMed search engine (in December 2009) it produced almost 2000 hits, including almost 300 reviews and with relevant research papers dating back over 50 years. Despite, in many cases, this long history of use and study, there is usually no consensus about the effectiveness of most of these substances. This may be partly because potential supplements that show the promise of providing large and immediate therapeutic benefits are likely to be recognised and developed by the pharmaceutical industry as orthodox medicines. However, it is also partly to do with the nature and quality of research studies on supplements: many studies are reductionist and those holistic trials that are conducted are often small and of low quality.

Testing: A summing up

The use of supplements and functional foods should be based on sound scientific evidence of their efficacy and safety. The methods outlined above must be used to gain or extend this evidence: double-blind, placebo-controlled trials of sufficient size and duration must be the ultimate aim in most cases. Unless usage of these substances is based on such evidence, then it is mere quackery.

Even if large and properly designed double-blind studies have been completed, there may still be arguments about the meaning and/or the applicability of the results, such as those listed below:

- A negative result may not be accepted as 'proof' of ineffectiveness because of claims that the dose used was insufficient or that the formulation of the product used for the test was not optimal, for example if a synthetic source has been used in a study it may be claimed to be less effective than a natural source. A single antioxidant preparation may be claimed to be 'unbalanced' and thus not an indication of what would happen if a balanced multisupplement or multiple supplements had been used. The supplement may contain indeterminate or inadequate levels of the bioactive components, for instance some garlic supplements may contain little of the compound (allicin) believed to be the active ingredient.
- Some trials may use combinations of supplements and it may be impossible to attribute any beneficial (or harmful) effects to any one component unless the study has been designed specifically to allow this from the outset.
- The results of a trial of a vitamin or mineral supplement might be different in subjects with low baseline intakes compared to those with high baseline intakes. Thus a trial with a positive outcome in a developing country where low intakes are common might not predict what would happen in a wealthy and well-nourished population in Europe or the USA.

- It may be argued that that the subjects used in a study are not those likely to gain most benefit from it (or most likely to be harmed by it) and thus the results are irrelevant to those at whom the advertising for the supplement is targeted.
- It may always be argued that the study was not big enough or of long enough duration for the benefits to manifest or become statistically significant.
- There may be other technical criticisms of the design and execution of a study that produces unfavourable results. Although these criticisms may be scientifically valid, often a (much) more sympathetic view is taken of similarly flawed studies that produce a favourable outcome.

Supplement suppliers have a commercial incentive to emphasise positive results from trials and to undermine the credibility of negative results; they often employ scientific consultants who can interpret scientific results in the most favourable way for the company. Such consultants may be less than objective and may emphasise the data and arguments that favour their employer's position. These consultants may be inherently sympathetic to the use of these products or may have careers and professional profiles based on supplement or functional food use; this may often do more to hinder their objectivity than any consultancy fees. In science, it is often extremely difficult to 'prove' a negative, for example to prove that a supplement or functional food is ineffective in all circumstances or, conversely, to prove that it has no adverse long-term effects.

Studies on the benefits and risks of β-carotene supplements illustrate several of these points (there is a more detailed, referenced discussion of this topic in Chapter 5). There is a mass of epidemiological evidence to suggest that people with naturally high β-carotene intakes (from coloured fruits and vegetables) have a reduced risk of dying prematurely from cancer and heart disease. This has precipitated a number of large scale trials of β-carotene-containing supplements. One large controlled study in China showed that subjects given a combination of β-carotene, vitamin E and selenium for an average of six years had significantly lower cancer and total mortality than those not receiving it. Even if one accepts the statistical evidence of benefit from the supplement, then there remain at least two major problems in interpreting these findings:

- The study design means that it is impossible to determine what element(s) of the combined supplement were responsible for the benefits seen. It could have been selenium, vitamin E, β-carotene as a precursor of vitamin A (people can convert carotene to vitamin A) or β-carotene *per se* as an antioxidant.
- This Chinese population had high cancer rates and had vitamin and mineral intakes that were low by western standards; the supplements were intended to correct existing deficiencies. Inadequate intakes of nutrients may increase susceptibility to cancer and so supplements would reduce this risk, but this does not mean that excess nutrients given to well-nourished populations will have the same effect. In this particular study, the effect of β-carotene as an antioxidant, the reason it is promoted as a supplement in industrialised countries, seems to be the least probable reason for the benefits attributed to the combined supplement.

- Several controlled studies of β-carotene containing supplements in industrialised countries have failed to reproduce the apparent benefit seen in the Chinese study. Studies with normal subjects have generally shown no benefit from the β-carotene supplements. Other studies have used subjects with an increased risk of lung cancer, such as smokers and asbestos workers, and these have suggested that β-carotene supplements may promote lung cancer growth in these susceptible people and increase total mortality.

The results of studies such as these have been widely interpreted thus:

- β-carotene supplements offer no overall benefit in reducing cancer or cardio-vascular disease in well-nourished populations in industrialised countries. Furthermore, there is some indication that they may actually increase the risk of lung cancer in high-risk groups (e.g. smokers and those exposed to asbestos) and may possibly have harmful effects in others. They may actually increase total mortality rather than decrease it.

This evidence led an official expert group reviewing dietary aspects of cancer on behalf of the UK Department of Health (COMA, 1998a) specifically to counsel against the use of β-carotene supplements. More recently, the Food Standards Agency expert group (FSA, 2003) recommended that the maximum daily dose of β-carotene in supplements should be 7mg, which was less than half that in many commercial supplements.

One argument used by proponents of the use of β-carotene supplements to refute these studies suggesting that it is ineffective and perhaps harmful is that the studies have used pure, synthetic β-carotene rather than natural preparations, which also contain other carotenoids (e.g. α-carotene, lycopene, lutein and cryptoxanthin). The implication is clearly that despite the negative evidence about pure synthetic β-carotene, these natural carotenoid preparations are safe and effective. While such arguments may be intellectually defensible, as there is no convincing direct evidence of their efficacy and fairly convincing evidence of the potential to do harm, it seems morally dubious to continue to market these supplements on health grounds. Some have even suggested that the doses used in these studies were insufficient!

2 An Overview of Micronutrient Adequacy

Introduction and scope of the chapter

The vitamins and minerals covered in this chapter are all proven essential nutrients. As they are required in relatively small amounts compared to the total weight of food eaten (mg or μg quantities), vitamins and essential minerals are often collectively termed the micronutrients; fats, proteins and carbohydrates are thus termed the macronutrients. It was the initial discovery of the essentiality of these micronutrients, and particularly the deficiency diseases that result from their absence in the diet, that started the fashion for dietary supplements and food fortification. The traditional reason for taking supplements of these micronutrients was to treat or prevent deficiency, but nowadays they may also be taken with the aim of treating or preventing non-deficiency diseases, or indeed for any of the other major purposes listed in Chapter 1.

In this chapter, the methods used to define and determine micronutrient adequacy are briefly reviewed. This review is followed by a discussion of the general micronutrient adequacy of diets in industrialised countries, with a particular focus on the micronutrient adequacy of different population groups within the UK. Discussion of individual vitamins, minerals and antioxidants is in Chapters 3, 4 and 5; the substances covered in these chapters account for a substantial proportion of the total spending on dietary supplements.

Judging the adequacy of micronutrient intakes

In order to assess the micronutrient adequacy of any individual or population's diet, one must first measure how much of different foods have been consumed and then estimate the micronutrient content of this food, usually by relying on tables of food composition. It is important to recognise that measurement of food and nutrient intake is a difficult business that is prone to large errors. It is also subject to factors that may completely undermine its validity, such as:

- Dishonest reporting by subjects.
- Subjects changing their eating habits during a period of dietary monitoring.

Dietary Supplements and Functional Foods, 2nd Edition. Geoffrey P. Webb.
© 2011 Blackwell Publishing Ltd.

- Factors that may make food tables an unreliable guide to the nutrient intake of food eaten, such as prolonged storage or warm holding of food or the addition of minerals from cooking utensils or water.

Discussion of these methods of measuring nutrient intakes is beyond the scope of this book, but much of the evidence used to justify supplement use is initially based on such dietary studies. Details of these methods and their sources of error may be found in Webb (2008) or other standard texts on nutrition.

Once estimates of micronutrient intakes have been made, clearly some published estimates of nutrient requirements or dietary standards are a key tool in making decisions about the adequacy of these intakes. The most-used standard in the UK is the reference nutrient intake (RNI), while in the USA, the rest of the EU and indeed on UK food labels it is the recommended dietary allowance (RDA). Full listings of dietary standards for micronutrients for all age groups in the UK may be found in COMA (1991) and for the USA in NAS (2004). The RNI in the UK is defined as 'the daily amount of a nutrient that is enough for almost every individual, even someone who has high needs for the nutrient' – it is therefore more than many people strictly need. These standards are generous estimates of the requirements of those people within a population group who have a high requirement for that nutrient. Any healthy person consuming an amount equal to or greater than the RDA/RNI is thus assumed to be receiving enough of that nutrient. Note that this means that an intake significantly below these values may be adequate for many people.

In order to set these standards, the average requirement of people within each of the population age groups must first be estimated (the estimated average requirement, or EAR). The criterion of 'need' used to make this estimate is that it is enough not only to prevent deficiency but also to allow for sufficient stores of the nutrient to be maintained, so that substantial periods of deficient intake or increased requirement (e.g. during illness) can be tolerated without immediately precipitating deficiency symptoms. Estimating the average requirement is difficult and in some cases is not much more than a reasoned guess by a panel of experts, so there is a marked but variable tendency to err on the safe (i.e. high) side.

The RNI is set at a notional two standard deviations above the EAR for the nutrient. The American RDA is also aiming for a similar target dose, but is often higher than the RNI; this is because of a tendency to assume lower absorption rates, aim for higher body reserves and ensure the adequacy of those with unusually high requirements (Harper and Rolls, 1992). If the RNI (or RDA) is set at a notional two standard deviations above the average value, then theoretically 2.5% of people require more than the RNI. However, given the fact that requirements are estimated generously and the equally generous criterion for requirement, it is safe to assume that the RNI (or RDA) is sufficient for any healthy person. Although these standards are set generously and allow for some storage of the nutrient, they do not usually take account of any increased need due to illness or injury or any claimed benefits from taking large supplemental doses of the nutrient. For example, the adult RNI for vitamin C in the UK is 40 mg/day;

this will certainly prevent any symptoms of scurvy and allow a person to accumulate sufficient stores of the vitamin to survive for some weeks of total deprivation before deficiency symptoms start to manifest. This RNI does not take account of the belief that doses of vitamin C more than 20 times greater than the RNI may help prevent infections like colds and flu or have beneficial effects on other illnesses.

Throughout this chapter an individual intake below the LRNI (see discussion and definition below) is taken as an indication of a high probability of insufficiency. Where average intakes are below the RNI, it suggests that it is likely that there will be many individuals with inadequate (below the LRNI) intakes, because even where average intake is well above the RNI, significant numbers of individuals may still have intakes below the LRNI. An individual intake below the RNI probably does not necessarily indicate a problem for that person, but means that adequacy is not assured.

The COMA panel considered that, for eight nutrients, it did not have sufficient information to estimate the rather precisely defined set of values discussed above. In these cases, therefore, it merely suggested a 'safe intake', which it defined as 'a level or range of intakes at which there is little risk of either deficiency or toxic effects'.

Most people come across these standards on food labels where nutrient contents are expressed as a percentage of the RDA (note that even British food labels use the term RDA because EU standards are used for food labelling). It is much more meaningful to consumers to quote nutrient levels in foods as a proportion of the 'requirement' than in absolute amounts – that is, in milligrams, micrograms or even millimoles – which would be very difficult for most people to interpret meaningfully. For example, 2 µg of vitamin B_{12} could be considered a substantial amount because it is 130% of the adult RNI, but 2 mg of vitamin C could be considered a small amount because it is only 5% of the RNI.

These standards vary according to age, and after puberty there are different standards for males and females. There are also separate standards for pregnant or lactating women (see Table 2.1 for an indication of how these standards are laid out).

In the UK, the lower reference nutrient intake (LRNI) is an amount that is estimated to represent the needs of those people within any population group who have a particularly low requirement for the nutrient. It can thus be assumed that anyone whose intake is close to or below the LRNI is receiving inadequate amounts of that nutrient, even though they may not be exhibiting obvious symptoms of deficiency. The LRNI is set at a notional two standard deviations below the EAR and so it should theoretically be enough for 2.5% of the population group. However, it seems improbable that those with the lowest needs will always be those with the lowest intakes, and so anyone whose intake is less than the LRNI is classified as deficient. Note that it is because of the generous estimates of average requirements and generous criterion for adequacy referred to earlier that intakes at or slightly below the LRNI do not necessarily result in overt symptoms of a deficiency disease.

Table 2.1 A plan of the layout of tables of dietary standards (e.g. RDAs or RNIs)

	Nutrient 1	Nutrient 2	Nutrient 3	Nutrient 4... etc.
Age group (examples)				
0–3 months				
10–12 months				
1–3 years				
7–10 years				
11–14 years (female)				
19–50 years (male)				
19–50 years (female)				
50+ years (female)				
Pregnant				
Lactating				

The British RNI and LRNI for adults for selected major nutrients are shown in Table 2.2 and the corresponding American RDA is included for comparison.

Note that dietary standards for energy are set at the estimate of average requirement for the age group (the EAR in the UK), not the estimate of people with the highest need.

Yates (2006) gives a referenced account of the origins and evolution of dietary standards and their theoretical basis.

A note about American standards

Since 1994 American and Canadian scientists have been collaborating on a programme to update and expand the concept of RDA. They have introduced a number of extra terms and a detailed listing and explanation of all current American (and Canadian) standards can be found in Appendix 2 of Shils *et al.* (2006). The term dietary reference intakes (DRI) is a collective term to cover all dietary standards and those terms that apply to micronutrients are listed below:

- The RDA, as discussed above.
- The estimated average requirement (EAR), which is essentially the same as that used in Britain since 1991 and discussed above.
- Adequate intake (AI) is the value used when an accurate RDA cannot be set and it is essentially the same as the 'safe intake' used in the British standards.
- The tolerable upper intake level (UL) is the highest average daily intake that is likely to pose no adverse risk to health to almost all individuals within the general population.

Table 2.2   The RNI, LRNI and American RDA for selected micronutrients for adults aged 19–50 years

Nutrient	Male			Female		
	RNI	LRNI	RDA	RNI	LRNI	RDA
Vitamin A (μgRE/day)	700	300	900	600	250	700
Thiamin (mg/day)	1.0	0.6	1.2	0.8	0.45	1.1
Riboflavin (mg/day)	1.3	0.8	1.3	1.1	0.8	1.1
Niacin (mgNE/day)	17	11	16	13	9	14
Vitamin B$_6$ (mg/day)	1.4	1.0	1.3	1.2	0.9	1.3
Folate* (μg/day)	200	100	400	200	100	400
Vitamin B$_{12}$ (μg/day)	1.5	1.0	2.4	1.5	1.0	2.4
Vitamin C (mg/day)	40	10	90	40	10	75
Vitamin D** (μg/day)	–	–	5	–	–	5
Vitamin E (mg/day)	above 4[#]		15	above 3[#]		15
Calcium (mg/day)	700	400	1000	700	400	1000
Chromium (μg/day)	above 25[#]		35	above 25[#]		25
Iron (mg/day)	8.7	4.7	8	14.8	8	18
Iodine (μg/day)	140	70	150	140	70	150
Magnesium (mg/day)	300	190	400	270	150	310
Potassium (mg/day)	3500	2000	4700	3500	2000	4700
Selenium (μg/day)	75	40	55	60	40	55
Zinc (mg/day)	9.5	5.5	11	7	4	8

Notes:
* It is now recommended that women of child bearing age take 400 μg/day supplements of folate.
** In Britain it is assumed that most adults can make sufficient vitamin when their skin is exposed to summer sunlight; the US value is for ages 25–50 years.
[#] Safe intake, used where the panel felt that they did not have enough information to set formal RNI and LRNI.

Recommended daily allowances on food labels

The RNI (and the RDA in the USA) vary according to age, sex and reproductive status and this makes it too cumbersome for routine use on food labels. In the UK and the European Union a single recommended dietary allowance is used for food labels; this has traditionally been based on the values for an adult male aged 19–50 years (except for iron, where the higher female value is used). These European food labelling RDA are listed in Table 2.3. A similar system is used in the USA, where the value used for food labelling is the higher of the male or female values for adults under 50 years.

Table 2.3 The recommended daily allowances used for food labelling within the European Union

Nutrient	'Labelling' RDA
Vitamin A (µgRE)	800
Thiamin (mg)	1.4
Riboflavin (mg)	1.6
Niacin (mg NE)	18
Vitamin B_6 (mg)	2
Folate (µg)	200
Vitamin B_{12} (µg)	1
Biotin (µg)	150
Pantothenic acid (mg)	6
Vitamin C (mg)	60
Vitamin D (µg)	5
Vitamin E (mg)	10
Calcium (mg)	800
Iodine (µg)	150
Iron (mg)	14
Magnesium (mg)	300
Phosphorus (mg)	800
Zinc (mg)	15

Measuring an individual's micronutrient status using clinical or biochemical observations

As an alternative to estimation of dietary intake, one can also make observations or measurements that give an indication of a person's current status for a particular micronutrient. One can:

- Look for clinical signs or symptoms that indicate a nutrient deficiency.
- Make biochemical measurements that indicate the individual's current status for the nutrient.

Clinical signs as indicators of micronutrient status tend to be insensitive, non-specific, subjective and qualitative:

- They are *insensitive* because they usually only become apparent after prolonged and/or severe inadequacy; that is, when the subject's stores of the nutrient are seriously depleted.

- They are *non-specific* because in many cases a particular sign or symptom may have multiple potential causes.
- They usually produce a *subjective* and *qualitative* assessment of symptom severity rather than an objective numerical value.

Some examples of clinical signs that can be associated with particular nutrient deficiencies are listed below:

- A swollen thyroid gland or goitre can be an indication of dietary iodine deficiency.
- Bowing of the legs and other skeletal abnormalities can be an indication of vitamin D deficiency (rickets).
- Pale pink conjunctiva may indicate iron deficiency anaemia.
- Spongy lesions at the corners of the mouth (angular stomatitis) may indicate riboflavin (vitamin B$_2$) deficiency.
- Spontaneous bruising or small subdermal haemorrhages (petechiae) may indicate vitamin C deficiency.
- Night blindness may be an early indication of vitamin A deficiency and a dry and infected cornea might be a later manifestation of this condition.

Biochemical tests of micronutrient status usually involve measurement of the nutrient or a metabolite in blood, although sometimes less direct measures or measurements with urine are used. In contrast to clinical signs, biochemical tests are sensitive, specific, objective and quantitative:

- *Sensitive* – changes in biochemical parameters like blood nutrient levels often reflect the level of bodily stores of a nutrient and these usually change well before any clinical signs of deficiency manifest.
- *Specific* – most biochemical tests are specific for a given nutrient, although for example blood haemoglobin level is not only dependent on iron status but is also affected by factors like altitude, pregnancy and physical training.
- *Objective and quantitative* – they usually produce an objective, numerical indicator of nutrient status.

The problems of using biochemical methods are that they usually involve invasive blood sampling and they are expensive and time-consuming to perform. Note also that although the measurements may be very precise and repeatable in some cases, it is difficult to interpret these results; that is, to decide whether a particular numerical value really indicates deficiency and/or the severity of that deficiency. This issue is well illustrated later in this chapter by the discussion relating to the improbably high incidence of biochemical evidence of deficiency of riboflavin and the absence of any biochemical evidence of vitamin A deficiency, despite evidence that many adults, especially younger adults, have unsatisfactory intakes of vitamin A (see Table 2.5 on page XX and the related discussion in the text). Some examples of biochemical indicators of status for particular micronutrients are listed below:

- *Iron* – blood haemoglobin levels have traditionally been used to assess iron status, but serum ferritin concentration is now regarded as a more sensitive and specific indicator of iron status. Haemoglobin levels are affected by other factors and only drop when iron stores have become depleted. Low blood haemoglobin indicates iron deficiency anaemia, whereas low serum ferritin indicates iron depletion, which may occur in the absence of anaemia.
- *Vitamin E* – total tocopherol in serum.
- *Thiamin B_1* – erythrocyte transketolase activation coefficient (ETKAC). Transketolase is an enzyme that requires thiamin pyrophosphate as a co-factor for activity; measuring the effect of adding extra co-factor on the red cell activity of this enzyme is used to indicate the donor's thiamin status. Large increases in enzyme activity when co-factor is added suggests that co-factor availability was limiting enzyme activity and thus that the blood donor had poor status for thiamin.
- *Riboflavin B_2* – erythrocyte glutathione activation coefficient. Glutathione reductase is an enzyme that requires riboflavin for activity and the logic is the same as in the previous example.
- *Vitamin D* – plasma concentration of 25-hydroxycholecalciferol, a metabolite of vitamin D that is the main circulating form.
- *Zinc, vitamin B_{12}, vitamin C, folic acid* – plasma or serum level of the nutrient.
- *Vitamin A* – plasma vitamin A, although clinical tests are often used because plasma levels of retinol are homeostatically controlled and decline only when liver reserves of retinol are considerably depleted (Ball, 2004).

Further information on these biochemical methods of assessment and values taken to indicate deficiency and normality may be found in Webb (2008).

Micronutrient adequacy of the UK population

Nutritionists and dieticians who are unsympathetic to the use of micronutrient supplements often state that they are unnecessary because:

- A varied and prudent diet that uses all of the major food groups and provides sufficient energy to meet current needs should also contain adequate amounts of all the essential micronutrients for a healthy person.
- Overt vitamin and mineral deficiencies are rarely seen among otherwise healthy people in affluent populations and almost everyone in these populations consumes adequate amounts of micronutrients.
- Vitamin and mineral supplements tend to be taken by those people in affluent populations who already have the highest intakes and are therefore the least likely to need them.

While the first of these statements is undoubtedly true, for it really to be used as an argument against supplement usage it must also follow that most people eat such a diet

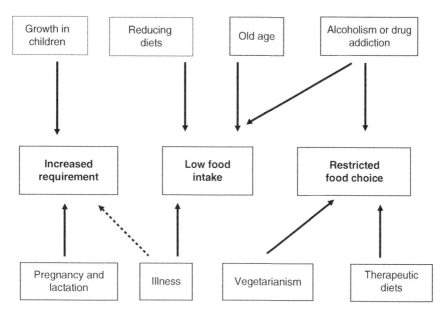

Figure 2.1   Circumstances that may increase the risk of a nutrient deficiency.
Source: Webb, G.P. (2001) Nutritional supplements: Benefits and risks. *Nursing and Residential Care*, 3, 477–81.

or can readily be persuaded to eat such a diet. It also follows that any circumstance that increases the requirement for a nutrient, or results in low food intake or in restricted food choice, may increase the risk of deficiency (see Figure 2.1). Few nutritionists or dieticians would dispute that a 'balanced diet' is the best way of achieving nutrient adequacy and that dietary supplements are no substitute for a varied and nutrient-rich diet. However, supplements may ameliorate some of the adverse consequences of a poor and inadequate diet; they may have a useful role where this 'balanced diet' is unlikely to be eaten. We have already seen evidence in Chapter 1 to support the third proposition in the above list, that those who need supplements least are the most likely to take them; surveys discussed later in the chapter will also support this proposition.

The rest of this chapter sets out to test the accuracy of the second and most critical of the above statements. It seeks to answer the question: 'Is almost everyone in the UK already getting sufficient of all the micronutrients from their current diet?' In order to answer this question I have largely relied on data from the rolling programme of National Diet and Nutrition Surveys (NDNS) in the UK. These surveys attempt to measure the nutrient intakes of the various subgroups of the UK population and compare them to the published standards for that population group. In many cases, other estimates of nutrient adequacy are also made using more sensitive and perhaps more reliable biochemical tests.

These NDNS surveys aim to provide comprehensive information on the dietary habits and nutritional status of Britons in all age groups and to monitor changes in these over time. These surveys include:

- The NDNS survey of children aged 1.5 to 4.5 years (Gregory *et al.*, 1995)
- The survey of adults aged 16–64 years (Gregory *et al.*, 1990)

- The survey of people aged over 65 years (Finch *et al.*, 1998)
- The survey of young people aged 4–18 years (Gregory *et al.*, 2000)
- The second adult survey of adults aged 19–64 years (summary 5th volume Hoare *et al.*, 2004; all five volumes can be accessed free online)

The latest survey of adults (summarised by Hoare *et al.*, 2004) consists of the following elements:

- A dietary interview that determines information on eating and drinking habits and socio-demographic information such as age, marital status, social class etc.
- A 7-day weighed inventory of all food and drink consumed.
- A 24-hour urine collection with analysis.
- Physical measurements such as height, weight, body mass index, waist and hip circumference and blood pressure.
- A 7-day activity diary.
- A blood sample, which was analysed for biochemical indicators of nutritional status and plasma cholesterol levels.

The data discussed in the rest of this chapter are for the main part only directly applicable to the UK, but it seems likely that they will also be a general barometer of the nutritional adequacy of the diets of affluent populations. While individual countries may have better or worse levels of nutritional adequacy than the UK, if there is evidence of widespread suboptimal nutrient intakes in the UK then it is likely that this also applies to many other affluent populations. If almost all people in the UK are consuming micronutrients in comfortably adequate amounts, this is alsolikely to apply widely across the industrialised world.

Young and middle-aged adults

In 1990, the first major survey of the NDNS programme was published (Gregory *et al.*, 1990). During 1986–87 a representative sample of British adults aged 16–64 years (well over 2000 people) completed a full weighed intake of everything they consumed for a seven-day period and energy and nutrient intakes were estimated from these records. Blood and urine analyses and other measurements were also made on these volunteers. This survey found that for most nutrients, average intakes were greater than the RNI, in many cases substantially greater. The exceptions were:

- the potassium intakes of men and women
- the magnesium intake of women
- the iron intake of pre-menopausal women

These apparently very satisfactory averages do, however, tend to obscure the fact that many individual adults recorded unsatisfactory intakes of some nutrients; that is, below the LRNI. Many women recorded unsatisfactory intakes of vitamin A, riboflavin (B$_2$), folic acid, iron and calcium; recorded vitamin A intakes were also unsatisfactory in many men. These intakes are total intakes, including any dietary supplements used, although it is noted that in most cases supplements made only a small difference to the recorded average intakes, with the major exception that supplements provided 15% of women's average iron intake. The nutrient intakes from food sources were higher in supplement users than those obtained from food by non-supplement users. This tends to confirm that those most likely to benefit are the least likely to use supplements. The larger nutrient intakes of men were entirely due to their higher total energy (food) intake; when expressed as amount of nutrient per 1000 kcal, the nutrient intakes of women were actually higher. The amount of nutrient per 1000 kcal is termed the *nutrient density*. No detailed discussion of the results of this survey are presented because it is now out of date. Its importance is that it was a model for other surveys in the series and it has also been compared to later data to see if any consumption trends are apparent or major individual changes have occurred.

In this survey the average recorded energy intake of the male sample was close to the EAR for energy (97%), whereas that for women was only 87% of the EAR, which could indicate some degree of under-reporting or widespread energy restriction in the women.

A similar survey was conducted with a representative sample of British adults aged 19–64 years in 2000–2001 and published in 2003 (all five volumes are available free online and the most useful for most readers is the fifth summary volume, Hoare *et al.*, 2004). Recorded energy intakes for both men and women were again below the EAR and slightly lower than the values recorded in 1986–87 (91% of EAR for men and 84% for women); 40% of the women in this sample reported using a dietary supplement, as did 29% of the men. Discussion of results from this survey focuses on the intake of micronutrients from food sources only, as this is a more useful indication of the case for widespread supplementation than the total intake including that from supplements. Despite the lower average energy intakes recorded in this second survey (and thus the real possibility of widespread underreporting of habitual intakes or energy restriction), the average intakes of most micronutrients from food sources were slightly higher than those recorded in the 1986–87 survey. Average recorded intakes of the following were higher in both sexes in 2000–2001 than in 1986–87:

- thiamin
- riboflavin
- niacin
- vitamin B_6
- folate
- vitamin B_{12}
- vitamin C
- vitamin D
- vitamin E
- calcium
- potassium

Table 2.4 Recorded average vitamin and mineral intakes of British adults as a percentage of the RNI from the Dietary and Nutritional Survey of British Adults data (collected 1986–87) and the National Diet and Nutrition survey (collected 2000–2001). Data from the latter survey also shown as a percentage of the American RDA

Nutrient	Men %RNI 1986–7	Men %RNI 2000–01	Men %RDA 2000–01	Women %RNI 1986–7	Women %RNI 2000–01	Women %RDA 2000–01
Vit. A	233	131	101	236	112	96
Thiamin	170	200	167	155	193	140
Riboflavin	160	162	162	143	145	145
Niacin	235	263	279	219	238	220
Folate	156	172	86	107	126	63
Vit. B_{12}	480	433	271	347	320	200
Vit. C	166	209	93	155	203	108
Vit. D	–	–	74	–	–	56
Vit. E	248*	265*	71	240*	270*	54
Calcium	134	144	101	104	111	78
Iron	157	152	165	71	68	56
Magnesium		103	77		85	74
Potassium		96	72		76	74
Zinc		107	93		106	93

Note:
* No RNI set, figure is percentage of minimum safe intake.

For magnesium and zinc, intakes in 2000–2001 were significantly lower than in 1986–87. Between the two surveys there was also a substantial reduction in the reported intake of vitamin A from food (44% reduction in men and 53% in women). This fall was largely due to reductions in the intake of pre-formed retinol rather than a reduction in that derived from carotene. Average intake of food iron also declined slightly in both sexes.

The average values recorded in these two British surveys are compared in Table 2.4. The recorded average intakes in each of these surveys are expressed as a percentage of the appropriate RNI; this confirms that the average intakes of most nutrients appear to be satisfactory. The American RDA are usually higher than British RNI and the values from the most recent survey are also shown as a percentage of this RDA. When judged against these American standards, the values for vitamin A, folate, vitamin E and calcium look less reassuring.

Further data from the later of these surveys (Hoare *et al.*, 2004) are also shown in Tables 2.5 and 2.6. These tables show the average intake of vitamins and minerals

Table 2.5 The vitamin and iron adequacy of the diets of British adults aged 19–64 (data from Hoare et al., 2004).

Vitamin	Average intake % RNI				% below LRNI				% below biochemical threshold			
	Men (aged)		Women (aged)		Men (aged)		Women (aged)		Men (aged)		Women (aged)	
	19–64	19–24	19–64	19–24	19–64	19–24	19–64	19–24	19–64	19–24	19–64	19–24
A (retinol equivalents)	130	80	112	78	7	16	9	19	0	0	0	0
Thiamin	214	160	193	181	1	2	1	0	3	0	1	0
Riboflavin	162	129	146	126	3	8	8	15	66	82	66	77
Niacin equivalents	268	232	257	246	0	0	1	2				
B_6	204	189	169	165	1	0	2	5	10	4	11	12
B_{12}	431	296	319	266	0	1	1	1	2	0	4	5
Folate*	172	151	125	114	0	2	2	3	4	13	5	8
C	209	162	202	170	0	0	0	1	5	7	3	4
D**	3.7 (µg)	2.9 (µg)	2.8 (µg)	2.3 (µg)	–	–	–	–	14	24	15	28
Iron#	151	131	82	60	1	3	25	42	3 (4)	0 (4)	8 (11)	7 (16)

Notes:
* Biochemical value is red cell folate, indicating marginal status.
** No adult RNI or LRNI for vitamin D – absolute values given.
# The two biochemical values are the value for haemoglobin indicative of anaemia and, in parentheses, the value for serum ferritin, indicative of iron store depletion.

Table 2.6 The mineral adequacy of the diets of British adults aged 19–64 (data from Hoare *et al.*, 2004).

Mineral	Average intake % RNI				% below LRNI			
	Men (aged)		Women (aged)		Men (aged)		Women (aged)	
	19–64	19–24	19–64	19–24	19–64	19–24	19–64	19–24
Calcium	144	123	111	99	2	5	5	8
Magnesium	103	86	85	76	9	17	13	22
Potassium	96	81	76	67	6	18	19	30
Zinc	107	95	105	98	4	7	4	5
Iodine	154	119	114	93	2	2	4	12
Copper	119	95	86	76	–	–	–	–

as a percentage of the RNI for selected age and sex categories; the percentage of the respondents in each of these categories with intakes below the LRNI; and, for vitamins and iron, the percentage of the sample below the panel's threshold values for biochemical measures of nutrient adequacy. Iron is listed in Table 2.5 for convenience because it is the only mineral for which biochemical estimates of adequacy are given.

For almost all the vitamins listed in Table 2.5, the average intake is in excess of the RNI and in most cases it is well in excess of the RNI. The only exception to this generalisation is the vitamin A intake of men and women in the 19–24-year age category, where it is 80% or less of the RNI. It was noted earlier that average recorded vitamin A intakes fell quite sharply between the two NDNS surveys of adults as a result of a reduced intake of pre-formed retinol. Milk fat, egg yolks, oily fish and offal are the major natural sources of retinol, although it is added to other foods, notably margarine and low-fat spread. Fewer whole milk, cheese, butter, liver and liver products were eaten by adults in the more recent survey, although oily fish consumption did increase between the two surveys. Significant numbers of those sampled had vitamin A intakes that are regarded as unsatisfactory (below the LRNI), with much greater numbers in the youngest age category (16% and 19% for men and women respectively). While no instance of unsatisfactory biochemical status for vitamin A was recorded, the measure used (plasma retinol concentration) is an insensitive indicator of vitamin A status; it is normally homeostatically controlled and only correlates well with dietary intake when it is very high or very low.

The average intakes of folate for both sexes look satisfactory when compared to the UK standard, although 4–5% of the whole sample and more than double this proportion of the younger age groups had red cell folate levels that indicate marginal folate status. It is also now recommended that all women of child-bearing age take supplements of 400 µg/day of folic acid. This is because of the demonstration that supplements of folic acid reduce the risk of babies developing a neural tube defect when they are given pre-conceptually and in very early pregnancy. Perhaps half of all pregnancies are unplanned, so targeting all women 'at risk' of becoming pregnant is thought to be an appropriate pro-phylactic measure (see Chapter 3). In practice, very few women within this group consumed 400 µg/day of folate from all sources; that is, only around 13% of women under 50 years.

Despite an increase in average intake since 1986–87, 3% of men and 6% of women still had inadequate riboflavin intakes, with substantially more in the younger age groups. Table 2.5 suggests that more than two-thirds of the sample showed biochemical evidence of riboflavin depletion, but this may be because of the high sensitivity of the assay used (see ETKAC earlier) and it may suggest a need to reconsider the level considered indicative of depletion.

For all of the other vitamins except vitamin C (0%), between 1 and 2% of women recorded unsatisfactory intakes, with 5% of 19–24-year-old women recording unsatisfactory intakes of vitamin B_6.

Other points of note from the biochemical analyses for vitamin status were the following:

- Despite the generally satisfactory vitamin C intakes, 5% of women (3% of men) showed biochemical evidence of vitamin C depletion. It is possible that food tables overestimated the amount of vitamin C in food as actually eaten. While supplements raised average intakes, they are unlikely to have been taken by those with the lowest intakes from food.
- 4% of women (2% of men) had unsatisfactory status for vitamin B_{12} despite high dietary intakes. Deficiency is most often due to poor absorption, including pernicious anaemia.
- Over 10% of the total sample showed biochemical evidence of vitamin B_6 deficiency.
- Around 15% of the sample showed biochemical evidence of vitamin D defi-ciency, with higher proportions in the younger age groups. Average intakes were only 3–4 µg/day, which is far less than the 10–15 µg/day recommended for those not getting regular exposure to sunlight. Eight times as many of those sampled in the winter months were below the biochemical threshold compared to those sampled in the summer months, emphasising the key role of sunlight in the endogenous production of vitamin D.

A quarter of women had inadequate iron intakes and this rose to over 40% in the under-35s (see Table 2.5). The iron intake of women receiving state benefits (the poorest) was substantially worse than the rest of the sample. Blood analysis indi-cated that 8% of the sample had haemoglobin levels indicative of anaemia and 11% had depleted stores of iron, as indicated by the serum ferritin levels. Levels were higher in the younger women and much lower in men.

All other mineral intakes are summarised in Table 2.6. These show that 4–19% of women recorded intakes below the LRNI for all of these minerals; numbers were higher in younger women and generally much lower in men. The long-term significance of the low recorded intakes for magnesium and potassium are unclear, although low potassium intake is an accepted risk factor for high blood pressure.

Overt micronutrient deficiency diseases are very rarely seen among otherwise healthy, young and middle-aged adults living in Britain and other industrialised countries (with the exception of iron deficiency anaemia in women). However, if the results of these surveys are a true indication of the normal habitual micronutrient intakes of British adults, it does suggest that substantial numbers of them are taking less than optimal amounts of several micronutrients. They are thus likely to have depleted stores of these nutrients, which will make them less able to withstand periods of further depressed intake or increased requirement, for example during illness or deliberate dieting. It may also lead to impaired physiological functioning or increase their susceptibility to infection or other illnesses in the short or long term, even though the deficiency may not be severe enough to result in overt and recognisable symptoms of a deficiency disease. Biochemical indicators of vitamin and iron status tend to confirm this image of substantial numbers of individuals with unsatisfactory nutritional status. Both Hoare *et al.* (2004) and the earlier survey of Gregory *et al.* (1990) clearly indicate that current supplement usage tends to be positively related to intake of nutrients from food, and so is concentrated among those who are relatively more affluent and whose intakes are already sufficient.

Some of the percentages of those with apparently 'inadequate' intakes of some nutrients seem small and thus reassuring, but this survey is intended to be representative of around 33 million people in the UK and so each percentage point of the total sample represents around 330 000 people; each percentage point in the youngest age category still represents over 30 000 people.

It is worth stressing the important qualification made to the comments in the previous paragraph; that is, 'if these survey results are a true indication of the normal habitual micronutrient intakes of British adults'. Is the sample truly representative? By analogy with other surveys, it is likely that the least educated and the most underprivileged, and thus those most vulnerable to dietary inadequacy, will be under-represented in this survey (the homeless or those without permanent homes are an obvious example). This would mean that these surveys might underestimate the extent of inadequate intakes. There are many other potential sources of error or bias in the weighed inventory methodology, for example:

- Subjects are more likely to forget to weigh and record something eaten or drunk than to weigh and record something not consumed.
- There may especially be under-recording of food and drink consumed outside of the home, especially casual drinks or snacks.
- Some people may deliberately change their eating habits to 'improve' their dietary record.

Table 2.7 Selected RNIs (EAR for energy) for various UK age groups, expressed as a percentage of the appropriate adult (19–50 years) value

	Pregnancy	Lactation	1–3 yrs Girls	4–6 yrs Girls	11–14 yrs Girls	15–18 yrs Boys	75+ yrs Men
Energy	100*	127	60	80	95	108	82
Protein	113	124	32	44	92	99	96
Vitamin A	117	158	67	83	100	100	100
Riboflavin	127	145	55	73	100	100	100
Folic acid	Supplements	130	35	50	100	100	100
Vitamin C	125	175	75	75	88	100	100
Calcium	100	179	50	64	114	143	100
Iron	100	100	47	41	100	130	100

Note:
* 1st two trimesters (110% last trimester).

- The weighing and recording process makes the subject more aware of what they are eating and drinking and so leads to subconscious avoidances or restrictions.
- Subjects may avoid eating or drinking something because they cannot be bothered to weigh and record it.
- Subjects who are temporarily dieting may eat more when not dieting and the recording process may make diet adherence more rigorous.

Most of these result in systematic underestimating of habitual intake and any systematic bias towards under-recording would of course tend to exaggerate the likely prevalence of inadequacy.

Children

Table 2.7 shows the estimated nutrient requirements (RNI) of several different sections of the UK population, expressed as a percentage of that of adults aged 19–50 years. The estimated average energy requirements (EAR) are also similarly represented. The energy values in this table can be used as a general indicator of the likely relative average food intakes of the groups. Thus one might expect a group with an energy value of 60% in Table 2.7 to take in around 60% of the energy (i.e. the amount of food) and thus, provided they are eating the same diet, also take in 60% of the amount of vitamins and minerals of adults. Using this logic, a group with 100% in the energy column would be expected to take in the same amount of essential nutrients as adults. This means that only where the value for an essential vitamin or mineral in Table 2.7 is substantially greater than the energy value for that group do they really require a diet that is richer in the essential nutrient (i.e. more nutrient dense).

Table 2.8 British RNI for selected micronutrients for selected age groups of children. All values are per day

Nutrient	Age and sex groups (years)					
			Boys		Girls	
	4–6	7–10	11–14	15–18	11–14	15–18
Vitamin A (µg RE)						
RNI	400	500	600	700	600	600
Riboflavin (mg)	.8	1.0	1.2	1.3	1.1	1.1
Folate (µg)	100	150	200	200	200	200
Vitamin C (mg)	30	30	35	40	35	40
Calcium (mg)	450	550	1000	1000	800	800
Iron (mg)	6.1	8.7	11.3	11.3	14.8	14.8
Zinc (mg)	6.5	7.0	9.0	9.5	9.0	7.0

Children have traditionally been seen as having high relative nutrient requirements, but Table 2.7 indicates that in many cases they can get all they need from a diet that has the same concentration of that nutrient (nutrient density) as adults; this is because of their higher relative requirement (i.e. per kilogram of body weight) for energy and thus higher relative food consumption. Perhaps the classic example of this assumption that children need a more nutrient-dense diet than adults is protein. Adults require only enough protein to replace what they use up each day, whereas children need enough to replace what they use up plus enough to allow for the growth of new tissue. Young children are therefore thought to require about twice as much as adults for every kilogram of body weight (at one time it was thought to be as much as five times more!). However, provided that these children eat freely of the same diets as adults, they are not at increased risk of being protein deficient because they require about three times as much food per kilogram of body weight. We can see in Table 2.7 that in all of the age groups shown, the protein value for children is less than the energy value – any diet that has enough protein for adults should also have enough for children. Of course, this logic only works if children's diets are basically similar to adult diets and would not apply if many of the calories are provided by low-nutrient but high-energy sweets, chocolate, fats, sugary drinks, cakes and so on. Selected UK RNI for different age groups of children are given in Table 2.8.

In a survey of the diets of a representative sample of British pre-school children aged 1.5 to 4.5 years, Gregory *et al.* (1995) found that energy intakes were below the EAR and they concluded that this was probably because the EAR was overestimated. The average intakes of most of the essential micronutrients were well above the RNI, with the exception of vitamin A, iron and zinc. Some of the micronutrient problems highlighted in this report were:

• The majority of these young children had iron intakes that were below the RNI and many had intakes below the LRNI. About 10% of the sample were anaemic and about 20% had biochemical evidence of depleted iron stores (serum ferritin below 10 µg/L).

- Around half of the sample had vitamin A intakes below the RNI and about 8% below the LRNI.
- Vitamin D intakes were only around 2 µg/day (RNI 10 µg/day), which is clearly inadequate for children unless they get adequate exposure to summer sunlight.

Adolescence is seen as a time when children may be particularly vulnerable to nutritional deficiencies. There is a marked and sustained growth spurt at this time, with major increases in lean body mass (protein), bone mass (calcium) and total body haemoglobin and myoglobin (iron) seen to put pressure on the supply of key nutrients. In a survey of the diets of British children aged between 10–11 years and 14–15 years carried out in 1983 (COMA, 1989), energy intakes were found to be close to those predicted by the EAR, adjusted for actual recorded weights, and average intakes of vitamins exceeded the RNI. Two problems with mineral intakes were highlighted by this survey:

- Average calcium intakes in the older age group were about 10% below the RNI.
- Around 60% of the girls had iron intakes below the RNI appropriate for the start of menstruation.

A more recent survey of the diets of British children aged between 4 and 18 years has since been conducted as part of the NDNS programme (Gregory *et al.*, 2000). Energy intakes in comparable groups were lower in this survey than those recorded by COMA (1989), even though the children were heavier. This may well reflect the continuing decline in activity and energy expenditure of children and indeed of the whole population. Such decreased activity decreases energy needs; this not only predisposes to weight gain and obesity, but also increases the risks of nutrient inadequacy if energy intake (i.e. total food intake) also falls to match the reduction in expenditure.

About 20% of all the children reported that they took a micronutrient supplement. About 10% of girls in the 15–18-year age band were vegetarian and about 16% were dieting (cf. 1% and 3% respectively of boys in the same age group).

Although average intakes of most nutrients were above the RNI, a number of problems with the micronutrient intakes of school-age British children were highlighted by the survey, namely:

- Average intakes of vitamin A were close to the RNI in younger children but below it in older children. Around 20% of older girls and 12% of older boys had intakes that were below the LRNI.
- A fifth of older girls had inadequate riboflavin intakes and biochemical evidence of poor riboflavin status was noted in some individuals in this survey (note the earlier caution about this biochemical test).

- Biochemical evidence of poor vitamin D status was found in 13% of 11–18 year olds, with a much higher proportion in winter than in summer samples.
- Biochemical evidence of poor nutritional status in some individuals was also found for thiamin, folate and vitamin C.
- There were substantial numbers of children with intake of at least one mineral that was below the LRNI: for zinc (well over 10% of all the children with three times this proportion in the youngest girls), potassium, magnesium and calcium in older children and iron in older girls.
- Some 50% of older girls had iron intakes below the LRNI and low ferritin levels, indicating low iron stores, were found in 27% of girls and 13% of boys.

Pregnant women

In casual conversation, pregnant and lactating women are often said to be 'eating for two' and so some readers may be surprised to see from Table 2.7 that the esti mated energy requirement (UK) of pregnant women does not increase during the first two trimesters and only increases by 10% in the final trimester, when the bulk of fetal growth occurs. Actual measurements of the food and energy consumption of pregnant women confirm that it does not increase except by a very small amount (c. 100 kcal) in the last few weeks. This means that any increased nutrient needs during pregnancy must be met from essentially the same amount of food that was eaten prior to pregnancy or be obtained from existing maternal stores of the nutrient. Morning sickness in the early weeks of pregnancy may depress the nutrient supply in some women.

In the case of some nutrients, there are widely divergent views on the extent of any extra nutrient needs in pregnancy. This is illustrated in Table 2.9, where the British RNI and the American RDA for pregnant and lactating women are shown for selected micronutrients. It is striking how similar the British values given in this table are to those for non-pregnant women of child-bearing age previously given in Table 2.4. A comparison of the UK RNI for pregnant and non-pregnant women is as follows:

- The mineral values are largely unaltered by pregnancy.
- The values for thiamin and niacin only increase marginally in the last trimester as a direct consequence of the increase in the estimated energy requirement.
- There are modest increases in the RNI for riboflavin, vitamin A and vitamin C during pregnancy.
- Supplements of folic acid of 400 μg/day are recommended for early pregnancy (4mg if there is a previous history of a neural tube defect); to be most effective this supplementation should start before conception. The evidence on which this recommendation is based is discussed in the section on folic acid in Chapter 3.
- There is an RNI for vitamin D of 10 μg/day for pregnant women, but no RNI for other women of child-bearing age. This RNI is almost four times the recorded

Table 2.9 The British RNI and American RDA for selected micronutrients in pregnant and lactating women. All values are per day

Nutrient	Pregnancy		Lactation	
	RNI	RDA	RNI	RDA
Vitamin A (μg RE)	700	770	950	1300
Thiamin (mg)	0.8	1.4	1.0	1.4
Riboflavin (mg)	1.6	1.4	1.8	1.6
Niacin (mg NE)	13	18	15	17
Vitamin B$_6$ (mg)	1.2	1.9	1.2	2.0
Folic acid (μg)	Supplements	600	260	500
Vitamin C (mg)	50	85	70	120
Vitamin D (μg)	10	5	10	5
Calcium (mg)	700	1000	1250	1000
Iron (mg)	14.8	27	14.8	9
Selenium (μg)	60	60	75	70
Zinc (mg)	7.0	11	13.0	12

intake of non-pregnant British women and so probably requires supplements or more food fortification to be realistically achievable.

Despite the modest increase in the RNI for vitamin A during pregnancy, the emphasis of health promotion in the UK has been to suggest that non-prescribed supplements of vitamin A (retinol) and even some very retinol-rich foods are contra-indicated in pregnancy. Large doses of retinol cause birth defects in animals and people, and even some vitamin A-rich foods like pâté and liver may contain enough to cause concern; no such problems are associated with carotene from vegetable foods, which can be converted into vitamin A.

The American RDA for pregnancy listed in Table 2.9 are generally higher than the British values. The British experts who set the RNI clearly took the view that most of any theoretical increase in nutrient needs during pregnancy could be met by the following means:

- Physiological adaptation such as increased intestinal absorption or reduced nutrient loss (e.g. reduced iron loss when menstruation ceases and increased absorption of iron and calcium).
- Utilisation of maternal nutrient stores without compromising the health of the mother (e.g. utilising calcium from the maternal skeleton because the fetal skeleton at delivery contains only about 25 g of calcium compared to around 1 kg in a healthy woman).

This British panel did make the point that the RNI might well be insufficient for women who had low stores at the start of pregnancy. For example, women with anaemia or depleted iron stores might require more iron and adolescent mothers whose own skeletons were still growing might require more calcium.

The American experts who set the RDA for pregnancy shown in Table 2.9 clearly took an alternate view. They considered that the extra nutrient requirements resulting from pregnancy should be met largely from an increased dietary supply. Several of the US values in Table 2.9 are substantially higher than the British RNI for non-pregnant women and in some cases more than double this value. For example:

- The American RDA for vitamin A for pregnant women is almost 30% higher than the British RNI for non-pregnant women
- Thiamin – 75% higher
- Riboflavin – 27% higher
- Niacin – 38% higher
- Vitamin B_6 – 58% higher
- Vitamin C – 112% higher
- Calcium – 43% higher
- Iron – 82% higher
- Zinc – 57% higher

The average intakes of non-pregnant women recorded in the 2000–2001 National Diet and Nutrition Survey are at or below the American RDA for pregnancy for several nutrients: vitamin A, riboflavin, folate, vitamin C, calcium, iron and zinc. Given that women eat almost the same amount of food whether pregnant or not, then unless they change the composition of their diet significantly when pregnant, this will also be true for pregnant British women. If some of these US target values are to be realistically achievable by most pregnant women, they imply the necessity for widespread use of supplements, for instance the value for iron. Earlier in this chapter it was also noted that even where average intakes exceed the RNI/RDA there will still be substantial numbers of individuals whose intakes are inadequate. This ultimately means that many British and American pregnant women consume amounts of some essential micronutrients that are a long way below the RDA set by American nutrition experts.

It has already been noted that large supplements of vitamin A (retinol) and even some retinol-rich foods suh as liver are contra-indicated in pregnancy and that most pregnant women are advised not to take retinol-containing supplements (including fish liver oil) without medical approval. Mathews (1996) suggests that high-dose vitamin A supplements in Africa have resulted in embryonic teratogenesis, an increased rate of malformations and birth defects; similar effects have been seen in animal studies. Mathews also reviews other studies, which suggest that:

- Concentrated protein supplements have been consistently associated with depressed average birth weights.

- Routine iron supplements in non-deficient women can increase rates of prematurity and low birth weight.
- Fetal malformations in zinc-deficient animals are much more frequent when calcium supplements are given than when both minerals are deficient, tending to support the proposition that supplementation with one nutrient can adversely affect the absorption and metabolism of others.

Such observations indicate that there is potential for harm if pregnant women are given unnecessary supplements. This possibility needs to be considered before universal supplementation is recommended; if the case for such supplements is accepted then dosage needs to be moderate.

The question of whether iron supplements should be routinely prescribed for pregnant women is something that has been debated for decades. The American RDA for iron increases substantially in pregnancy, but this high iron intake is only practically achievable for most women with supplementation. In contrast, the British RNI is not increased at all, leading to no need for routine supplementation. One complicating factor in this ongoing debate is that blood haemoglobin concentration naturally declines during pregnancy due to a haemodilution effect. Increases in plasma volume during pregnancy are greater than increases in red cell mass, so haematocrit and haemoglobin concentration decrease despite an increase in the total amount of haemoglobin in the circulation. This physiological drop in haemoglobin concentration has, in the past, been interpreted as evidence of very widespread anaemia in pregnancy and iron supplements have been used in an attempt to bring the haemoglobin concentration back up to the non-pregnant level. Mathews (1996) reviews convincing evidence that:

- Iron deficiency anaemia is associated with increased risk of low birth weight and prematurity.
- High haemoglobin levels are associated with similar outcomes, although this may not be a simple cause-and-effect relationship.
- Routine iron supplementation does not produce measurable benefits.

At least in developed countries, where this is a feasible option, iron supplements should probably be targeted at those women identified as iron deficient by screening.

Lactating women

Table 2.7 indicates that the estimated average energy requirement (EAR in the UK) of women rises by about a quarter during lactation, implying that food intake also increases by about a quarter and therefore that nutrient intake increases by a similar amount unless the diet changes significantly during lactation. According to COMA (1991) this 25% increase in the EAR reflects the real increases in energy consumption by lactating women. Table 2.9 shows the British RNI and American RDA for lactating women for selected micronutrients. This table indicates that the increased RNI for some nutrients is substantially more than a quarter; that is, the RNI for vitamin A, riboflavin, vitamin C, calcium and zinc. If one assumes that the nutrient density of the diet of lactating women is essentially similar to that of other women of child-bearing age, then the problems noted earlier with the intakes of vitamin A, riboflavin, calcium and zinc will be markedly worse during lactation.

In general, if there is low maternal intake of a micronutrient, milk content is maintained at the expense of maternal stores of the nutrient. If maternal stores become depleted, the milk content of vitamins and some trace minerals will be affected by continuing low maternal intake.

The elderly

Table 2.7 suggests that elderly men are a potential high-risk group for nutrient deficiency because their estimated energy requirement is substantially less than that of younger men, but their estimated nutrient needs are usually similar; that is, they require the same amount of nutrients from less food. The same arguments apply to elderly women, although they are not specifically listed in Table 2.7.

The figures in the table may well understate the true decline in energy and thus food intake that occurs in the elderly because of the way the energy standards were set. COMA (1991) set the dietary standards for energy by calculating the expected average basal metabolic rate from average weight and then multiplying this by a factor that reflected the level of extra energy expended due to all of the day's activity – the physical activity level, PAL. In younger adults it used a PAL multiple of 1.4, which it deemed appropriate for a population that is largely sedentary both at work and during their leisure time. For older adults it used a multiple of 1.5 times the BMR, despite clear evidence that activity levels tend to decline with age (e.g. Allied Dunbar National Fitness Survey, 1992). The committee made this decision because its members did not want to encourage the belief that energy intakes and energy expenditure should fall sharply with age.

The only differences between the micronutrient RNI/RDA for older people and younger adults are those listed below:

- Slight reductions in the RNI for thiamin and niacin, because they are set per 1000 kcal and thus reflect the drop in estimated energy requirement.
- Reductions in the RNI/RDA for iron for older women to the same value as that of men, because of the perceived reduction in iron need when menstruation ceases.
- An RNI/RDA of 10 µg/day of vitamin D set for elderly people (no RNI for young adults), because it can no longer be assumed that sunlight exposure will be sufficient to manufacture all the required vitamin D (many people become increasingly housebound as they become elderly). The American RDA increases to 15 µg/day in the over-70s age group.
- A substantial increase in the American RDA for vitamin B_6.
- A 20% increase in the American RDA for calcium.

It may well be that the actual requirement for a number of nutrients is increased in old age, although this is difficult to quantify and so the dietary standards for younger adults are often used for older adults partly by default. For example, the efficiency of absorption of some nutrients may decrease in the elderly and some medical conditions that increase nutrient requirements become more prevalent in older people.

If elderly people become immobile and largely housebound, this will reduce their energy expenditure to well below the standard values used to construct Table 2.7. Similarly, actual energy (food) intake will be depressed if they are underweight and losing weight; that is, not even eating enough to maintain an energy balance. Under such circumstances, it may become difficult for them to obtain all of the nutrients they need from the relatively small amount of food being consumed. The problem will be compounded if their diet is not nutrient dense and they are consuming a large proportion of their energy in the form of energy-rich but nutrient-depleted foods, such as sugary drinks or foods, alcoholic drinks or fatty foods. Being largely housebound will restrict the exposure of some elderly people to summer sunlight and so compromise their ability to make vitamin D in their skin. The case for micronutrient supplements strengthens in the elderly especially if they are inactive, underweight and/or housebound. According to Mintel (2001), supplement usage does increase with age and almost half of Britons over 65 years report using supplements. The elderly housebound, and indeed anybody not regularly exposing at least their hands and faces to summer sunlight, is at high risk of vitamin D deficiency. Dietary intakes of vitamin D are unlikely to be sufficient to meet physiological needs fully and so supplements are strongly indicated.

Finch *et al.* (1998) published the results of the National Dietary and Nutrition Survey of Britons aged over 65 years. This was similar in scope and design to that for young and middle-aged adults discussed earlier. The sample included both elderly people living independently in their own homes and those living in residential care accommodation. As with the surveys of younger adults, the recorded energy intakes were below the estimated average requirements. The average intakes of the free-living men were 82% of the total recorded for the 2000–2001 survey of younger adults; the corresponding figure for the free-living women was 87%. Average energy intake declined with age in free-living men. The recorded intakes were higher for those living in residential care than those living in their own homes; this was especially marked in women. The prevalence of underweight was low in the free-living samples, suggesting that energy intakes *per se* were generally sufficient. This survey's results suggest that the theoretical reduction in the energy needs of elderly men shown in Table 2.7 do probably give a reasonable indication of the actual reduction in energy and food intake in the elderly of both sexes.

The average recorded intakes of most nutrients in this sample of elderly British people were close to or above the RNI and in some cases well above the RNI. As noted earlier, such apparently satisfactory averages may well obscure substantial numbers of individuals with inadequate intakes. In general, the average intakes of elderly men and women were lower in this survey than the average recorded in younger adults in the 2000–2001 survey; this was true for both those living freely and those living in institutions. The only major exceptions were average vitamin A intakes, which were substantially higher than those in younger adults, and only around 5% of the free-living sample reported intakes from food that were below the LRNI and only 1% of the institutionalised sample. Intakes of vitamin D from food were also higher in the elderly sample, although as one might expect almost all of them were below the RNI of 10 µg/day set for older adults. For other micronutrients, the numbers recording inadequate intakes (below the LRNI) were generally 5% or less, with the following exceptions:

- Riboflavin intakes were inadequate in 7% of those living freely but in only 3% of those living in institutions.
- Calcium in 5% of men and 9% of women living freely but less than 1% of the institutionalised sample.
- Iron in 5–6% of all women and institutionalised men but only 1% of free-living men.
- Magnesium and potassium in around a quarter of the total samples.
- Zinc in 8% of free-living men and 13% of institutionalised men (5% and 4% respectively for women).

Supplements had little effect on the average total intake of those living in institutions with the exception of vitamin C (7% increase for men and 15% for women); corresponding vitamin C figures for the free-living samples were 5% for men and 12% for women. Supplements also made a significant difference to the intake of a few micronutrients in the free-living sample, as listed below:

- Big increases in average intakes of thiamin, riboflavin and B_6 for women only.
- A 10% increase in vitamin A intake.
- Around a 15% increase in average vitamin D intake.
- Big increases in vitamin E intake (12% for men and 53% for women).
- Increases in total iron intake of 5% for men and 3% for women.

Despite generally lower average intakes than younger adults, the percentages of elderly people reporting inadequate intakes of key micronutrients is generally small, although as noted earlier this may represent substantial numbers of individuals.

Biochemical status was also measured for several key nutrients and some particular causes for concern noted by the authors of this report were:

- About 10% of the sample showed biochemical evidence of poor iron status (i.e. a low serum ferritin level).
- About 8% of the free-living sample and 37% of those living in care accommodation had biochemical evidence of poor vitamin D status.

- Around 40% of the total sample had biochemical indication of low riboflavin status, although this may be an indication that the test itself overestimates deficiency.
- Around 40% of the institutionalised group had low biochemical status for folate and vitamin C as well as around 15% of the free-living group.
- Low biochemical status for thiamin was found in 10–15% of both the free-living and the institutionalised sample.
- Recorded intakes of zinc were at or below the RNI and 15% of men and 7% of women in institutions had biochemical evidence of zinc deficiency.

The relatively high numbers with biochemical evidence of insufficiency for some nutrients compared with the smaller numbers reporting frankly inadequate intakes tend to give some support to the case that the requirement for some micronutrients may be increased in the elderly, for instance because of a decrease in the efficiency of absorption. These figures represent the numbers whose biochemical status is deemed to be low even with current supplement use. These relatively high percentages do seem to provide a *prima facie* case for more widespread use of either selected micronutrient supplements or multinutrient supplements among the elderly population of Britain.

In the previous edition of this book, studies published by R. K. Chandra were discussed as evidence that micronutrient supplement improved immune function in elderly people. Some work of this author has now been discredited and so even though these studies are still in the literature, they have been omitted from this discussion. This issue was raised in Chapter 1 and further information can be found in Smith (2005) and Hamblin (2006).

Mowe *et al*. (1994) assessed the diets and nutritional status of a large sample of elderly people admitted to hospitals in the Oslo area for an acute cause like a stroke or myocardial infarction. They compared these results with those obtained from a matched sample of well elderly people living within the same area. They concluded that there were several indicators suggesting that the food and nutrient intake of the hospitalised group had been inferior to that of the well group in the three months prior to admission. They raised the possibility that poor food and nutrient intake might be a contributory factor in the acute illnesses that led to hospitalisation.

Athletes in training

Athletes in training expend considerably more energy than the average person targeted by dietary standards; they may expend more than double their basal metabolic rate (BMR) compared with the 1.4–1.5 times BMR expended by the average sedentary adult and perhaps even less by an elderly housebound person. This means that provided they eat enough to satisfy their appetite and to maintain a constant body weight, they should also consume more calories than the average person. If their diet is similar in nutrient density to that of the rest of the population, it also follows that they should also take in more essential micronutrients than the average person. Increased total food intake should therefore make micronutrient inadequacy less likely in athletes.

There are at least two potential problems with this logic and these are outlined below:

- First, some female athletes in particular may perceive the need to be very lean and thus restrict their energy intake. In practice, they have much lower energy intakes than would be predicted from their activity levels (see Wilson, 1994). In some sports, being lean may have or be seen to have a favourable influence on judges, for example in gymnastics and figure skating. In other sports, athletes may be divided into weight categories or being light may offer a clear advantage, such as with jockeys and boxers.
- Secondly, there is a widely held belief among athletes and coaches that training increases the requirement for protein and micronutrients. This remains a contentious issue, but it may well be that there are small increases in the requirement for certain water-soluble vitamins, protein and iron, although these increases should be more than offset by increases in energy intake in most athletes who are not deliberately and severely restricting their energy intake.

While deficiencies of essential micronutrients would certainly impair the ability of an athlete to train and compete, equally there is no substantial evidence that supplemental intakes of micronutrients improve performance in athletes who are already well nourished. This view is supported by a joint position statement by three North American organisations (ACSM, ADA and DC, 2000) that athletes who obtained sufficient energy from a variety of sources would get adequate amounts of vitamins and minerals from their food. They further suggested that supplements might be necessary in athletes who restrict their energy intake, indulge in severe dieting, avoid whole food groups or consume a high-carbohydrate diet with low micronutrient density.

Deficiencies of iron and iron deficiency anaemia have been claimed to be relatively common among athletes, particularly female endurance athletes. Training may lead to some small increases in iron losses and impair the increase in iron absorption that normally occurs when iron stores are low, but as with other micronutrients this should be more than compensated for by the increase in total food intake during training. Note, however, that it was seen earlier in the chapter that many ordinary women and girls have marginal or inadequate iron intakes and anaemia would certainly have an adverse effect on training and performance.

One confounding problem here is that endurance training tends to lower the haemoglobin concentration in blood because it increases plasma volume more than red cell mass; the concentration of haemoglobin in blood falls even though the actual amount of circulating haemoglobin is increased. As noted earlier, this haemodilution effect is also seen in pregnancy, where a natural decline in haemoglobin concentration has also often been misinterpreted as evidence of widespread iron deficiency anaemia. True anaemia with low circulating haemoglobin and low iron stores (as measured by serum ferritin) is much less common among athletes.

Iron deficiency, particularly among female athletes, is primarily due to poor intake of available iron. Those who restrict their energy intake to keep their body weight low would seem to be particularly at risk, although very low body weight can lead to a cessation of menstruation, which would paradoxically result in considerable iron savings.

Summing up

Since the 1950s there has been a general tendency in the UK and other wealthy industrialised countries to regard micronutrient inadequacies as largely diseases of the past, which now really only affect those with unusual or bizarre dietary choices or special medical and social risk factors, such as:

- the frail elderly
- those with certain chronic medical conditions
- those at the extremes of social deprivation, such as the homeless unemployed
- those with highly restrictive, 'fad' dietary choices
- those who abuse alcohol or illegal drugs

However, the in-depth analyses of the data provided by the UK's ongoing programme of National Diet and Nutrition Surveys suggest that the assumption that 'almost everyone in the UK consumes adequate amounts of all the essential nutrients' is probably overoptimistic. Even where average intakes of nutrients are reassuringly high compared to the RNI, there may be substantial numbers of individuals in all age groups who have apparently inadequate intakes of one or more micronutrients. In a few cases, even average intakes appear to be unsatisfactory; if one uses American standards as the benchmark then this position would look significantly worse. The increasingly sedentary nature of the population has led to apparently large decreases (c. 25%) in average energy intakes since the 1950s. This declining food intake must clearly reduce nutrient intakes, especially if it is coupled with the consumption of increasing amounts of energy-rich but nutrient-depleted sugary or fatty snacks, drinks and convenience foods.

As suggested at the start of this chapter, the ideal way to provide good amounts of all the essential nutrients is to eat reasonable amounts of a well-balanced diet. To achieve these ends without encouraging excessive energy consumption may require substantial changes in both diet and lifestyle (through increased activity and energy expenditure). Of course, health promotion and nutrition education must in the longer term seek to encourage and facilitate such changes. However, supplements may be a useful, immediate and practical adjunct to these long-term programmes if micronutrient deficiencies are currently impairing or threatening the health and physiological functioning of substantial numbers of people. Supplements may be very much a second-best option in the eyes of most nutritionists and dieticians, but if the first-choice option is becoming for many only a long-term aspiration, they may be the only realistic choice in the immediate future.

It should also be borne in mind that health-promotion programmes aimed at encouraging supplement use may have limited impact on those who would most benefit; that is, those with the lowest intakes from food. Such programmes would need to be carefully targeted and might require the distribution of free supplements, in schools for example. Experience with the recommendations regarding the use of folic acid supplements in women of child-bearing age discussed in Chapter 3 suggests that they have been largely ineffective in Europe even 10 years after they began. In contrast, food fortification with folic acid in North and South America has had an immediate measurable effect.

In a controversial and thought-provoking article, Horrobin (2003) argues that multinutrient supplements should be universally prescribed. He argues that micronutrient deficiencies are common and that current supplement usage tends to be concentrated among the affluent middle classes who largely do not need them; this latter point has been made several times already in this chapter. He quotes and references studies purporting to show the following:

- Micronutrient and macronutrient deficiencies are common among hospital admissions and nutritional status tends to deteriorate during time spent in hospital (e.g. Hall *et al.*, 2000; Cunha *et al.*, 2001).
- Multinutrient supplements reduce hospital stay and improve outcome compared to placebos in hospital patients (Keele *et al.*, 1997; Vlaming *et al.*, 2001).
- He quotes work of R. K. Chandra suggesting that micronutrient supplements improve immune function and reduce infection times in elderly people, although some of this author's work has now been discredited (see Chapter 1).
- In controlled studies, micronutrient supplements reduced violent behaviour among prison inmates (e.g. Gesch *et al.*, 2002).

Horrobin used these studies and observations to support his claim that many people would benefit from this universal supplementation. He argues that universal supplementation would be a rapid, cheap and effective of way of ameliorating these problems. It would also help reduce the apparent widespread levels of marginal or inadequate intakes of micronutrients highlighted by the National Diet and Nutrition Survey programme.

3 The Individual Vitamins

Vitamins are a group of organic substances that are essential for survival, growth and normal body functioning. They are only required in small amounts (mg or µg quantities) and do not act as sources of dietary energy. They are not synthesised in the body or are only synthesised from specific dietary precursors. Inadequate intake of a vitamin (and any precursor) results in characteristic adverse signs and symptoms, which, provided that irreversible damage has not occurred, are cured by administration of sufficient amounts of the vitamin. At least some of the precise biochemical and physiological functions have been established for each of the vitamins and detailed, referenced accounts of vitamin functions can be found in Ball (2004). Detailed information on maximum UK intakes from food and other sources as well as the effects of vitamin overdoses and estimates of safe maximum intakes can be found in FSA (2003); references for the primary studies on the effects of high vitamin intakes can be found in this report. Much of the information in this chapter on dietary sources of vitamins, their functions and the effects of deficiency can be found in standard nutritional texts (e.g. Webb, 2008) and so is not specifically referenced here.

Table 3.1 shows estimates of the doses of vitamins found in single-vitamin and multinutrient supplements; the RNI for an adult man and the FSA (2003) indication of maximum 'safe' doses and maximum exposure from food are also included for comparison. These figures for dose levels are those in products sold in 1998–99. Table 3.2 shows estimates for the same period of the number of tablets/capsules sold in the UK that contained the vitamin, either as a single vitamin or in a multiple-nutrient preparation.

The vitamins are subdivided into those that are water soluble and, first, those that are soluble in fat or lipid solvents.

The fat-soluble vitamins

Vitamin A (retinol)

The chemical structure of retinol is shown in Figure 3.1. The UK RNI for vitamin A is 700 µg (RE)/day for adult men and 600 µg/day for women; the corresponding American RDA are 900 and 700 µg/day respectively. Pre-formed vitamin A (retinol)

Dietary Supplements and Functional Foods, 2nd Edition. Geoffrey P. Webb.
© 2011 Blackwell Publishing Ltd.

Table 3.1 The adult male RNI for vitamins, the range of doses* in single and multiple-nutrient supplements and the 'safe maximum' as interpreted from FSA (2003); other vales are from EVM (2000). Values in brackets are the most commonly used doses. Estimated and approximate maximum intakes from food are also shown

Vitamin	RNI	Single vitamins	Multiple nutrients	'Safe' maximum	Food maximum
Retinol (µg)	700	2250–2400	200–2300 (750–800)	2400**	6000
β-carotene (mg)	n/a	1.3–15	0.4–20 (3–15)	7	7
Vitamin D (µg)	n/a	10	1.25–12.5 (5)	12.5	9
Vitamin E (mg)	4	50–670 (200–670)	2–268 (10–40)	500+	18
Vitamin K (µg)	70#	n/a	10–200 (30–95)	1000	n/a
Thiamin (mg)	0.9	50–100	0.3–100 (1.4–3.9)	100+	3
Riboflavin (mg)	1.3	100	0.2–100 (1.6–50)	40	3.5
Nicotinamide§ (mg)	16	100–250	0.25–150 (18–50)	500	60NE
Vitamin B_6 (mg)	1.4	10–200 (10–80)	0.35–100 (2–82)	10+?	4
Vitamin B_{12} (µg)	1.5	5–1000 (100)	0.5–3000 (1–50)	2000	20
Folic acid (µg)	200	400–800 (400)	0.7–500 (200–500)	1500	500
Biotin (µg)	10–200#	300–1000 (300)	0.5–2000 (50–150)	900+	70
Pantothenic acid (mg)	3–7#	50–550 (200)	0.7–140 (6–50)	200+	10
Vitamin C (mg)	40	60–3000	10–1000 (50–150)	1000+	160

* Note that figures for doses used were current in the UK in 2000; i.e. before the effect of the publication of FSA (2003). These vales are the manufacturers' declared levels and in some cases it is routine to overformulate to compensate for any possible losses during manufacture.
** Legal maximum for pregnant women a total intake from food and supplements not exceeding 1500 µg/day.
# The safe intake – no RNI.
§ Nicotinic acid is sometimes used in multiple nutrient supplements – most common dose 10 mg/day (NE is niacin equivalents).

Table 3.2 Annual sales (millions of capsules/tablets) of single-vitamin and multiple-nutrient supplements containing individual vitamins. Figures are taken from EVM (2000) and should thus only be taken as a guide to current relative popularity. Internet sales were not included, although some other mail-order sales are

Vitamin	Single-vitamin sales	Multiple-nutrient sales
Retinol	2.1	1053
β-carotene	4.4	270
Vitamin D	1.1	1216
Vitamin E	79	564
Vitamin K	not sold	137
Thiamin	8	514
Riboflavin	0.8	548
Nicotinamide	n/a	175
Nicotinic acid	not sold	375
Vitamin B_6	18.5	391
Vitamin B_{12}	4.7	433
Folic acid	13.7	414
Biotin	1.04	12
Pantothenic acid	1.8	250
Vitamin C	252	522

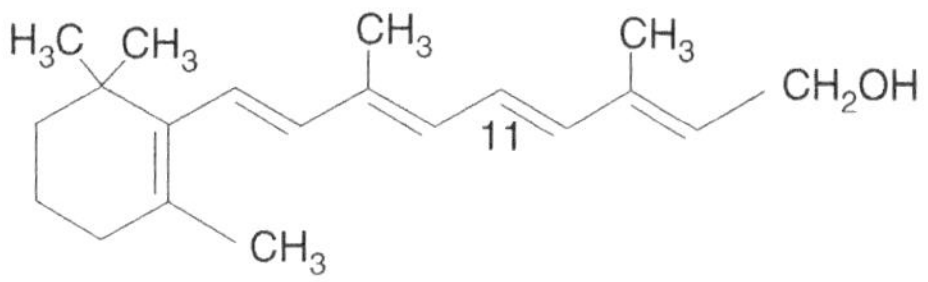

Figure 3.1 The structure of vitamin A (all trans retinol).

is only found naturally in foods of animal origin such as egg yolks, dairy fat, liver, fatty fish and fish liver oil; there is little retinol in muscle meat or white fish, but it is added to margarine, some breakfast cereals, some processed milks and to infant foods. Retinol is present in many multinutrient supplements in amounts up to 2400 μg per day. Fish liver oils also contain high concentrations of retinol.

Humans are capable of converting the plant pigment β-carotene and a few other carotenoid pigments into retinol; these carotenoids are found in dark green, yellow, orange and red fruits and vegetables and in palm oil. The efficiency of absorption of these plant pigments is less than that of retinol itself and so 6 μg of β-carotene and 12 μg of the other carotenoids with pre-vitamin A activity are said to be equivalent to 1 μg of retinol. When estimating the dietary intake of

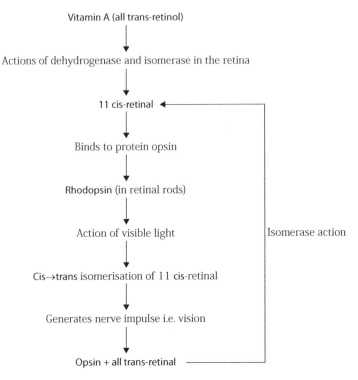

Figure 3.2 Scheme for the visual function of vitamin A in the rods of the retina
Source: Reproduced with permission from G.P. Webb (2008) *Nutrition: A Health Promotion Approach*, 3rd edn, Hodder Arnold, London.

vitamin A, one must convert intakes of β-carotene and other carotenoids into retinol equivalents (RE):

$$1 \text{ μg retinol, } 6 \text{ μg β-carotene or } 12 \text{ μg of other active}$$
$$\text{carotenoid} = 1 \text{ μg retinol equivalen (RE)}$$

A derivative of retinol (11-*cis*-retinal) is the light-sensitive component (chromophore) of all known visual pigments, including those of the human eye. The rods of the retina are responsible for black-and-white vision at low-intensity light, whereas the cones are responsible for colour vision in higher-intensity light. The visual system in the rods has been extensively studied and is the best understood. In the rods, vitamin A (all-trans-retinol; that is, retinol with all double bonds in the trans-isomeric configuration) is converted to 11-*cis*-retinal, which combines with a protein called opsin to produce rhodopsin or visual purple. It is the interaction between rhodopsin and visual light that initiates the nerve impulses in the rods that we perceive as vision. Light induces a cis-trans-isomerisation of 11-*cis*-retinal, which causes dissociation from opsin, and these events ultimately lead to the opening of sodium ion channels and the generation of a nerve impulse (see Figure 3.2 for a diagrammatic summary). The difference between cis and trans isomers is illustrated in Figure 6.1g in Chapter 6 and discussed in the corresponding text. A reduced ability to see in low-intensity light (night blindness) is the first symptom of vitamin A deficiency.

Retinol and its metabolites, especially retinoic acid, play an important role in the regulation of gene expression and via these mechanisms control many aspects of cell division and differentiation, growth, development and homeostasis. There are nuclear receptors for retinoic acid and other retinoids and these receptors are of the same type as those that mediate the actions of steroid and thyroid hormones.

Adequate intakes of vitamin A are necessary to maintain the integrity of epithelial tissues in, for example, the eye, the respiratory tract and the alimentary tract. In vitamin A deficiency pronounced pathological changes occur in these epithelial tissues, which, among other things, reduce their effectiveness as a barrier to infection. There is overgrowth of improperly developed epithelial cells, which become hard and dry with reduced secretion of mucous. When this occurs in the cornea, it can ultimately lead to permanent blindness. Initially overgrowth of the corneal epithelium results in white spots (Bitot's spots) on the surface of the cornea due to clumps of epithelial cells; this progresses to hardening and drying of the cornea, with frequent infections. Eventually the corneal tissue becomes necrotic, the front of the eye 'melts' and the lens may fall out. These ocular manifestations of vitamin A deficiency are collectively termed xerophthalmia.

Loss of integrity of epithelial tissue reduces its effectiveness as a non-specific barrier to infection and thus increases the risk of infection. Vitamin A deficiency also reduces the effectiveness of both antibody-mediated and cell-mediated immunity. In vitamin A deficiency:

- Production of many antibodies is impaired.
- There are reduced numbers of natural killer cells in the circulation.
- Neutrophils show an impaired ability to ingest and kill pathogenic organisms.

Macrophages also show an enhanced phagocytic and killing capacity when treated with retinoic acid; they may also show an enhanced ability to kill tumour cells (see Ball, 2004).

Increased susceptibility to infection is a major reason for child mortality being high in areas where vitamin A deficiency is prevalent.

Vitamin A deficiency occurs wherever people, and especially children, rely largely on a starchy staple for most of their calorie intake, without substantial input of either dairy products or coloured fruits and vegetables. Vitamin A is normally absorbed with fat, so a very low fat intake can precipitate vitamin A deficiency because it impairs absorption of both retinol and carotene; any condition that impairs fat absorption can also precipitate vitamin A deficiency, for example cystic fibrosis. According to the World Health Organisation, up to 7 million new cases of xerophthalmia occur each year and around 10% of these will have permanent corneal damage. High risk of blindness and increased child mortality, due primarily to increased infection risk, are features of areas where vitamin A deficiency is common, such as South East Asia, the Indian subcontinent, and some developing countries in Africa and South America. Vitamin A deficiency is the most common cause of non-congenital blindness in children.

We have seen in Chapter 2 that substantial numbers of both adults and children in the UK have marginal or frankly inadequate vitamin A intakes. Average vitamin A intakes of adults have fallen sharply in the past decade or so. This would seem to make a reasonable *prima facie* case for the targeted use of supplements containing moderate amounts of vitamin A as a second-best option to dietary improvement. On the other hand, there are serious safety issues concerning the overuse of supplements of retinol. There are also concerns about the chronic use of large β-carotene supplements, despite its low acute toxicity. These toxicity issues will be dealt with separately.

The adult dietary standards for vitamin A vary between the UK RNI for women of 600 µgRE/day and the American RDA for men of 900 µgRE/day. According to the Food Standards Agency (FSA, 2003), the top 2.5% of UK adults consume more than 6000 µgRE/day of retinol from food and in some cases supplements might add up to a further 2400 µgRE/day (the legal maximum for general sales in the UK). This means that the maximum intake of retinol may be close to ten times the normal dietary standard for total vitamin A. Many of these high consumers of retinol from food are people who regularly eat liver or products made from liver. While single doses of 100 times the dietary standard may be required to produce acute toxicity in adults, chronic consumption of amounts that are close to the maximum UK adult intake may produce subacute or chronic toxicity, and some vulnerable individuals may be harmed by doses that are only a fifth of this.

Acute vitamin A poisoning can cause abdominal pain, anorexia, vomiting, blurred vision, irritability and headaches, while chronic toxicity leads to cracked lips, dry and hardened skin, conjunctivitis, hair loss, red skin lesions, liver damage, raised intracranial pressure, headaches, bone-mineral loss and joint pain. Retinol intakes of only three times current average intakes in post-menopausal women may double the risk of hip fracture. High doses of retinol are known to increase the risk of birth defects when given to pregnant laboratory animals and, although epidemiological evidence suggests that this is also true in humans, it is difficult to establish the threshold dose for this effect in humans. These observations led the FSA (2003) to support the view that women who are or intend to become pregnant should take vitamin A-containing supplements only if medically advised to do so. They further suggest that total intakes of greater than 1500 µgRE/day as retinol may be ill advised (cf. average intakes of c. 500 µgRE/day). Many people who regularly consume liver will get considerably more than this from their food and some supplements contain more than this tentatively suggested maximum total dose. FSA (2003) also notes that some supplements may contain more than the amount on the label to compensate for possible losses of retinol during the intended shelf life of the product.

While β-carotene is not an essential nutrient *per se* and so has no specific dietary standards, it does contribute to the total vitamin A content of the diet, as noted earlier. β-carotene has generally been considered to be a non-toxic substance for humans, although high consumption does lead to a yellowing of the skin. It has been administered chronically in doses of up to 300 mg/day to people with a condition known as erythropoeitic protoporphyria without any obvious ill-effects (their skin is extremely sensitive to light and the β-carotene is intended to reduce their sensitivity to light).

A high intake of fruits and vegetables has been shown on numerous occasions to be associated with a reduced risk of cancer and heart disease and this means that high β-carotene intakes are also associated with these benefits. While high β-carotene intakes may contribute to these beneficial effects, this association does not necessarily mean that β-carotene prevents cancer. Several studies completed in the last decade have in fact suggested that doses of 20–30 mg/day of β-carotene may increase the risk of lung cancer in smokers and asbestos workers, without providing any clear evidence of benefit for the population as a whole. Studies with ferrets as an animal model have suggested that exposure to high doses of β-carotene may lead to overgrowth of epithelial cells in the lung (metaplasia) and that this effect is amplified by concurrent exposure to cigarette smoke, but is not caused by exposure to cigarette smoke alone. There is a more detailed and referenced account of studies on the effects of β-carotene supplements in Chapter 5.

Average adult intakes of β-carotene from food in the UK are just over 2 mg/day, with the top 2.5% of consumers taking in excess of 7 mg/day. Supplements may provide up to a further 20 mg/day. The expert working group of the Food Standards Agency (FSA, 2003) suggested a safe upper level for β-carotene supplements of only 7 mg/day. The COMA expert working group on diet and cancer (COMA, 1998a) went even further and recommended 'the avoidance of β-carotene supplements as a means of protecting against cancer'. This latter group highlighted the need for caution in the use of other purified supplements, which they emphasised could not be assumed to be without risk. It is difficult to reconcile the apparent protective effect of foods rich in carotenoids with the suggestion that purified supplements of β-carotene may promote cancer growth in some people. One of several possibilities is that fruits and vegetables contain a mix of carotenoids, whereas single supplements produce an imbalance in the body's carotenoid profile (see Chapter 5).

Vitamin D (cholecalciferol)

The chemical structure of vitamin D_3 and its precursor 7-dehydrocholesterol are shown in Figure 3.3. Vitamin D_3 or cholecalciferol is produced in the skin of humans, animals and birds by the action of ultraviolet light (from sunlight) on 7-dehydrocholesterol, a compound synthesised in the skin from the ubiquitous steroid cholesterol by the action of a dehydrogenase enzyme that inserts an extra double bond in ring B (see Figure 3.3). Vitamin D would thus fail a strict application of one of the criteria of Harper (1999) for establishing that a nutrient is essential, namely the criterion that 'the substance is not synthesised in the body and is required throughout life'. Vitamin D can be synthesised in the skin provided that it is regularly exposed (at least the hands and face) to the correct wavelengths of ultraviolet light, which in the UK are only found in summer sunlight. For most adults and school-aged children, there is no RNI given for vitamin D in the UK because it was assumed by COMA (1991) that they would normally manufacture sufficient of the vitamin in their skin during the summer to last the whole year. RNI are given for babies and younger children, the elderly and pregnant and lactating women,

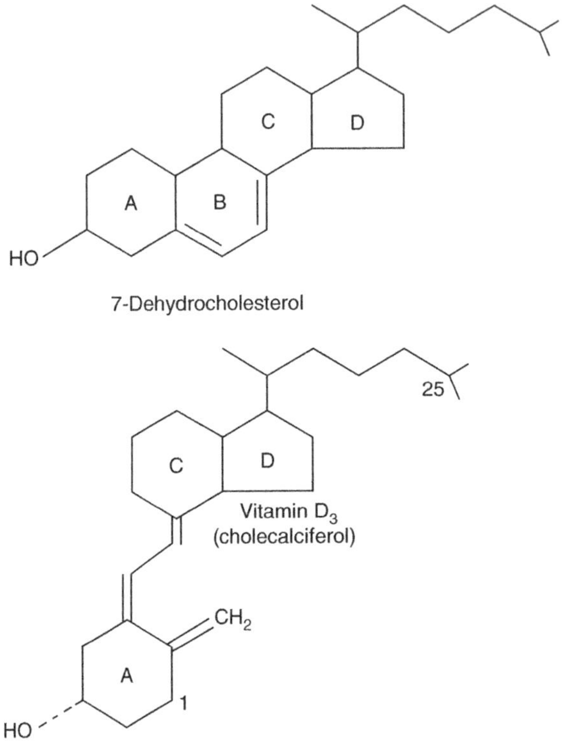

Figure 3.3 The structures of 7-dehydrocholesterol and vitamin D_3 (cholecalciferol).

and these vary between 7 and 10 µg/day as compared with a typical average UK dietary intake of only 2–3 µg/day.

Clearly, anyone whose skin is not regularly exposed to summer sunlight is unlikely to obtain enough vitamin D from their diet to satisfy the level of physiological need for the vitamin indicated by these RNI. In America an RDA is set for all age groups, varying from 5 µg/day for most adults up to 10 µg/day for most children, elderly people and pregnant and lactating women, and this rises to 15 µg/day in those aged over 70 years who are not regularly exposed to sunlight. Holick and Chen (2008) suggest even higher supplementary intakes of 20–25 µg of vitamin D for both adults and children where production from sunlight cannot be assured. Even the official dietary standards are thus an implicit recommendation for the widespread use of vitamin D-containing supplements or fortified foods, and many experts believe that these standards are too low.

Vitamin D is only found naturally in foods of animal origin and has a similar distribution to retinol, for example it is found in egg yolk, dairy fat, liver and other offal, oily fish and fish liver oil. Some other foods are fortified with added vitamin D, such as some breakfast cereals, some processed milks, infant foods and margarine. Vitamin D_2 (calciferol) is an alternative form of vitamin D that is formed when a fungal steroid called ergosterol is irradiated with ultraviolet light. Irradiated yeast has been a convenient source of vitamin D for therapeutic use and for use in food fortification. Holick and Chen (2008) suggest that despite earlier concerns, the potency of vitamin D_2 and vitamin D_3 is the same.

In order to become physiologically active within the body, vitamin D must undergo two hydroxylation reactions (addition of hydroxyl or OH groups). First, a hydroxyl group is added to carbon 25 in the liver and a second hydroxyl added at carbon 1 in the kidney to give 25-hydroxy vitamin D and 1,25-dihydroxy vitamin D respectively (see Figure 3.3). The 25-hydroxy vitamin D is the main circulating form of the vitamin and measures of its level in blood are used as a biochemical indicator of vitamin D status. A plasma concentration of <25 nmol/L (OH) D (25 hydroxycholecalciferol) is taken as the cut-off point for vitamin D deficiency in the UK NDNS (Hoare et al., 2004). Holick and Chen (2008) suggest that a level of <50 nmol/L should be the criterion for deficiency and that <75 nmol/L indicates some degree of insufficiency, because in post-menopausal women these levels are necessary to minimise parathyroid hormone (PTH) levels (an elevated level of PTH is an indicator of vitamin D insufficiency). The 1,25-dihydroxy vitamin D produced in the kidney is also called calcitriol and it behaves like a steroid hormone. It could be said that the function of vitamin D is to act as a precursor to enable the kidney to synthesise this hormone.

The primary function of calcitriol and thus of vitamin D is to induce the synthesis of proteins in the gut that are essential for the efficient absorption of calcium and thus the maintenance of the body's calcium homeostasis. It is also necessary for the efficient reabsorption of filtered calcium in the kidney. Calcitriol induces key proteins that are found in bone matrix and is necessary for normal bone development, mineralization and remodelling. Calcitriol also stimulates bone resorption by osteoclasts.

Acute vitamin D deficiency leads to a condition known as rickets in children and osteomalacia in adults. At the start of the twentieth century, rickets was very prevalent among poor children living in the industrial towns of Britain and other parts of northern Europe. Reduced calcium absorption leads to low blood levels of calcium and thus to reduced bone calcification, ultimately leading to skeletal abnormalities like bowing of the legs and overgrowth of cartilage in the wrist and ribs. Muscle weakness and high prevalence of infections are also seen in children with rickets.

It is also suggested that prolonged vitamin D deficiency and the compensatory increase in parathyroid hormone, which releases calcium from bone to maintain blood levels, may be an aetiological factor in the genesis of osteoporosis (brittle bones) in elderly people who are wholly or largely housebound. It was noted in Chapter 2 that large numbers of children (13% of 11–18 year olds sampled in the winter), adults (c. 26% of 19–24 year olds) and elderly people (37% of those living in institutions) in Britain show biochemical evidence of vitamin D deficiency. Not only are elderly and largely housebound people less exposed to the sunlight that is vital for production of vitamin D in the skin, they are also less efficient at synthesising the precursor substance in their skin, and declining kidney function may also impair their ability to produce the active compound calcitriol from its vitamin D-derived precursor. Holick and Chen (2008) suggest that the capacity to produce vitamin D in the skin may be reduced by as much as 75% in those who are over 70 years. Sunscreens also reduce the production of vitamin D and, if applied properly to all exposed skin, a sunscreen of SPF15 or more may reduce vitamin D production by up to 99%. When levels of solar radiation are low, skin pigmentation also reduces vitamin D production; those people of African descent with the darkest skin may have their capacity to produce vitamin D in the skin reduced by up to 99%.

Vitamin D and osteoporosis

Some, but not all, studies have suggested that supplements of vitamin D and calcium can reduce fracture risk in elderly people. For example, Chapuy et al. (1994) reported that calcium and vitamin D supplements given to elderly institutionalised women in France over a period of three years substantially reduced the risk of fractures, including hip fractures, compared to a placebo. There was biochemical evidence of widespread vitamin D deficiency among these women prior to the supplementation. Dawson-Hughes (2006) summarises trials of oral supplements of vitamin D in elderly people (some also included calcium supplements) and found that there was a considerable reduction of 25–50% in non-vertebral fracture risk in four studies that used 17.5–20 µg/day, whereas those that used lower doses of 7.5–10 µg did not find a significant effect. It should also be noted in the light of the meta-analysis of Avenell et al. (2009), discussed below, that three of the four high-dose trials gave supplemental calcium along with the vitamin D (two involved institutionalised elderly people) and the fourth high-dose study used a monthly oral bolus of vitamin D that averaged out at 20.5 µg/day.

A Finnish study that used annual injections of vitamin D eliminated the problems of patient compliance and poor intestinal absorption and it also achieved a substantial reduction in fracture risk. It is common practice to prescribe supplements of vitamin D and calcium to people who have had a fracture attributed to osteoporosis. However, a large controlled trial (Record Trial Group, 2005) found no indication that either vitamin D or calcium supplements alone or in combination are any more effective than placebos in preventing new fractures in elderly people who have already experienced a low-trauma fracture. This placebo-controlled study involved over 5000 people aged over 70 years (85% female) with a previous occurrence of a low-trauma fracture and the follow-up period was between two and five years.

A very recent Cochrane review (Avenell et al., 2009) of the effects of vitamin D (and some of its analogues) in preventing post-menopausal fractures due to osteoporosis found the following effects from meta-analyses of eligible studies:

- Nine trials (c. 25 000 participants) of vitamin D alone versus a placebo found no statistically significant effect of vitamin D on fracture risk.
- Eight trials (c. 47 000 participants) found that vitamin D plus calcium did significantly reduce hip-fracture risk and the significance of this effect was primarily due to the effect on frail elderly people living in institutions.
- Vitamin D analogues seemed to offer no advantage over vitamin D itself and may increase the risk of adverse effects.

Avenell *et al.* (2009) appear not to have attempted a differential analysis according to dosage and indeed they suggest the need for the effects of dose to be investigated and for ways to ensure patient compliance with the prescribed dosing schedule.

Clinical trials currently completed would thus suggest that vitamin D and calcium supplements of sufficient dose do reduce first fracture risk in elderly people, especially those who are frail and living in institutions for the elderly. There is as yet no evidence that they reduce fracture recurrence in those with established osteoporosis and previous fracture history.

Vitamin D and incidence of non-bone diseases

Some cells that are not obviously involved in calcium homeostasis have receptors for the active metabolite of vitamin D (1,25-hydroxy vitamin D or calcitriol). These include T and B lymphocytes, monocytes, skin cells and many cultured tumour cell lines, including those from some cancers of the breast, colon, lung and prostate. In those cultured tumour cells that have calcitriol receptors, calcitriol has an antiproliferative effect. The presence of calcitriol receptors on cells of the immune system has led to suggestions that it may have a role in regulating immune responses, and thus that poor vitamin D status may be a significant aetiological factor in the development of some autoimmune diseases such as multiple sclerosis and type 1 diabetes. It has also been suggested that calcitriol, which is produced in the kidney, reduces the output of renin from the kidney and this would lead to reduced blood pressure.

Observations such as these have led to numerous claims that vitamin D deficiency may increase the risk of type 1 diabetes, multiple sclerosis, hypertension and certain cancers and, conversely, that vitamin D supplements may help to prevent or perhaps may even be useful in the treatment of some of these conditions. Some of the evidence supporting these suggestions is briefly summarised below:

- The incidence of some cancers, type 1 diabetes, multiple sclerosis and hypertension increases with increasing latitude. This is consistent with the proposal that reduced solar radiation and consequent vitamin D insufficiency may be implicated as a factor in their development.
- There have been several case-control and cohort studies that have reported a reduced risk of several types of cancer in those who have received vitamin D supplements or in those with good biochemical status for the vitamin. A major international report on all aspects of food, nutrition and cancer (WCRF/AICR, 2007) concluded that the evidence is inconsistent, but that there is limited evidence that good vitamin D status protects against colorectal cancer.
- Many studies have reported that either calcitriol or vitamin D itself can reduce the incidence of diabetes in non-obese diabetic (NOD) mice (e.g. van Etten *et al.*, 2002). NOD mice are used as an animal model of type 1 human diabetes, where a high proportion of the mice spontaneously develop autoimmune diabetes during their first year of life.
- Some epidemiological studies suggest an association between poor vitamin D status and the risk of type 1 diabetes. Zipitis and Akobeng (2008) found four

case-control and one cohort study that had assessed the effect of vitamin D supplementation on the risk of developing type 1 diabetes. They concluded from these studies that early childhood vitamin D supplementation may offer protection against the development of type 1 diabetes, but they highlighted the need for large, well-designed trials to test this hypothesis.

- Parker *et al.* (2010) identified 28 studies of various types (100 000 patients) that had investigated the relationship between vitamin D status (by serum 25 OH vitamin D levels) and various cardiometabolic diseases, including cardiovascular disease and diabetes in adults. They found that the highest levels of 25 OH vitamin D in serum were associated with a substantial reduction (about 40%) in cardiometabolic disorders, including cardiovascular diseases, type 2 diabetes and metabolic syndrome. If this association could be shown to be causal, it would suggest that improved vitamin D status in middle-aged and elderly people could lead to a substantial decrease in these conditions.
- Several cross-sectional studies have reported that low vitamin D status is associated with increased risk of hypertension. Forman *et al.* (2008) conducted a prospective case-control study using stored blood samples from middle-aged obese women who did not have hypertension when the samples were collected and frozen. They found that levels of 25 hydroxyvitamin D were significantly lower in 750 of these women who developed hypertension in the subsequent six to eight years than in a matched sample who did not.
- Pilz *et al.* (2009), in an analysis of clinical studies, found that they generally but not consistently favoured the hypothesis that vitamin D sufficiency promoted blood pressure lowering, particularly in vitamin D-deficient hypertensive patients.
- In reviews of the suggested link between vitamin D deficiency and multiple sclerosis (MS) risk, Smolders *et al.* (2008) and Hayes (2000) reported that multiple sclerosis incidence is lower in areas where solar radiation is higher. This seems to be true even where genetically similar populations living in the same country but at different altitudes are compared. Changes of multiple sclerosis rates in migrant populations seem generally to change in directions that are consistent with a protective effect of solar radiation. Most MS patients exhibit long-term vitamin D deficiency, although this could be a consequence of the MS as well as a potential cause. Calcitriol reduces development of symptoms in experimental murine models of multiple sclerosis, which is induced by immunising mice with spinal cord homogenates containing myelin.
- Human epithelia cells have nuclear receptors for calcitriol, which inhibits proliferation and increases differentiation in these cells. Oral supplements of vitamin D have been used in the treatment of psoriasis, but these carry the risk of toxicity and topical application of creams containing less toxic analogues of vitamin D is widely used to treat psoriasis. These are effective enough to have been granted a medicinal licence.

This evidence, while interesting and suggestive, is by no means conclusive about any of these putative links between poor vitamin status and disease risk. It does, however, amplify the case for trying to reduce the prevalence of vitamin D insufficiency in all groups of the population. The fact that insufficiency is widespread and that good status is necessary for good bone health is in itself sufficient justification for this aim. This evidence suggests that broader benefits may result from improved levels of vitamin D sufficiency and that the adverse effects of vitamin D insufficiency are probably not restricted to the skeleton.

Improving the vitamin D status of the population

The vitamin D status of many people of all age groups in the UK, and especially of many institutionalised elderly people, is unsatisfactory. This probably has adverse effects on bone health and the adverse effects may not be restricted to bone. Holick and Chen (2008) suggest that vitamin D deficiency is now recognised as a global pandemic, with prevalence as high as 30–50% in North America, Europe, the Middle East, India, Asia and Australasia. Methods that could be used to address this problem are listed below:

- Trying to increase skin exposure to sunlight by encouraging outdoor activity in children and improving access to sunlight for the elderly. Excessive sunlight exposure, especially where it causes burning, is associated with an increased risk of skin cancer and melanoma and so a difficult balance needs to be struck. Morning or late-afternoon sunlight exposure may be good for vitamin D production and at these times the sunlight is less damaging to skin.
- Targeted supplements of vitamin D (perhaps in combination with calcium).
- The fortification of staple foods(s) with moderate amounts of vitamin D.
- Encouraging the traditional daily moderate dose of cod liver oil in all age groups of the population.

Vitamin D toxicity

Vitamin D is the most acutely toxic of the vitamins. Overdoses of this vitamin lead to an elevated concentration of calcium in blood and urine. This results in the calcification of soft tissues, including the heart and kidneys, and there is an increased risk of kidney stones. The FSA (2003) report found one study suggesting that some cases of hypercalcaemia occurred in elderly people given doses of only 50 µg/day for six months. FSA (2003) estimated that those consuming the highest amounts of the vitamin may obtain more than 9 µg/day from food and that supplements may contain up to a further 12.5 µg/day (i.e. a total maximum of 22 µg/day). They suggested that long-term intakes of up to 25 µg/day should be safe for the general population, but that doses even more than this safe maximum might need to be used under medical supervision in some cases. Holick (2006) suggests that Vitamin D_3 is sensitive to photodegradation, which may help to explain why overexposure to sunlight does not cause vitamin D toxicity.

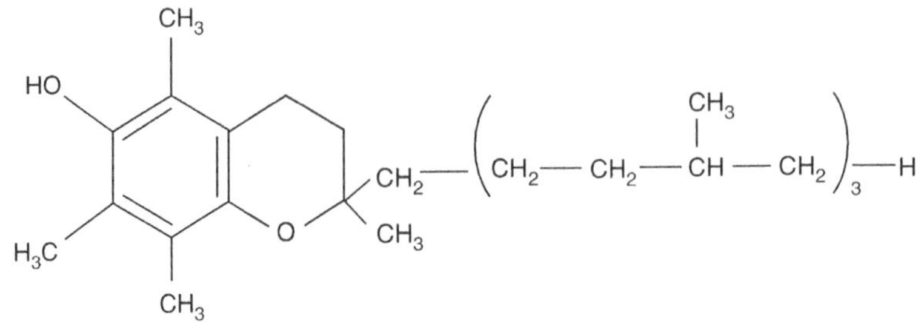

Figure 3.4   The structure of vitamin E (α-tocopherol).

Vitamin E (α-tocopherol)

The structure of alpha-tocopherol is shown in Figure 3.4. Alpha-tocopherol is one of several compounds synthesised by plants that have vitamin E activity. It is found in vegetable oils in concentrations that typically lie within the 10–50 mg/100 g range and is also found in lower concentrations in animal fats. Overt vitamin E deficiency is rarely seen in humans and where it occurs it is usually associated with some medical disorder that impairs fat absorption. COMA (1991) felt that it did not have sufficient data to enable it to set the full set of dietary reference values, so it merely suggested that in men more than 4 mg/day and women more than 3 mg/day should represent a 'safe intake'. In the USA, the RDA set for vitamin E in the 1989 revision of the RDA were 10 mg/day for men and 8 mg/day for women, which has subsequently been raised to 15 mg/day for both men and women. It is ironic given the rarity of overt deficiency that vitamin E-containing supplements are among the most common vitamin supplements (see Table 3.2). Although in most cases supplements make little difference to average vitamin intakes, it was noted in Chapter 2 that supplements of vitamin E raise the average intake of free-living elderly women by over 50%.

Vitamin E is one of the antioxidants and these are discussed as a group in Chapter 5. Its primary function is to prevent the oxidation of polyunsaturated fatty acid residues in membrane phospholipids by oxygen free radicals. Vitamin E protects against atherosclerosis by preventing the oxidation of low-density lipo-protein (LDL), which would make it more damaging to arterial walls. Vitamin E itself is readily oxidised and so can 'soak up' these reactive oxidative species before they interact with other cellular components and produce cellular damage.

Experimental vitamin E deficiency in animals and spontaneous cases of vitamin E deficiency in people result in nerve degeneration, muscular atrophy and retinopathy. In studies in rats, deficiency of vitamin E has been shown to produce sterility and the death and reabsorption of fetuses in pregnant animals.

FSA (2003), in its review of the toxic effects of high doses of vitamins and minerals, discussed two relatively small studies on the toxic effects of vitamin E supplements. These indicate that no apparent biochemical or physiological ill-effects were seen in healthy people who were given the equivalent of 540–970 mg/day of vitamin E. FSA (2003) suggested that prolonged intakes of 500 mg/day of vitamin E should be generally safe; in fact, the data it reviews gives no indication of any general ill-effects at double this intake. One small study did suggest a possible increase in risk of brain haemorrhage in hypertensive smokers with much smaller doses, but this has not been supported by other evidence. There is some evidence from animal studies that high doses of vitamin E may interfere with vitamin K and that this may be a potential problem for patients taking warfarin-type anticoagulants.

Vitamin K (phylloquinone)

The structure of phylloquinone is shown in Figure 3.5. Natural dietary vitamin K_1 (phylloquinone) is of plant origin; intestinal bacteria also produce an alternate form, vitamin K_2 (menaquinone), which is absorbed and contributes to total vitamin K intake. There are also two synthetic water-soluble forms of vitamin K, menadione (K_3) and menadiol (K_4). COMA (1991) set a safe intake for vitamin K intake of 1 µg/kg body weight/day; it felt that there was insufficient data to set a full range of dietary reference values, one uncertainty being the contribution made by the vitamin K produced by the gut flora. In the USA, an RDA of 120 µg/day is set for men and 90 µg/day for women. Green leafy vegetables are the main dietary sources of vitamin K and some vegetable oils like rapeseed oil, soybean oil and olive oil are also good sources of phylloquinone. Vitamin K is not usually used as a single supplement, but is present in many multivitamin supplements at doses of up to 200 µg/day. True dietary deficiency of vitamin K is rarely seen in adults and any deficiency of vitamin K is usually the result of poor absorption as a secondary consequence of some disease process, such as biliary obstruction.

Vitamin K plays an essential role in the production of active prothrombin and several of the other clotting factors. These factors only become functional when certain residues of the amino acid glutamic acid within their primary structure are carboxylated (i.e. the addition of a carboxyl or COOH group). The enzyme responsible for these carboxylations (γ-glutamyl carboxylase) requires vitamin K as a co-factor. Proteins with these carboxylated glutamate residues are referred to as Gla proteins. These Gla proteins bind calcium much more readily than those that have not been carboxylated and calcium binding produces the correct conformation for their biological activity. Proteins that undergo similar carboxylations are also found in other tissues, including bone, although the role of these proteins and the importance of the carboxylation process to their functioning has not been clearly established.

Ball (2004) reviews evidence suggesting that vitamin K plays an important role in bone metabolism and that perhaps vitamin K insufficiency may be a contributory factor in osteoporosis. A brief summary of this evidence is given below, although it must be stressed that these reported associations do not necessarily mean that there is a cause-and-effect relationship. Vitamin K status could, for example, be an indicator of fat-soluble vitamin status generally.

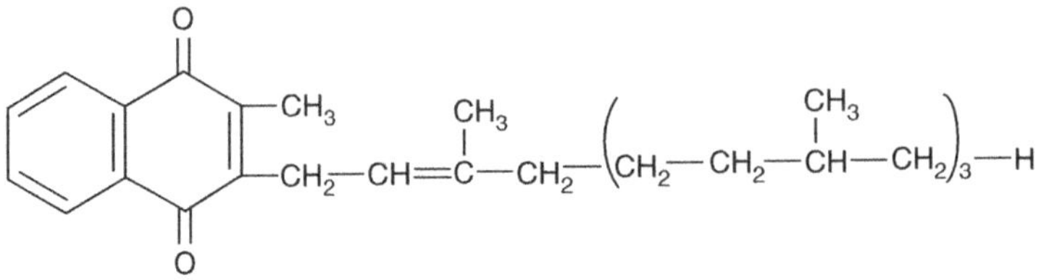

Figure 3.5 The structure of vitamin K (phylloquinone).

- There are three Gla proteins in bone: osteocalcin (which also circulates in blood), matrix Gla protein and protein S. The precise functions of these three proteins are not clearly established.
- On a normal diet, with normal blood clotting, circulating osteocalcin is not fully γ-carboxylated and substantial supplements are required to achieve 100% carboxylation. The clinical significance of this undercarboxylation is not clear.
- In very elderly women, γ-carboxylation of circulating osteocalcin is impaired and high concentrations of undercarboxylated circulating osteocalcin are associated with low bone density at the hip and increased risk of fracture.
- Low vitamin K intakes in women have been associated with increased risk of hip fracture.
- Women in the lowest quartile of vitamin K intakes have been reported to have lower bone density at the hip and spine than those in the highest quartile of intakes.

A Cochrane review of the effectiveness of vitamin K in treating and preventing osteoporosis is currently underway and the protocol of this review has been published (Sangkomamhang *et al.*, 2010), but no data was available when this edition was written.

Newborn babies, especially premature babies, have low biochemical status for vitamin K and this has been linked to the intracranial haemorrhages that occasionally occur shortly after birth and may result in death or permanent disability. It has thus been common practice to give prophylactic vitamin K to newborn babies (especially premature babies) immediately after delivery and this reduces the risk of post-natal brain haemorrhage. Earlier concerns that post-natal injections of vitamin K might be associated with an increased risk of childhood cancer now appear to be unfounded (Eklund *et al.*, 1993). There is no evidence that vitamin K given to pregnant women has any beneficial effects for premature babies (Crowther *et al.*, 2010).

There is little evidence of natural vitamin K_1 toxicity in humans or in experimental animal studies. High doses of the synthetic forms do cause adverse effects in animals and humans and have some mutagenic activity in bacteria. FSA (2003) considered it undesirable to use these synthetic forms in dietary supplements. The EU Food Supplements Directive gives phylloquinone and menaquinone as the only permitted forms of vitamin K and so these alternate synthetic forms cannot now be used in vitamin supplements. Supplements in the UK may provide up to 200 μg/day

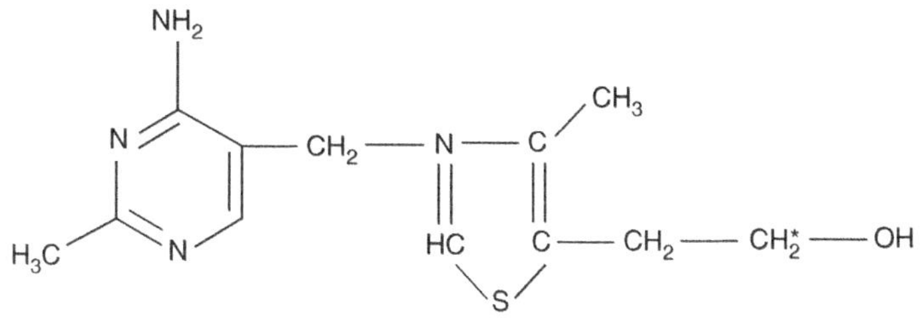

Figure 3.6   The structure of thiamine (vitamin B₁).

of vitamin K to go along with the average of around 70 μg/day obtained from food. On the basis of very little data, FSA (2003) considered that supplements containing up to 1 mg/day of natural vitamin K_1 are unlikely to produce any adverse effects. Note that coumarin anticoagulant drugs such as warfarin work by antagonising the effects of vitamin K and so large doses of vitamin K will interfere with this therapy.

The water-soluble vitamins

Vitamin B₁ (thiamin)

The chemical structure of thiamin is shown in Figure 3.6. Thiamin is one of the vitamins that comprise the so-called B complex. It was originally thought that yeast extract contained a single essential 'accessory food factor' or vitamin, which was designated vitamin B. As it became clear that vitamin B was in fact made up of several essential vitamins, so the term B complex was used and the individual compounds that make up this mixture designated B_1, B_2, B_3 and so on. Each of these is a vitamin in its own right.

One of the main functions of thiamin is in energy metabolism and the metabolism of carbohydrate has a greater thiamin requirement than that of fat. The requirement for thiamin is related to the rate of energy metabolism and so COMA (1991) set the RNI for thiamin for all groups except very young children at 0.4 mg/1000 kcal. This translates to 1 mg/day for men consuming the energy EAR and 0.8 mg/day for women; corresponding American RDA are 1.2 mg/day for men and 1.1 mg/day for women. COMA (1991) suggested that even those consuming very low-calorie diets should not have thiamin intakes of less than 0.4 mg/day.

Thiamin is present in the bran and germ layers of whole-grain cereals and is also found in pulses, vegetables, milk, offal and pork and added to many breakfast cereals. It is mandatory in the UK and the USA to fortify white flour with added thiamin; that is, to add back what is removed during the milling process and removal of the bran and germ layers of the wheat grain. Rice, even whole-grain rice, is relatively low in thiamin and white or polished rice is particularly low in this vitamin. This means that diets where most of the calories are derived from white rice are likely to be deficient in thiamin.

Thiamin can be converted to thiamin pyrophosphate and this is an important co-factor for several key enzymes:

- Pyruvic oxidase, the enzyme that converts pyruvic acid to acetyl co-enzyme A, a reaction that is essential to allow the aerobic metabolism of carbohydrate.
- α-Ketoglutaric acid oxidase, an enzyme of the tricarboxylic acid (Krebs) cycle where the acetyl co-enzyme A produced from all substrates undergoes oxidative metabolism to produce most cellular energy.
- Transketolase, an enzyme of the pentose phosphate pathway that generates $NADPH_2$ for fat synthesis and/or ribose for nucleic acid synthesis.

Thiamin deficiency results in a functional block in the oxidative metabolism of carbohydrate and a consequential rise in blood levels of pyruvic acid and lactic acid from the anaerobic metabolism of carbohydrate. Thiamin deficiency leads to a potentially fatal disease called beriberi that was, until a few decades ago, very prevalent among some of the populations of the Far East where white rice was the dominant staple. The symptoms of beriberi include:

- Acidosis due to build-up of lactic acid.
- Peripheral neuropathy, a degeneration of peripheral nerves that starts with a loss of sensory function, then degeneration of motor nerves and eventually wasting of muscles that lose their nerve supply. This starts with a tingling sensation at the extremities and leads ultimately to progressive paralysis (if this is the major feature it is called dry beriberi).
- Oedema and heart failure (where this occurs it is called wet beriberi).

Wernicke-Korsakoff syndrome is the name given to a myriad of neurological symptoms that result from thiamin deficiency. It is prevalent among alcoholics in affluent countries and is an important and sometimes overlooked cause of dementia-like symptoms. There is progressive demyelination and necrosis of parts of the brain, which results in abnormal eye movements, difficulty with standing and walking, loss of existing memories and an inability to make new memories as well as other neurological disturbances. Alcoholics are generally prone to deficiency of micronutrients because of their often low food intake and the poor quality of their diet. However, high alcohol intake may increase the requirement for thiamin, impair its absorption and decrease the activity of the enzyme that converts thiamin to its active form (thiamin pyrophosphate). Thiamin deficiency and Wernicke-Korsakoff syndrome seem to be a particular problem associated with alcoholism. Thiamin deficiency may also contribute to a condition called fetal alcohol syndrome, in which babies born to alcoholic mothers are small with characteristic facial abnormalities, are often mentally retarded, immunodeficient and show poor postnatal growth.

It may well be that supplemental doses of thiamin could reduce the risk of these manifestations of thiamin deficiency in high alcohol consumers. There does seem to be a theoretical case for recommending thiamin supplements for those who

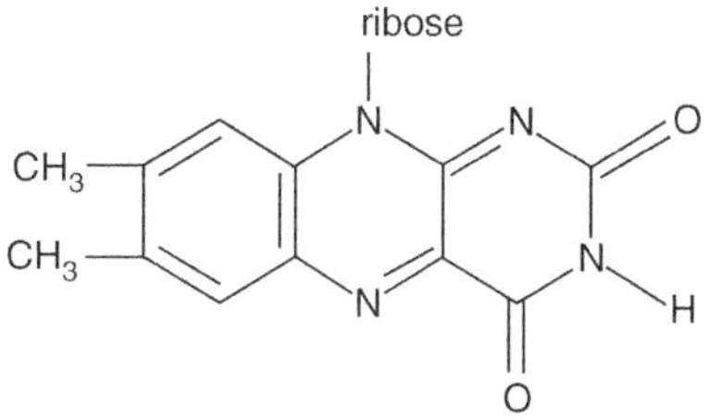

ribose

Figure 3.7 The structure of riboflavin (vitamin B$_2$).

cannot be persuaded to reduce their alcohol consumption. Of course, high alcohol consumption has many harmful effects over and above those due to thiamin deficiency and focusing on this problem may well divert attention from the primary cause of the problem – alcohol abuse. It is strongly advised that women either avoid alcohol completely during pregnancy or confine themselves to small, occasional amounts.

Thiamin is a component of many multinutrient supplements, where it would normally provide 1–5 mg/day; thiamin-only supplements are available and these may provide up to 300 mg/day. FSA (2003) concluded from an analysis of available data that daily supplemental doses of 100 mg of thiamin should be safe, although amounts well in excess of this may well be without hazard and there is always the possibility of individual idiosyncratic reactions.

Vitamin B$_2$ (riboflavin)

The structure of riboflavin is shown in Figure 3.7. COMA (1991) set the adult RNI for riboflavin at 1.3 mg/day for men and 1.1 mg/day for women; corresponding American RDA are the same as the UK RNI. Riboflavin is widely distributed in foods, with dairy products, meat, fish, eggs, liver and some green vegetables being good dietary sources. Prolonged exposure to light (e.g. milk left on a doorstep) destroys riboflavin, as does heating in alkaline solution (e.g. by adding bicarbonate of soda when boiling vegetables). If high doses of riboflavin are consumed then it is excreted unchanged in the urine, which reduces the potential for toxicity. Riboflavin is a permitted (yellow) colouring agent for foods or pharmaceuticals, but because of its light sensitivity is used relatively infrequently for this purpose. High intakes of riboflavin may lead to a harmless yellow discolouration of the urine.

Riboflavin is the precursor of flavin nucleotides FMN (flavin mononucleotide) and FAD (flavin adenine dinucleotide), which are prosthetic groups essential for the functioning of several enzymes involved in the oxidative reactions that produce cellular energy. A riboflavin derivative is also necessary for the functioning of one of the key enzymes involved in the quenching of oxidative free radicals (glutathione reductase).

Mild riboflavin deficiency is relatively common, but a major deficiency syndrome has not been described for this vitamin. It was noted in Chapter 2 that significant

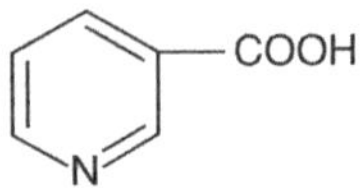

Figure 3.8 The structure of niacin (nicotinic acid).

numbers of adults, children and elderly people were found to have apparently inadequate riboflavin intakes and in some cases there was biochemical evidence of poor riboflavin status. There is no clearly defined riboflavin deficiency disease, but symptoms of riboflavin deficiency that have been described in volunteers deprived of riboflavin include skin lesions, various lesions in and around the mouth and anaemia.

Average daily intakes of riboflavin in the UK are around 1.8 mg/day, with top consumers taking in around double this amount. Additionally, multinutrient supplements may contain as much as 100 mg/day of riboflavin. FSA (2003) suggests that supplemental intakes of around 40 mg/day are unlikely to produce any harmful effects, but it had insufficient data to set a safe upper maximum and it may well be that doses well in excess of this level produce no adverse effects. There is little evidence of riboflavin having toxic effects in humans. At low intakes riboflavin is very efficiently absorbed, but this active absorption process has a limited capacity and absorption is less efficient when large amounts are taken in.

Vitamin B$_3$ (niacin)

The structure of nicotinic acid is shown in Figure 3.8. The term niacin covers nicotinic acid, its amide nicotinamide and the co-enzyme forms of this vitamin present in plant and animal tissues (NAD and NADP). The adult RNI for niacin is 17 mg of niacin equivalents (NE)/day for men and 13 mg NE/day for women; the corresponding American RDA are 16 mg/day and 14 mg/day respectively. Niacin can be obtained from the diet in the forms noted above or it can be synthesised in the body from the essential amino acid tryptophan. When calculating the total niacin content of a food or diet, it is assumed that 60 mg of tryptophan is equivalent to 1 mg of niacin, so:

$$1 \text{ mg niacin equivalents (NE)} = 1 \text{ mg niacin or } 60 \text{ mg tryptophan}$$

Around 1% of the dietary protein in typical British and American diets would be tryptophan. There is therefore some validity to early suggestions that the niacin deficiency disease pellagra was a manifestation of protein deficiency. High protein foods alleviate pellagra because they supply tryptophan, which acts as a source of niacin. Pre-formed niacin is found in red meat, liver, pulses, eggs, milk and wholegrain wheat flour and is added to many breakfast cereals. It is mandatory in both the UK and the USA to add niacin to white flour.

Niacin is a component of the important co-enzymes NAD (nicotinamide adenine dinucleotide) and the phosphorylated form NADP. These co-enzymes are essential for many enzyme reactions involved in oxidation/reduction reactions. NAD 'accepts' hydrogen in many oxidation reactions of metabolism to become $NADH_2$ and it is the reoxidation of $NADH_2$ in oxidative phosphorylation that is responsible for producing most of the ATP in the oxidative metabolism of food. $NADPH_2$ is an important hydrogen 'donor' in many reduction reactions of synthetic processes, for example in fatty acid and steroid synthesis.

Pellagra is a potentially fatal disease that results from niacin deficiency. It is characterised by symptoms referred to as the 3Ds – dermatitis, diarrhoea and dementia – and ultimately the fourth D, death. Epidemics of pellagra have usually been associated with poor populations subsisting on a diet based on maize. Maize protein is low in tryptophan and the niacin present is in a bound from that cannot be absorbed. Note that this bound niacin is released when maize is heated under alkaline conditions, as in traditional tortilla production among Central American Indians where maize originated. In some parts of India and China pellagra has been associated with sorghum-based diets. Primary deficiency of niacin rarely occurs in industrialised countries, although alcoholics may have poor niacin status.

Some multivitamin preparations contain up to 100 mg/day of nicotinic acid, but most contain nicotinamide at doses of up to 150 mg/day in multivitamins and as much as 250 mg/day in single preparations of the vitamin. Average intakes from food are around 30 mg/day in the UK (from tryptophan as well as pre-formed niacin), with the highest consumers receiving as much as double this amount.

High doses of nicotinic acid have been used successfully to reduce high plasma cholesterol and to reduce coronary heart disease mortality. Some symptoms of toxicity have been reported when it has been used for this purpose, such as flushing, itching, nausea and vomiting. Other more serious symptoms have been reported when very high doses have been consumed for extended periods (more than 100 times the RNI).

Flushing has been reported to occur with doses of nicotinic acid as low as 50 mg/ day when it is taken as a single dose. FSA (2003) suggests that daily doses of nicotinamide of up to 500 mg/day would not be expected to have any adverse effects.

Vitamin B_6 (pyridoxine)

The structures of the three major forms of vitamin B_6 are shown in Figure 3.9. Vitamin B_6 is a generic term that covers three biologically active and interconvertible substances found in food, namely pyridoxine, pyridoxal and pyridoxamine as well as their phosphorylated derivatives (note that the only forms of B_6 permitted by the EU Food Supplements Directive are pyridoxine hydrochloride and pyridoxine phosphate). This vitamin is widely distributed in animal and plant foods, for example in liver, eggs, meat, fish, green leafy vegetables, pulses, fruits and whole-grain cereals. Some glycosides of vitamin B_6 found in plant foods have very little biological activity in humans. The adult RNI for vitamin B_6 is 1.4 mg/day for men and 1.2 mg/day for women; corresponding American RDA are 1.3 mg/day for both men and women. Pyridoxine is present in many food supplements and multivitamin

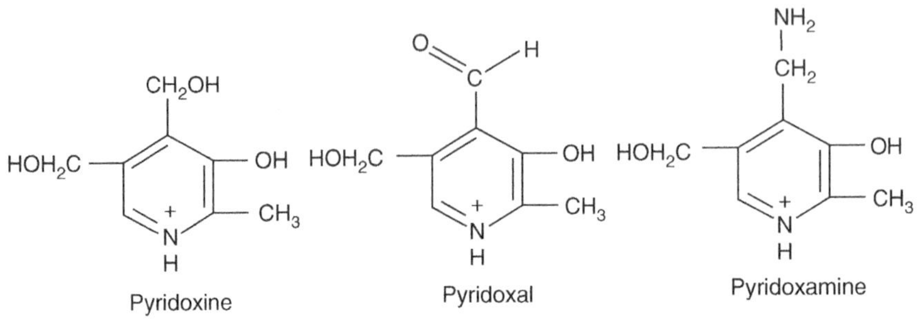

Figure 3.9   The structure of the three forms of vitamin B$_6$.

preparations generally at doses of up to 10 mg/day, but some supplements and single-vitamin preparations may contain as much as 100 mg/day.

The substances that comprise vitamin B$_6$ are the precursors of pyridoxal phosphate, a co-enzyme that is important for a number of important enzymes, including those involved in the following:

- The transfer of amino groups from one amino acid to make another (transamination).
- The decarboxylation of amino acids and the production of several important nerve transmitters such as dopamine, serotonin (5HT), histamine and GABA (gamma amino butyric acid).
- The conversion of the amino acid tryptophan to niacin.
- The breakdown of glycogen.
- The synthesis of haem.

It is because of its role in the production of nerve transmitters and so in the functioning of the nervous system that it has been suggested that vitamin B$_6$ might have the potential to affect mood and it has been widely used for the treatment of pre-menstrual tension. This is the single most important motivation for taking supplements that are specifically marketed as being high in vitamin B$_6$. Most women of reproductive age report that they experience some adverse symptoms in the period prior to the onset of menstruation. The physical symptoms of this pre-menstrual syndrome include bloating, weight gain, breast tenderness, abdominal discomfort, lethargy and headache, while the psychological symptoms include anxiety, irritability, aggression and loss of control. In up to 5% of women in this age group the symptoms can be severe enough to markedly disrupt everyday life.

In a systematic review of randomised and placebo-controlled trials of vitamin B$_6$ in the treatment of pre-menstrual syndrome, Wyatt *et al.* (1999) found some limited evidence to support the view that at daily doses of 100 mg (and perhaps 50 mg), vitamin B$_6$ had some benefits on both the physical and psychological symptoms of this syndrome. The effects did not appear to be dose dependent and so the trials reported up to this point did not support the use of doses greater than 100 mg/day.

These authors did note that the general size and quality of the studies that they reviewed did not allow them to draw definite conclusions and highlighted the need for a large, high-quality study to be undertaken. Pyridoxine is one of a number of treatments used to help control morning sickness in early pregnancy and, according to Jewell and Young (2003), there is some evidence that it reduces the severity of nausea but does not reduce frequency of vomiting. However, this conclusion was based on the results of only two controlled trials of pyridoxine.

A more restricted use of vitamin B_6 supplements has been for the treatment of carpal tunnel syndrome, which produces pain, tingling, numbness in the fingers and thumb and loss of grip strength. It is due to compression of the median nerve in the 'carpal tunnel', a narrow space at the front of the wrist through which the tendons that control the fingers and thumb also pass. Anything that causes swelling or inflammation in this region can lead to nerve compression, for example arthritis, fluid retention, mechanical injury or repetitive strain injury, or hormonal imbalances and changes, including those of pregnancy. According to Viera (2003), up to 3% of Americans may suffer from this condition. It is treated by using anti-inflammatory drugs, wrist splints, diuretics or, if the symptoms are severe and prolonged, by minor surgery. Viera (2003) references several randomised controlled trials indicating that vitamin B_6 is no more effective than a placebo in treating this syndrome and a systematic review comes to the same conclusion (Gerritson et al., 2002)

Overt deficiency of B_6 is rare in humans. In the 1950s a fault in the processing of some infant formula in the USA led to some infants being fed B_6-depleted formula. These infants exhibited weakness, irritability, weight loss and insomnia. Adult volunteers who have been made deliberately B_6 deficient become depressed and irritable, have cracked lips and tongue and some other dermatological symptoms.

It has been suggested that women taking oral contraceptives may have an increased requirement for B_6. Certain drugs such as isoniazid, used in the treatment of TB, may increase the requirement for B_6 and supplements are usually given when these drugs are used. Supplements of B_6 interfere with the actions of L-Dopa, used in the treatment of Parkinson's disease, probably by increasing its peripheral conversion to dopamine; pyridoxal phosphate is a co-factor for the decarboxylase enzyme that converts dopa to dopamine.

FSA (2003) suggests that average UK intakes of B_6 from the diet are around 2 mg/day, with the highest consumers taking in around double this amount. At the extremes some supplements may provide as much as 100 mg/day, although most provide up to 10 mg/day. In animal studies, it has been shown that B_6 has the potential to be neurotoxic. Very high doses cause abnormalities of gait and balance and can produce permanent, histologically verified peripheral nerve damage. Largely on the basis of animal studies, FSA (2003) suggested that a lifetime dose of 10 mg/day should have no harmful effects. It was unable to judge the risk posed to humans of taking up to 200 mg/day. It suggested that while this might well be negligible in the short term, it did not have sufficient data to offer that assurance. There are several reports of people developing sensory neuropathy, manifested initially by a tingling sensation in the hands and feet, when taking large supplemental doses of B_6 (FSA, 2003).

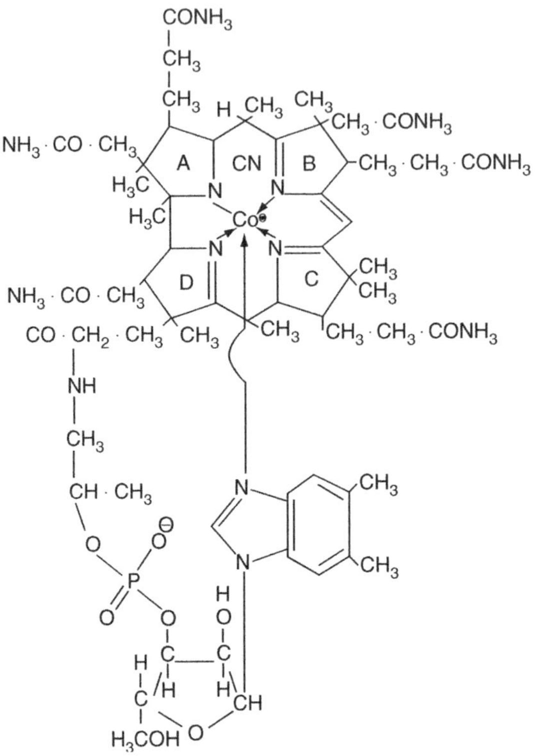

Figure 3.10   The structure of cyanocobalamin (vitamin B$_{12}$).

Vitamin B$_{12}$ (cobalamins)

The structure of cyanocobalamin is shown in Figure 3.10. Vitamin B$_{12}$ is comprised of several complex, cobalt-containing compounds that are present in animal foods. The synthetic compound cyanocobalamin is widely used in vitamin supplements and so less frequently is hydroxocobalamin; these two forms are the only ones on the permitted list of the EU Food Supplements Directive. The vitamin is initially synthesised in micro-organisms (bacteria, fungi and algae) and is present in meat (especially offal), fish, eggs and milk. Plant tissue contains no B$_{12}$ *per se*, but anything that is contaminated with micro-organisms, such as mould, will contain B$_{12}$ and so will the root nodules of some legumes where it is synthesised by the bacteria they contain. A strict vegetarian or vegan diet will theoretically contain no B$_{12}$, although contamination by micro-organisms, insect remains or faecal matter will provide some. Healthy, young omnivorous adults will have several years supply of vitamin B$_{12}$ stored in their livers.

The adult RNI for vitamin B$_{12}$ is extremely small at 1.5 µg/day; the American RDA is 2.4 µg/day. This means that even the amounts present in contaminants of food, coupled with some contribution from intestinal bacteria, may be sufficient to prevent overt symptoms of deficiency in people whose diet theoretically does not contain any of the vitamin. Algal preparations like spirulina and chlorella are often marketed as sources of vitamin B_{12} that are suitable for strict vegetarians (see Chapter 8); the B_{12} in spirulina is almost certainly not biologically active in humans.

Vitamin B_{12} and folic acid are essential for synthesis of the nucleotide thymidylate, which is a component of DNA. This means that deficiency of either of these vitamins interferes with normal cell division and this leads to a megaloblastic anaemia, in which large, unstable red cells enter the circulation – this ultimately causes a severe and potentially fatal anaemia. B_{12} is also a co-factor for the enzyme that converts methyl malonyl CoA to succinyl CoA in the metabolism of fatty acids with odd numbers of carbon atoms and in the metabolism of certain amino acids.

Apart from the megaloblastic anaemia, prolonged B_{12} deficiency causes irreversible damage to the spinal cord due to demyelination: combined subacute degeneration of the spinal cord. This initially manifests as tingling of the fingers and toes, but can lead to progressive paralysis and eventually to neuropsychiatric symptoms if the demyelination progresses to areas of the brain. One explanation for these neurological changes is that vitamin B_{12} deficiency impairs the production of s-adenosyl methionine, which in turn reduces myelin production (see Chapter 7 for a discussion of s-adenosyl methionine).

At levels of intake from food sources, absorption of B_{12} requires the presence of intrinsic factor produced in the parietal cells of the stomach. This absorption system becomes saturated at high intakes, say greater than 2 µg in a single meal/dose. A small proportion (c. 1%) of the ingested vitamin can be absorbed by simple diffusion and so when large pharmacological doses are consumed the amount absorbed by this route may be sufficient to meet physiological needs.

B_{12} deficiency is rare in younger people; strict vegans and some Asian lactovegetarians who only consume milk depleted of B_{12} by boiling with tea are at potential risk. Most cases of deficiency arise because of impaired absorption of the vitamin due to a lack of intrinsic factor, a condition called pernicious anaemia. This can be congenital or acquired and becomes more common in elderly people. True dietary deficiency of B_{12} would be treated by oral supplements, whereas when symptoms arise because of severely impaired absorption it is treated by regular injection of the vitamin. Note that the original treatment for pernicious anaemia was to feed sufferers doses of raw liver that were very rich in the vitamin and enough was absorbed by diffusion to alleviate the symptoms. Partly because of the neurological roles of B_{12} and the neurological consequences of deficiency, vitamin B_{12} supplements have been suggested as possibly beneficial for elderly people with low serum levels of B_{12} and cognitive impairment or dementia. Malouf and Sastre (2003) found that the limited studies to date provide no suggestion that any significant benefit results in cognitive function from using these supplements.

Average UK intakes of B_{12} from food are around 6 µg/day, with the highest consumers taking in more than 20 µg/day. Supplements may provide up to 3 mg/day. The vitamin is water soluble, high oral intakes are poorly absorbed and excessive amounts in blood are excreted in urine. This means that oral supplements have low potential for toxicity and long-term consumption of 2mg/day should not produce any adverse effects (FSA, 2003).

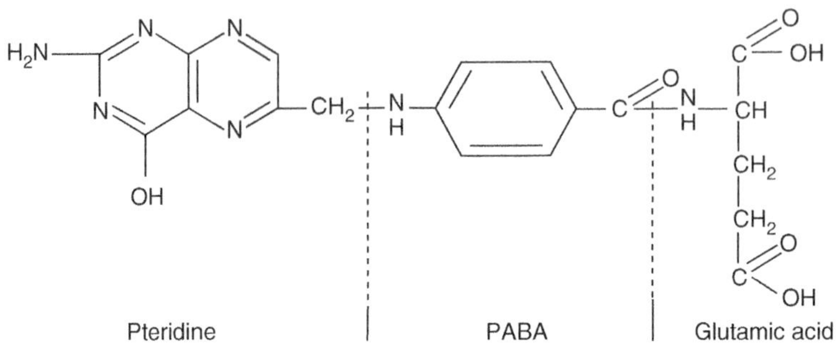

Figure 3.11   The structure of folic acid.

Folic acid (folate, folacin)

Folate is a collective term that covers several derivatives of the parent compound folic acid (pteroylmonoglutamic acid), whose structure is shown in Figure 3.11. Folic acid itself is not present in food but it is the form of the vitamin that has usually been used in supplements and food fortification. Folate is present in most natural foods: green vegetables, liver, yeast extract, mushrooms, nuts and whole grains are good sources. In food the pteridine ring of folic acid is usually reduced to dihydrofolate or tetrahydofolate and there are various single-carbon units that can be attached to the nitrogens of this ring. In food, most folate is present as polyglutamates with five to seven glutamic acid residues attached. Details of the different structures of folate compounds may be found in Ball (2004). Very controversially, the only form of folate that is permitted by the original EU Food Supplements Directive was folic acid itself, rather than the forms more usually found in food (in 2009 calcium L-methylfolate was also added as an alternative permitted form of folate).

The RNI for folate is 200 μg/day for men and women; the RDA in the USA is 400 μg/day for both men and women. It is also recommended in the UK that women of child-bearing age should take an additional supplemental dose of 400 μg/day if there is any chance that they might become pregnant. Women who are pregnant or are planning a pregnancy are strongly recommended to take this supplemental dose of folic acid. Folic acid is present in many multivitamin preparations and is also available as a single-vitamin preparation at daily doses of up to 800 μg/day. Preparations providing up to 5 mg/day may be prescribed to women known to be at high risk of having a baby affected by a neural tube defect (anencephaly or spina bifida), for example because of a previously affected pregnancy.

Folic acid is involved in biochemical reactions that involve the transfer of methyl groups. It interacts with vitamin B_{12} in the methyl transfer reactions that are involved in the synthesis of DNA and are essential for proper cell division. Rapidly dividing cells in the bone marrow are thus some of the first to be affected by deficiency and, as with vitamin B_{12} deficiency, this manifests as a megaloblastic anaemia, characterised by large, unstable and immature red cells being released into the circulation. Very high doses of folic acid will mask the haematological consequences of B_{12} deficiency, but will not prevent its neurological consequences. It is thus important that B_{12} deficiency is excluded before folic acid therapy is used to treat megaloblastic anaemia.

Some degree of folate deficiency is relatively common among people subsisting on a low-folate starchy staple with few green vegetables or other foods that might provide folate. Some drugs increase folate requirement (some anti-epileptics) and alcoholics often have poor folate status. As noted in Chapter 2, folate insufficiency is widespread in the UK, with 4–5% of young and middle-aged adults and 30–40% of elderly people showing biochemical evidence of marginal or poor folate status and 16% of institutionalised elderly people showing evidence of severe deficiency; young adults (19–24 years) also showed high incidence of marginal folate status (13% for men and 8% for women).

Folic acid in pregnancy

There is now very persuasive evidence that consumption of folic acid supplements by women immediately prior to conception and in the first 12 weeks of the pregnancy greatly reduces the risk of the baby developing a neural tube defect (NTD). The term 'neural tube defect' covers several developmental defects in which the brain, spinal cord, skull and/or vertebral column fail to develop normally. In some cases, there is almost complete failure of brain and skull development (anencephaly) and these babies die before or shortly after birth. Spina bifida is a failure of the spinal canal to close and so the spinal cord bulges out of the back. Children born with spina bifida suffer from a range of physical disabilities such as paralysis and incontinence, and may have neurological damage caused by a build-up of cerebrospinal fluid around the brain (hydrocephalus). About 1:250 UK pregnancies are affected by these conditions and about 1:4000 babies are born with an NTD; many affected foetuses are detected by pre-natal screening and aborted.

Studies dating back to the 1960s have suggested a link between folate insufficiency and the occurrence of NTD (see Department of Health, 1992 for details and references to these early studies). MRC (1991) reported the results of a double-blind trial using over 2000 women with a previously affected pregnancy that was set up specifically to test whether large peri-conceptual doses of folic acid reduced the recurrence rate of this condition. Women with a previous history of an affected pregnancy are 10 times more likely to have another affected pregnancy than the general female population. Half of these women took 4 mg/day of folic acid (with or without other vitamins) when they were planning to conceive and in the first three months after conception. There was a 72% lower recurrence in women taking folic acid than in those who did not take it; other supplemental vitamins had no measurable effect. Subsequent studies (e.g. Czeizel and Dudas, 1992) have shown that lower doses of folic acid (800 µg/day in this 1992 study) reduced first occurrence of NTD in women with no previous history of an affected pregnancy.

It is not thought that folate insufficiency *per se* is a major cause of NTD. One suggestion for the effect of folic acid is that some women have a genetically determined variation in the enzyme methionine synthase, which reduces its activity. Methionine synthase is a folate-requiring enzyme and it thought that the supplemental folic acid helps to ameliorate the effect of this low enzyme activity (Eskes, 1998).

There now seems to be a general acceptance that increased peri-conceptual intake of folic acid reduces the incidence of NTD. In a review of experience in Hungary of using supplements containing 800 µg of folic acid, it was found that the rate of primary NTD fell by up to 90% (Czeizel, 2009). Furthermore, there is increasing evidence that folic acid supplements may also reduce the incidence of other birth defects. Czeizel (2009) suggested that incidence of other congenital defects had decreased significantly in Hungarian women receiving large folic acid supplements, especially congenital defects of the heart and urinary tract. A large case-control study of Norwegian women concluded that folic acid supplements in early pregnancy reduced the incidence of cleft lip by around a third. In the Canadian province of Quebec, there was a significant and sustained decrease in the incidence of severe congenital heart defects in the years immediately after fortification of flour and pasta with folic acid was made mandatory (Ionescu-Ittu et al., 2009).

In 1992, an expert advisory group in the UK (DH, 1992) advised that women who were planning to become pregnant should take 400 µg/day folic acid before becoming pregnant and during the first 12 weeks of pregnancy. High-risk women who had already experienced an affected pregnancy were advised to take a much higher dose (5 mg/day). The current advice is that all women of child-bearing age in the UK should take supplements of 400 µg/day of folic acid if there is any chance that they might become pregnant. This is because many pregnancies are unplanned and folic acid is most effective when taken prior to conception or very early in the pregnancy. However, over 85% of women of child-bearing age fail to take in this much, even when supplement and food intakes are combined. More than a decade ago an expert group (COMA, 2000) recommended that all flour in the UK should be supplemented with 240 µg/100g of folic acid. Although many breakfast cereals and some bread are voluntarily supplemented with folic acid, at the time of writing (2010) this recommendation has still to be implemented in the UK, although it has been in the USA, Canada and about fifty other countries.

An international study (Botto et al., 2005) strongly suggests that widespread food fortification with folic acid may be necessary to achieve measurable reductions in the incidence of NTD. An analysis of the incidence of these defects in several European countries and Israel between 1988 and 1998 found that recommendations to take peri-conceptual supplements of folic acid had had no discernible effect on the incidence of this group of birth defects. This is despite the fact that these recommendations have been in existence for some years in some of the surveyed countries, for example since 1992 in England and Wales and since 1993 in Ireland. In contrast to this lack of impact of supplements, in the comparatively small number of countries where fortification with folic acid had then been introduced there had been highly significant falls in the incidence of these birth defects (see below). This may exemplify a general weakness of any health promotion programme that relies on use of supplements, because as we have already seen there is substantial evidence that supplements tend to be taken by those who need them least; that is, those with the highest nutrient intakes from food.

- In the USA, fortification of enriched cereal products with folic acid became mandatory in January 1998. Incidence of NTD in the period October 1998–December 1999 was 19% lower than in the period October 1995–December 1996 (Honein *et al.*, 2001).
- In Canada, most cereal grain products have been fortified with folic acid since January 1998. The resultant estimated increase in folic acid of 100–200 µg/day was associated with an approximate halving of the incidence of neural tube defects in the province of Ontario in the period after fortification was introduced (Ray *et al.*, 2002).
- In Chile, NTD incidence dropped by 31% after the fortification of flour began and it reached the $P < 0.001$ level of significance in the twentieth month after fortification began (Castilla *et al.*, 2003).

Possible wider benefits of folic acid fortification

Food fortification should reduce the prevalence of folate deficiency in the UK, especially among elderly people. Experience from the USA found that following mandatory fortification of flour with 140 µg/100 g flour, there was an approximate twofold increase in adult plasma folate levels. This rise in folate levels was higher than predicted and this is probably the result of substantial overfortification by food manufacturers to ensure that their product contained the mandatory minimum amounts (see Mason *et al.*, 2007).

Observational studies have suggested that a folate-rich diet is associated with a reduced risk of several cancers, including bowel cancer. WCRF/AICR (2007) assessed this evidence and confirmed that the epidemiological evidence was indeed suggestive of an association between high folate intake from food and reduced risk of developing colorectal cancer, although they noted the difficulty of completely excluding the confounding effects of, for example, high dietary fibre intake. Their conclusion was that there is limited evidence to suggest that foods containing folate protect against colorectal cancer and, on the basis of much less available evidence, made similar conclusions for pancreatic and oesophageal cancer. As noted earlier, folate is involved in methylation reactions in DNA synthesis, including the formation of the pyrimidine base thymine, which is found only in DNA. In folate deficiency, there may be incorporation of the RNA base uracil into DNA in place of thymine and other abnormalities of methylation, which if not repaired may lead to cancerous changes in cells (see Mathers, 2009).

Homocysteine is a sulphur-containing amino acid that is an intermediate in the conversion of methionine to cysteine. It is not present in the diet in significant amounts as it is not incorporated into protein. In the inherited condition homocystinuria, there is an increased accumulation of homocysteine in blood, which predisposes these individuals to premature heart disease. Excess homocysteine is toxic to vascular endothelial cells, promotes LDL oxidation and increases the risk of thrombosis (COMA, 1994). Folate deficiency can lead to more moderate elevation of blood homocysteine levels, as a folate-derived co-factor is involved in the conversion of homocysteine to methionine (see Ball, 2004). Both case-control and cohort studies show that an elevated blood homocysteine level and low folate intake are associated with increased risk of diseases linked to atherosclerosis. The suggestion is therefore that folic acid supplements may help to protect against cardiovascular disease by lowering levels of homocysteine. Despite this observational evidence, there is as yet no supporting evidence from several large clinical trials that folic acid supplementation reduces all-cause mortality or cardiovascular events in people with or without existing cardiovascular disease (Bazzano *et al.*, 2007; Marti-Carvajal *et al.*, 2009).

There have been suggestions from epidemiological studies that high folate intake may be protective against Alzheimer's disease and that raised blood homocysteine levels may be associated with increased risk. In a 10-year study of almost 600 elderly people in Baltimore, Corrada *et al.* (2005) suggested that a high total folate intake from food or supplements was associated with a significantly decreased risk of developing Alzheimer's disease. Malouf and Grimley Evans (2008), in an update of an earlier (2003) systematic review, found that there is as yet no evidence from controlled trials that folic acid supplements (with or without vitamin B_{12}) had any preventive or beneficial effects on the course of dementia in elderly people. However, they found some preliminary evidence that folic acid supplements might enhance the response to some drug treatments and that folic acid supplements might improve cognitive function in elderly people with raised homocysteine levels.

Potential hazards of folic acid fortification of food

There has been considerable debate about whether the relatively small numbers of definite beneficiaries justifies the supplementation of everyone's food with folic acid, especially as it is know that there are some who might be theoretically at risk from large supplemental doses of this vitamin.

Those people who might be at increased risk from high folate intakes are:

- People (especially elderly people) at risk of vitamin B_{12} deficiency, because a high intake would mask the haematological effects but not stop the neurological consequences of B_{12} deficiency.
- People taking drugs that work by interfering with folate metabolism, because a high intake might reduce the effectiveness of their therapy.
- There is also a more recent suggestion that folic acid might stimulate the growth of bowel adenomas, increase their recurrence in people treated for this condition and stimulate the development of benign adenomas into malignant tumours (reviewed by Mathers, 2009).

The first two possibilities were taken into account by FSA (2003) when it concluded that an intake of 1500 µg/day of folic acid would not be expected to have any adverse effects. According to Carmel (2006), most cases of neurological deterioration as a result of folic acid supplements in misdiagnosed vitamin B_{12} deficiency have occurred with daily doses of more than 5 mg of folic acid. These figures should be considered in the light of current average intakes of less than 250 μg/day in free-living elderly people, with even lower intakes in those living in institutions.

Recent concerns about a possible link between folic acid and bowel cancer risk have been triggered by a report that a small rise in colorectal cancer rates occurred in the USA and Canada at around the time that folic acid fortification of flour became widespread (Mason et al., 2007). These authors show evidence that prior to fortification rates of colorectal cancer had been falling steadily in both countries, but at the time of fortification a small rise in rates occurred, which peaked in 1998 in the USA and 2000 in Canada. After this 'blip' the incidence continued to decline at the previous rate, but remained above the number that would have been predicted from the 'pre-blip' trends (around 4–6 additional cases per 100 000 people).

This observation seems anomalous in the light of previous evidence that folate-rich foods seem to have a protective effect against bowel cancer (WCRF/AICR, 2007). One suggested reason for this apparent anomaly is that free folic acid, which is not found in food, is used to fortify foods and in supplements. The liver may have a limited capacity to convert folic acid to the normal circulating form of folate (5-methyl tetrahydrofolate) and at high folic acid intakes this might result in the presence of free folic acid in the circulation. Free folic acid may reduce the ability of natural killer cells to kill emerging tumour cells (see Mathers, 2009). Note that antifolate drugs such as aminopterin and methotrexate have been used in cancer chemotherapy for over 50 years. They work by reducing the effects of folate in rapidly dividing tumour cells that have a high folate requirement; there is therefore some theoretical basis for a possible growth-stimulating effect of folic acid on tumour cells.

In October 2009 the Food Standards Agency again advised the British government to make folic acid supplementation of flour mandatory. The Scientific Advisory Committee on Nutrition, which advises the Food Standards Agency, took into account the reports of an increased incidence of bowel cancer in the USA and Canada immediately after fortification was introduced in these countries, but decided that this was insubstantial and could simply be as a result of better screening.

Average intakes of folate from food in the UK are around 260 μg/day, with the highest consumers receiving around twice this amount. Over-the-counter supplements may provide an additional 500 μg/day for men and up to 800 μg/day in some women. This means that some women may have a total intake of around 1.3 mg/day. FSA (2003) concluded that a total intake of 1.5 mg/day would not be expected to have any adverse effects.

Biotin

The chemical structure of biotin is shown in Figure 3.12. Biotin is one of the vitamins where the expert committees in both the USA and the UK felt that there was insufficient data available to set a detailed set of dietary standards. COMA (1991) concluded that adult intakes of 10–200 μg/day should be sufficient with no risk of toxicity (in the USA 30 μg/day is recommended). One reason for uncertainty about

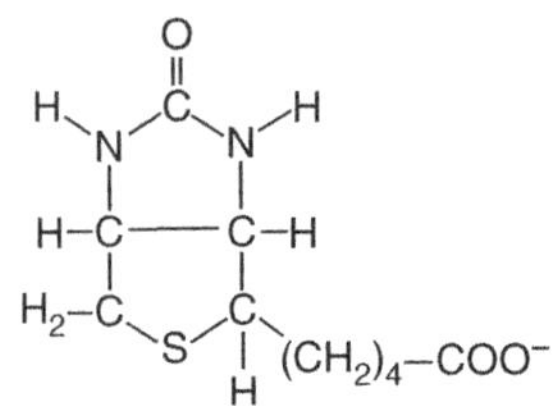

Figure 3.12   The structure of biotin.

biotin requirements is because it is not known whether or how much biotin is available from synthesis by intestinal bacteria. Biotin is widely distributed in foods at low concentrations and is present in good amounts in liver and other offal, egg yolk, whole-grain cereals and yeast. It is present in brewer's yeast and many multinutrient supplements and is added to infant formula. Over-the-counter preparations may provide up to 2 mg of biotin per day.

In the past, biotin was referred to as the 'anti egg white injury factor', because raw egg white contains a protein that interferes with biotin absorption and so eating large amounts of raw egg white can precipitate symptoms due to biotin deficiency. Biotin deficiency results in dermatitis and a range of other symptoms, but it is rarely caused by a simple dietary deficiency. It has been reported to occur as a consequence of some medical therapies (e.g. total parenteral nutrition and dialysis) and in some individuals who have defective absorption or a genetic abnormality in a biotin-associated enzyme.

Biotin is a co-factor for several carboxylase enzymes that add carboxyl (COOH) groups, such as pyruvate carboxylase and acetyl coenzyme A carboxylase. These enzymes are important in gluconeogenesis (glucose synthesis) fatty acid synthesis and in the metabolism of certain branched chain amino acids. Biotin therapy is an accepted treatment for some congenital defects in biotin-associated enzymes and it has been claimed to be of value in the treatment of brittle nails and abnormal glucose tolerance.

Average intakes of biotin from food are around 33 µg/day in the UK, with the highest consumers getting double this amount. Over-the-counter supplements may provide up to a further 2 mg/day. There is little evidence of toxicity associated with oral consumption of biotin supplements. Doses of up to 10 mg/day have not been associated with any reported toxic effects. FSA (2003) concluded that doses of biotin of up to 0.9 mg/day should not have any adverse effects, because no toxic effects had been reported with doses ten times this amount.

Pantothenic acid

The chemical structure of pantothenic acid is shown in Figure 3.13. Requirements for pantothenic acid are difficult to establish with confidence and COMA (1991) set a 'safe intake' for adults of 3–7 mg/day (5 mg/day in the USA). Pantothenic acid is a precursor of coenzyme A (CoA) and CoA-containing moieties (e.g. acetyl

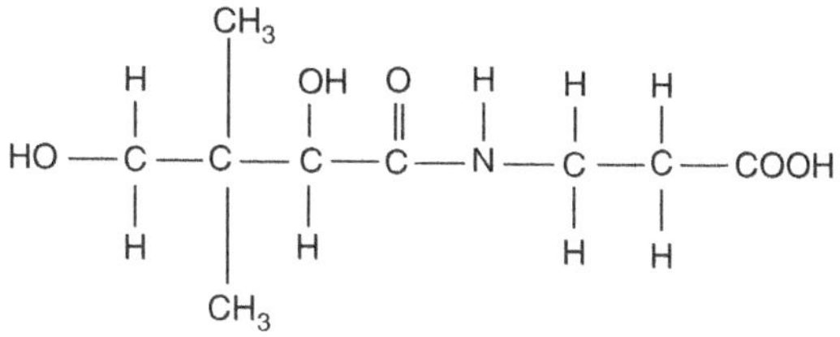

Figure 3.13   The structure of pantothenic acid.

CoA and succinyl CoA) are key intermediaries in many metabolic pathways. Pantothenate is present as CoA in most animal and plant cells and so is widely distributed in foods.

Spontaneous cases of pantothenic acid deficiency do not occur. Average UK intakes from food are around 5.5 mg/day, with the highest consumers taking almost double this amount. Over-the-counter supplements may provide a further 550 mg/day. Pharmacological doses of calcium pantothenate have been suggested as a possible treatment for rheumatoid arthritis and lupus erythromatosis and doses of 2000–10 000 mg/day have been used in trials of its efficacy in this regard, with almost no reports of toxic effects. FSA (2003) suggests that a supplemental dose of 200 mg/day would not be expected to produce any harmful effects.

Vitamin C (ascorbic acid)

The chemical structure of ascorbic acid is shown in Figure 3.14. Vitamin C exists as ascorbic acid and its oxidised form dehydroascorbic acid, which are interconvertible in animal tissues. Most species of animals can make vitamin C from glucose, but primates, guinea pigs and a few exotic species lack a key enzyme on the pathway (gulanolactone oxidase) and so are dependent on a dietary source of the vitamin. COMA (1991) set an adult RNI for vitamin C of 40 mg/day (RDA in the USA is 90 mg/day for men and 75 mg/day for women). It is well established that doses of around 10 mg/day will prevent overt symptoms of the deficiency disease scurvy. Cigarette smokers seem to have an increased requirement for vitamin C on the basis of measurements of plasma vitamin levels.

Vitamin C is found in fruit and vegetables (including potatoes) and these are traditionally regarded as the main sources of the vitamin. It is also present in liver and kidney and fresh unprocessed milk. Vitamin C is prone to oxidation and so some is lost during cooking or heat processing (especially under alkaline conditions) and it may leach into cooking water from vegetables. Vitamin C is found in many multinutrient supplements, is widely used as a single-vitamin supplement and is present in many over-the-counter medicinal products such as cold remedies. Ascorbic acid is used as an antioxidant additive in some foods and maximum levels of use are not specified. People living for extended periods on dried cereals and dried meat have in the past been at risk of scurvy, for example sailors and passengers undertaking long sea voyages by sail and explorers to places where there was no access to fresh foods.

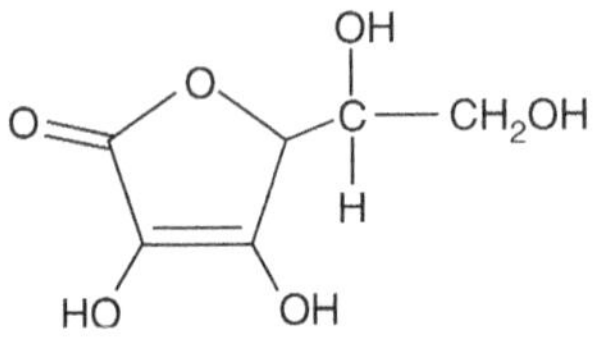

Figure 3.14 The structure of vitamin C (ascorbic acid).

Ascorbic acid is an antioxidant and helps to protect tissues from the damaging effects of free radicals (see Chapter 5). Vitamin C is a co-factor involved in the synthesis of collagen; it acts as a co-factor for enzymes involved in the post-translational hydroxylation of amino acids, which are essential for it to fulfil its structural roles in connective tissue. Vitamin C also acts as a co-factor in the synthesis of carnitine (necessary for cellular handling of long-chain fatty acids and discussed as a supplement in Chapter 7) and the synthesis of several nerve transmitters and peptide hormones, including noradrenalin. The presence of vitamin C in the gut increases the absorption of non-haem iron.

Vitamin C deficiency leads to the condition scurvy, which is characterised by symptoms caused by a general breakdown of connective tissue, such as bleeding gums, loose teeth, small haemorrhages under the skin and poor wound healing. In severe cases there will be large areas of spontaneous bruising and bleeding into the brain or heart muscle, with a risk of sudden death from haemorrhage or heart failure. Scurvy was recognised as a disease of dietary origin in the eighteenth century and in 1795 the regular provision of lime juice or a suitable alternative was given to British naval personnel to prevent it (the origin of the term 'limey').

Vitamin C is one of the most widely used of the single-vitamin preparations. In a popular book (*Vitamin C and the Common Cold*) published in 1972, the Nobel Prize winner Linus Pauling claimed that large supplemental doses of vitamin C could boost the immune system and help prevent infections like the common cold. In the succeeding decades there have been dozens of trials to test whether vitamin C can prevent colds and these generally show no benefit in preventing colds, although some have suggested that it may have some effect on the duration and severity of the symptoms. Earlier suggestions that very high doses of vitamin C might be of use in treating advanced cancers have also proved to be unfounded (see Coulter *et al.*, 2003, which is summarised in Chapter 5).

In a meta-analysis of 30 trials involving over 11 000 participants, Hemila *et al.* (2007) found no evidence that vitamin C prophylaxis (at least 200 mg/day) reduced the risk of developing a cold. A subgroup of six trials involving participants who were marathon runners, skiers or soldiers on subarctic exercises did find evidence of preventive benefit under these circumstances. These reviewers concluded that 'routine mega-dose prophylaxis is not rationally justified for community use'. There was evidence from these prophylaxis studies that vitamin C has a small but statistically significant effect in reducing the duration of cold symptoms, but these authors concluded that this small effect may be of little clinical value. Four trials using up to 8 g/day of vitamin C found no significant evidence that it had any benefits when it was taken at the onset of cold symptoms.

It has been suggested on the basis of epidemiological evidence that low intakes of vitamin C are associated with increased risk of cancer and coronary heart disease. Much of this evidence relates to the apparent protective effect of fruit and vegetables that contain vitamin C, but the effect could be related to other components of fruit and vegetables, or indeed a high intake of fruit and vegetables may simply be a marker for a relatively healthy diet and/or lifestyle. Vitamin C is known to be an antioxidant and so one possible mechanism by which it could protect against degenerative diseases like cancer, heart disease and cataracts is by reducing the oxidative damage to tissue components caused by free radicals. The antioxidants are discussed in Chapter 5 and this discussion includes a review of evidence suggesting that vitamin C supplements do not reduce mortality from cardiovascular diseases or cancer. It is also suggested that the presence of vitamin C in the stomach reduces the formation of carcinogenic nitrosamines from food proteins and this could reduce the risk of stomach cancer. Impaired wound healing and dental problems are symptoms of vitamin C deficiency and it has been suggested that vitamin C supplements might be beneficial in these circumstances, especially for people with poor baseline status. In a Cochrane review of nutritional interventions (including zinc and vitamin C) for preventing and treating pressure sores, Langer *et al.* (2003) found some evidence that nutrition interventions may have some effect on their frequency. They found that there were not enough quality studies to identify which dietary interventions were likely to be effective, however.

Mean intakes of vitamin C from food in the UK are around 65 mg/day, with the highest consumers taking close to treble this amount. Supplements may provide as much as a further 3 g/day.

If doses of several grams of vitamin C are taken this can cause diarrhoea and other gastrointestinal symptoms due to the presence of unabsorbed vitamin C in the large bowel. It has been suggested that high intakes increase urinary oxalate excretion (a metabolite of the vitamin) and that this may increase the risk of kidney stones composed of calcium oxalate. According to FSA (2003), the data on oxalate excretion after high doses of vitamin C is conflicting and some of the claims may be due to experimental artefact. People with certain (genetic) disorders that make them prone to iron overload may potentially be at risk from high supplemental doses of vitamin C because it increases the absorption of non-haem iron. FSA (2003) concluded that a supplemental dose of up to 1 g/day was unlikely to have significant adverse effects, even in those who may be in potential higher-risk groups. Doses well in excess of this are widely used without any apparent ill-effects. At high doses, the efficiency of absorption from the gut decreases and being water soluble, vitamin C is also excreted in urine when high doses are taken.

4 The Minerals

It is difficult to put an exact figure on the number of minerals that are essential nutrients. Several minerals such as calcium, iron and zinc are required in relatively large (mg) daily quantities. Some others are clearly essential but are required in much smaller (µg) quantities, including chromium and selenium, and these are often referred to as the trace elements. Cobalt is essential only in the sense that it is a component of an essential organic compound, vitamin B_{12}. There are several others where there is some evidence of them being essential or claims that they are essential, but there is still doubt about whether they are true essential nutrients. Legislation in 2003 based on the EU Food Supplements Directive originally listed 15 minerals that may be used in food supplements:

- calcium
- magnesium
- iron
- copper
- iodine
- zinc
- manganese
- sodium
- potassium
- selenium
- chromium
- molybdenum
- fluoride
- chloride
- phosphorus

The absence of certain minerals such as boron, vanadium and silicon from this initial positive list was the subject of some controversy in the UK, as these have been used in supplements in the past; at the end of 2009, boron and silicon were added to the positive list. This does not, however, mean that the Commission has

Dietary Supplements and Functional Foods, 2nd Edition. Geoffrey P. Webb.
© 2011 Blackwell Publishing Ltd.

Table 4.1 The adult male RNI for selected minerals, the range of doses* in single- and multiple-nutrient supplements and the 'safe maximum' from supplements as interpreted from FSA (2003); other vales are from EVM (2000). Values in brackets are the most commonly used doses. Estimated and approximate maximum intakes from food are also shown

Mineral	RNI	Single range	Multiple range	'Safe maximum'	Food maximum
Calcium (mg)	700	400–2000 (400–1000)	20–1200 (60–500)	1500	1500
Chromium (µg)	>25**	200–600 (200)	10–200 (25–200)	10 000	170
Copper (mg)	1.2	2	0.2–2 (0.5–2)	7+	3
Iodine (µg)	140	490	40–200 (50–200)	500	430
Iron (mg)	8.7	5–51 (14–18)	2–60 (10–18)	17	24
Magnesium (mg)	300	150–750 (150–250)	0.5–500 (60–300)	400	510
Manganese (mg)	>1.4**	0.04–10 (10)	1–9 (1–2.5)	12#	8.2
Molybdenum (µg)	50–400	333	2–140 (20–50)	none	210
Potassium (mg)	3500	200	0.5–80 (0.5–50)	3700	4700
Selenium (µg)	75	50–300 (200)	10–200 (25–100)	450§	100
Zinc (mg)	9.5	15–50 (30)	2–20 (10–15)	25	17

* Note that figures for doses used were current in the UK in 2000, i.e. before the effect of the publication of FSA (2003).
** Safe intake.
# Total intake from all sources, reduced to 8.7 mg in elderly people.
§ Total intake from all sources.

accepted that these two minerals are essential nutrients, as the following quote from the Directive makes clear:

> Only vitamins and minerals normally found in, and consumed as part of, the diet should be allowed to be present in food supplements although this does not mean that their presence therein is necessary.

In general, even if they are confirmed to be essential, deficiency of some minerals would be unlikely to occur except on an experimental diet designed to produce deficiency, or when patients are fed totally by intravenous infusion for extended periods (total parenteral nutrition, TPN). I have restricted discussion in this section to minerals where a deficiency syndrome is well documented or where the mineral has been widely promoted as having potential value as a dietary supplement and is on the original positive list above. Information in this

Table 4.2 Annual sales (millions of capsules/tablets) of single-mineral and multiple-nutrient supplements containing individual minerals. Figures are taken from EVM (2000) and should thus only be taken as a guide to current relative popularity. Internet sales were not included, although some other mail-order sales are

Mineral	Single-mineral products	Multiple-nutrient products
Boron	0.8	123
Calcium	7.42	276
Chromium	0.41	152
Copper	0.03	112
Iodine	n/a	136
Iron	n/a	373
Magnesium	5.7	226
Molybdenum	n/a	152
Nickel	not sold	122
Potassium	n/a	149
Selenium	n/a	167
Silicon	0.02	91
Tin	not sold	122
Vanadium	not sold	n/a
Zinc	0.43	157

Note: Nickel, tin and vanadium are not on the positive list of approved minerals that came into force in 2005.

chapter that is likely to be found in a standard textbook of nutrition is not specifically referenced.

Table 4.1 shows the range of doses of minerals found in single-mineral and multiple-nutrient supplements sold in the UK in 2000 (from EVM, 2000). The adult male RNI and the maximum safe supplemental dose as interpreted from FSA (2003) are also given, as is the estimated normal maximum UK intake from food sources. Note that the doses in supplements represent the UK market in 2000 and do not reflect any more recent changes, for instance due to the influence of the publication of the Food Standards Agency report on maximum safe levels in supplements (FSA, 2003), or the voluntary code on reformulation and label advisory statements agreed between the FSA and the food supplements industry in 2004 (see Chapter 1 for details).

Table 4.2 shows the relative sales of supplements of single minerals and multiple-nutrient supplements containing individual minerals at the start of 2000. Figures for several minerals not regarded as essential nutrients are also given in this table to indicate the potential impact of the EU Food Supplements Directive. These figures do not include internet sales; although some mail-order sales may be included, at the time these data were collected these outlets were relatively minor contributors to total sales (EVM, 2000).

Calcium

The adult RNI for calcium in the UK is 700 mg/day. The RNI for adolescents is higher than that for adults, as is that for lactating women but not for pregnant women in the UK. In the USA, the Institute of Medicine has designated 1000 mg/day as an adequate intake of calcium for adults aged 19–50 years, with higher vales for the elderly and older children (up to 1300 mg/day), including pregnant and lactating girls less than 19 years. The earlier discussion of the dietary micronutrient adequacy of different life-cycle groups in the UK suggested that substantial numbers of individuals, especially older children, younger adults, free-living elderly people and lactating women, had intakes of calcium that would be regarded as inadequate; that is, below the LRNI. Dairy products are the richest and most readily absorbed source of calcium in the diet and probably account for two-thirds of average calcium intakes in the UK. Other useful sources of dietary calcium are green leafy vegetables, nuts and white flour, which must be fortified with calcium in the UK.

Calcium is a frequent component of dietary supplements; it may be taken as a single supplement or in combination with other minerals and/or perhaps vitamin D for bone health. Many multinutrient supplements also contain calcium. It may be present as relatively insoluble calcium carbonate or in some other more soluble and more readily available form. Antacid preparations contain calcium carbonate.

An adult human body contains more than a kilogram of calcium and almost all of it is concentrated in the mineral component of the skeleton as the calcium phosphate compound hydoxyapatite. Bone mineral gives much of the mechanical strength to bones and teeth. The 1% or so of calcium that is outside of the skeleton has a number of very important functions, for example:

- It serves as an intracellular regulator.
- It is involved in the release of nerve transmitters and hormones.
- It is a co-factor for some enzymes, including some involved in blood clotting.
- It is an important link between electrical excitation and contraction in muscles.
- It is important in nerve and heart function.

The blood calcium concentration is hormonally regulated and is normally kept within narrow limits. Adverse symptoms result from either too low or too high a plasma calcium concentration. The skeletal calcium can thus be seen to serve a dual purpose: not only to give mechanical strength to bones and teeth, but also to act as a very large sink or reservoir of calcium, which can be hormonally induced to release calcium to maintain blood calcium if it is falling or can accept surplus calcium to prevent the blood level rising too high. The hormonal and dietary influences on calcium homeostasis are summarised in Figure 4.1; vitamin D and calcitriol, the hormone which is produced from it in the kidney, were discussed in Chapter 3.

High calcium intakes, whether from food or supplements, have been widely promoted for the maintenance of bone health and the prevention and/or treatment of osteoporosis. In the USA, people over 50 are recommended to increase their calcium intake to 1200 mg/day. Even though the British RNI for elderly adults is the

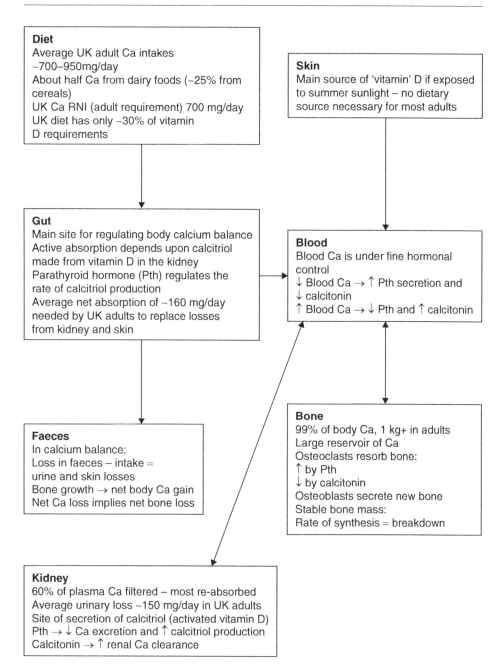

Diet
Average UK adult Ca intakes
~700–950mg/day
About half Ca from dairy foods (~25% from
cereals)
UK Ca RNI (adult requirement) 700 mg/day
UK diet has only ~30% of vitamin
D requirements

Skin
Main source of 'vitamin' D if exposed
to summer sunlight – no dietary
source necessary for most adults

Gut
Main site for regulating body calcium balance
Active absorption depends upon calcitriol
made from vitamin D in the kidney
Parathyroid hormone (Pth) regulates the
rate of calcitriol production
Average net absorption of ~160 mg/day
needed by UK adults to replace losses
from kidney and skin

Blood
Blood Ca is under fine hormonal
control
↓ Blood Ca → ↑ Pth secretion and
↓ calcitonin
↑ Blood Ca → ↓ Pth and ↑ calcitonin

Faeces
In calcium balance:
Loss in faeces – intake =
urine and skin losses
Bone growth → net body Ca gain
Net Ca loss implies net bone loss

Bone
99% of body Ca, 1 kg+ in adults
Large reservoir of Ca
Osteoclasts resorb bone:
↑ by Pth
↓ by calcitonin
Osteoblasts secrete new bone
Stable bone mass:
Rate of synthesis = breakdown

Kidney
60% of plasma Ca filtered – most re-absorbed
Average urinary loss ~150 mg/day in UK adults
Site of secretion of calcitriol (activated vitamin D)
Pth → ↓ Ca excretion and ↑ calcitriol production
Calcitonin → ↑ renal Ca clearance

Figure 4.1 Typical calcium fluxes in UK adults, with summary of the main dietary and hormonal influences on calcium homeostasis. Reproduced (with minor revisions) with permission from Webb (2001) What is osteoporosis? Nursing and Residential Care, 3 (9), 434–8.

same as that for younger adults (700 mg/day), the National Osteoporosis Society recommends a 'bone-friendly' diet rich in calcium and a calcium intake of 1200 mg/ day for those with osteoporosis (NOS, 2010).

At birth, babies have around 30 g of calcium in their skeletons and this increases to a maximum of around 1–1.5 kg in the third decade (the peak bone mass) depending on skeletal size. Thereafter total bone mineral mass and calcium content declines with age and there is an accelerated loss in women during the years around the menopause; this is due to reduced sex hormone (oestrogen) production by the ovary. In elderly people, particularly in older women, the loss of bone mineral may reach a point, termed the fracture threshold, at which some bones are liable to fracture when subjected to relatively minor trauma such as a simple fall. This high propensity to fracture due to thinning of the bones is called osteoporosis and results in many tens of thousands of wrist, hip and vertebral fractures each year in the UK and other industrialised countries. Hip fracture (breaking off of the neck of the femur) is a major public health problem; many people never fully recover their mobility after a hip fracture and many die in the weeks and months after the initial fracture and surgical repair.

Given that osteoporosis is associated with a depletion of skeletal calcium, it is not surprising that boosting calcium intakes should be seen as a potentially useful way of treating or preventing this disabling and costly condition. It is suggested that high calcium intakes in childhood and early adulthood will help to maximise the 'peak bone mass' and so extend the amount of bone mineral that can be lost before the fracture threshold is reached. In older people it is said that a high calcium intake will help slow the loss of bone mineral. However, the evidence that calcium deficiency *per se* is a major contributory cause of the condition or that supplemental calcium has a major preventive role is inconclusive and controversial.

Does a high calcium intake during childhood increase the peak bone mass? This would theoretically raise the amount of mineral that can be lost during old age before the fracture threshold is reached and thus delay, perhaps beyond a person's life span, the onset of osteoporosis. The absorption of calcium from the intestines is hormonally regulated; when calcium intakes are low then a higher proportion of the dietary load is absorbed than when calcium intakes are high. Only when calcium intakes are below those likely to be seen in western countries is bone growth noticeably impaired by lack of dietary calcium.

Double-blind placebo-controlled studies of calcium supplements in childhood suggest that for the first few months they do cause a small increase in measured bone density, but that this effect disappears after the supplements are stopped (reviewed by Prentice, 1997 and Phillips, 2003). In contrast, there is substantial evidence that weight-bearing exercise during childhood and indeed throughout life does significantly increase bone density. A recent meta-analysis has been conducted of 19 trials (c. 3000 total participants) of calcium supplements and measured bone density in healthy children (Winzenberg *et al.*, 2006). The minimum duration of supplementation considered was three months and the minimum duration of follow-up on bone density was six months. These authors found no effect of calcium supplements on bone density in the femoral neck or lumbar spine, although at six months there was a small effect on bone density in the upper limb, which they considered would have no clinically significant benefit.

There is also little evidence of any relationship between bone density and calcium intake in young and middle-aged adults. Osteoporosis is more common in western countries where adults drink milk and so have relatively high calcium intakes than it is in countries where adults do not drink milk. There have been a number of reports (e.g. Hegsted, 1986) of a *positive* correlation between calcium intake and the incidence of osteoporosis fractures. This would suggest that calcium intake is not a major determinant of bone density or fracture risk in these adults, although it does not preclude the possibility that calcium supplements may have some beneficial effect. According to Phillips (2003), there is now an emerging consensus that calcium intake slows the rate of bone loss in post-menopausal women, especially those whose habitual intakes from food are low.

Many individuals in the UK and probably in other western countries have habitual intakes of calcium from food that are considered to be unsatisfactory. There is evidence that large calcium supplements in children initially lead to small but measurable increases in bone density, although the effectiveness seems to decline with continued usage and there is no indication that this effect is sustained in the long term once supplementation ceases. It is important that children are encouraged to maintain good intakes of readily available food calcium, usually by ensuring that they consume enough milk products (low-fat milk products are just as rich in calcium as full-fat products). There is little convincing evidence that high calcium intakes in adulthood prior to the menopause have a significant influence on bone density, and indeed osteoporosis is more common among milk-drinking adult populations with internationally high calcium intakes.

In the elderly, calcium supplements do seem to slow bone loss in women whose habitual calcium intake is low, so calcium supplements may be a useful alternative if improvements in dietary intakes of available calcium cannot be achieved. In elderly people at high risk of osteoporosis or already diagnosed with this condition, calcium supplements are frequently prescribed or advised. In Chapter 3, it was noted that a recent large trial (Record Trial Group, 2005) suggested that neither calcium supplements nor vitamin D supplements (alone or in combination) prevent fracture recurrence in elderly people with a history of osteoporosis. Of course, good vitamin D status is essential for efficient absorption of calcium and combined vitamin D and calcium supplements are often used. Some beneficial effects of very high calcium intakes may be because they compensate for poor vitamin D status; at high calcium intakes, more calcium is absorbed by non-vitamin-D-dependent mechanisms. In general, any (elderly) person not regularly exposed to summer sunlight should consider taking a supplement containing vitamin D and calcium. It was noted in Chapter 3 that supplements of vitamin D and calcium can reduce fracture risk in frail elderly people with no previous history of fractures.

There have been suggestions that high calcium intakes or calcium supplements might reduce blood pressure in primary hypertension, but there is as yet no substantial evidence to support this (Beyer *et al.*, 2006).

FSA (2003) suggests that the average calcium intake from food in the UK was around 830 mg/day, with the highest consumers taking in near twice this amount. Drinking water may provide a further 600 mg/day in some areas and over-the-counter supplements up to 2400 mg/day, giving an estimated maximum exposure of up to 4500 mg/day. For guidance purposes, FSA (2003) suggested that supplemental doses of 1500 mg/day would not be expected to produce any adverse effects. At higher doses gastrointestinal symptoms may occur and in some people taking medicinal calcium supplements a milk-alkali syndrome has sometimes been found. Milk-alkali syndrome can result in hypercalcaemia, calcification of tissues, alkalosis, hypertension, neurological symptoms and renal impairment.

Chromium

Chromium has been shown to be essential in rats and humans, but overt human deficiency is only observed in patients undergoing long-term TPN. COMA (1991) felt that it had insufficient data to set formal LRNI and RNI for chromium, but rather indicated that the 'safe intake' of chromium for adults was above 25 μg/day; in the USA, the RDA is 35 μg/day for men and 25 μg/day for women. Relatively large amounts are present in processed meats, whole-grain cereals and pulses. It is also present in multinutrient supplements and may be used as a single-component supplement with does of up to 600 μg/day in the UK. In nature chromium only exists in the trivalent state and this is the form present in food. Together with the organic form chromium picolinate, these are the only forms permitted in supplements within the EU.

In animal studies and in individual patients receiving long-term total parenteral nutrition, it has been shown that chromium deficiency leads to impaired glucose tolerance due to insulin resistance; under these circumstances, chromium supplements improve insulin sensitivity and glucose tolerance. It is postulated that chromium is a component of a 'glucose-tolerance factor' that also contains nicotinic acid and several amino acids. It has been suggested that because of the presence of nicotinic acid in this complex, chromium supplements may be more effective if administered with nicotinic acid.

Given its apparent role in insulin response and normal glucose tolerance, it has been suggested that chromium supplements might have beneficial effects in the management of type 2 diabetes mellitus, where the primary pathological change is a decline in insulin response; that is, insulin resistance. Some reports have suggested that there are some grounds for believing that chromium supplements may increase insulin sensitivity, and improve glucose tolerance and other measures of diabetic control in patients with type 2 diabetes.

Althuis et al. (2002) performed a meta-analysis of randomised controlled trials of the effects of chromium supplements on insulin responses in both healthy individuals and those with type 2 diabetes. They identified 15 trials that met their inclusion criteria, involving a total of 193 participants with type 2 diabetes and 425 in good health or with impaired glucose tolerance (pre-diabetes). They found no evidence of any significant effect of the chromium supplements in the non-diabetic subjects. Most of the diabetic subjects (155) were in a single trial of diabetics in China. Data from the other 38 diabetic subjects did not show any beneficial effects of the chromium supplements, whereas the Chinese data suggested that chromium supplements did reduce both glucose and insulin concentrations and also reduced the concentration of glycosylated haemoglobin; blood concentration of glyco- sylated haemoglobin is regarded as an indicator of average blood glucose concen- trations over the previous few weeks. Althuis *et al.* concluded that the data for the effect of chromium supplements in type diabetes is inconclusive.

It is worth noting that in an analysis of controlled trials, Vickers *et al.* (1998) found no trial published in China or the USSR/Russia that established a test treatment to be ineffective and suggested the likelihood of publication bias (see Chapter 1) in studies originating from these countries. There seems to be no justification for non- diabetics to take chromium supplements and only weak evidence to support its use in diabetics, although as noted below these supplements are probably harmless.

The average UK intake of chromium from food is around 100 µg/day and the highest consumers get close to double this amount. Supplements in the UK may provide up to a further 600 µg/day, giving a total maximum exposure of almost 800 µg/day. FSA (2003) suggests that daily doses of chromium of up to 10 000 µg should not have any adverse effects. One reason why natural chromium compounds are relatively non-toxic is because of their poor absorption.

Copper

Copper is clearly established as an essential mineral; COMA (1991) set an adult RNI in the UK of 1.2 mg/day (0.9 mg/day in the USA). Nuts, shellfish and offal have particularly high concentrations of copper. Drinking water may contain significant amounts of copper because some copper will dissolve from copper piping, particularly if the water is acidic. Most water in the UK contains less than 1 mg/L, although it may contain up to 3 mg/L.

There are several important copper-containing enzymes and proteins in the body, including:

- Ceruloplasmin, which is involved in the transport and oxidation of iron prior to haemoglobin synthesis.
- Tyrosinase and dopamine hydroxylase, involved in the synthesis of catecho- lamine nerve transmitters and the pigment melanin from tyrosine.
- Cytochrome c oxidase in the electron transport system in mitochondria.
- Extracellular copper-zinc superoxide dismutase, involved in the removal of the damaging superoxide radical.

As copper is a co-factor for some types of superoxide dismutase, it is one of the antioxidant nutrients discussed in Chapter 5, but *in vitro* it acts as a pro-oxidant.

Dietary deficiency of copper has been characterised in animals and it results in anaemia, low levels of neutrophils and in osteoporosis and skeletal abnormalities. Copper deficiency rarely occurs in humans, but it has been described in patients receiving TPN and in premature and low-birth-weight babies fed on milk diets. The symptoms seen in human copper deficiency are similar to those seen in animals. It has been suggested but not established that marginal copper deficiency can lead to high blood cholesterol, reduced skin pigmentation and impaired glucose tolerance. A rare sex-linked inherited condition, Menke's disease, is associated with reduced copper uptake and low activity of copper-containing enzymes. This disease results in death in early childhood and even parenteral administration of copper does not alleviate the symptoms or prevent death. Copper bracelets are worn by many people in the belief that they offer some relief from the symptoms of arthritis, but there is no substantial evidence that copper supplements have beneficial effects in arthritis. There is speculation that copper supplements may protect against hypercholesteraemia, although there is little evidence to support this.

A detailed account of copper nutrition may be found in Turnlund (2006). There seems to be no justification for specifically taking copper supplements other than to ensure adequacy. High doses of supplemental iron, zinc or ascorbic acid may reduce copper uptake and can produce indications of copper deficiency in animal studies.

The average intake from food in the UK is around 1.4 mg/day, with the highest consumers taking in more than double this amount. In the UK, copper is present in many mineral and multinutrient supplements at levels of up to 2 mg/day and licensed medicines purchased from pharmacies may contain double this amount. FSA (2003) set a safe upper level for lifetime consumption of copper of 10 mg/day. Those UK consumers with the highest intake of copper from food and drinking water may theoretically slightly exceed this figure if they also take supplements, but the panel included a tenfold safety margin to allow for uncertainties when it set this level.

Acute systemic copper poisoning is rare, because copper compounds have an unpleasant taste and emetic effects and also cause abdominal pain and diarrhoea. There is normally good homeostatic regulation of copper uptake in the gut, which reduces the likelihood of chronic copper overload. A couple of rare inherited conditions, Wilson's disease and Indian childhood cirrhosis, both lead to excessive accumulation of copper in the body. In both of these conditions, accumulation of copper in the liver leads to cirrhosis, and in Wilson's disease accumulation of copper in the brain causes neurological damage.

Fluoride

The expert panels that set the current dietary standards in the UK (COMA, 1991) and the USA (NRC, 1989) both concluded that while fluoride is not strictly an essential nutrient, it can, in the correct dose, be a beneficial dietary substance that reduces the risk of dental caries (tooth decay) in children. A level of 1 mg/kg (1ppm) is widely regarded as an optimum level in drinking water, enough to halve the risk of dental caries in children but not enough to produce serious or widespread tooth mottling. COMA (1991) supported the recommendation that drinking water should be fortified with fluoride to make the concentration up to this level. In the USA, more than half of the population drink fluoridated water (concentration ranges from 0.7–1.2 mg/L). Tea and seafood are the richest sources of fluoride in the diet and tea provides up to 70% of the fluoride in the UK diet. Adults who consume large amounts of tea made with fluoridated water may consume three times the average intake.

Fluoride reacts with the hydroxyapatite of bone mineral and tooth enamel to form fluorapatite, which is less soluble and more resistant to demineralisation. Fluoride in saliva may also reduce the growth of acid-producing bacteria in the mouth and it may stimulate the remineralisation of newly forming caries by accelerating recrystallisation. It is generally accepted that moderate intakes of fluoride reduce the incidence of dental caries and there has been speculation about whether it might also reduce the risk of osteoporosis. There is little persuasive evidence for an anti-osteoporosis effect of fluoride, however; Dawson-Hughes (2006) suggested that it may increase the radiographic density of bone, but not increase its quality or tensile strength and thus not reduce fracture risk.

It was recognised more than 60 years ago that the incidence of dental caries is substantially lower in areas where the concentration of fluoride in drinking water is naturally high. Conversely, a mottling of the tooth enamel occurs increasingly in high fluoride areas, which in mild cases manifests as white flecks on the surface of the enamel, but severe fluorosis manifests as brown stains and pitting of the enamel. Severe chronic fluoride overdose also has other effects such as joint pain, osteoporosis, muscle wasting and neurological problems. Very high doses, such as might occur through acute accidental exposure, can have fatal consequences.

In the UK, fluoride supplements are sold as licensed medicines although they can also be included in dietary supplements. The recommended dose of fluoride depends on the local level of fluoride in the drinking water and fluoride supplements should only be given in the light of this local water concentration, which can be obtained from the local water-supply company. British dental authorities, including the British Dental Association, recommend that supplements should not be given before six months of age and should not be given if the water concentration exceeds 700 µg/L.

If the water concentration is less than 300 µg/L, then they recommend:

- 250 µg/day at 6 months–3 years
- 500 µg/day at 3–6 years
- 1 mg/day over 6 years until puberty

If the water fluoride concentration is between 300 µg/L and 700 µg/L, then they recommend:

- 250 µg/day for 3–6 year olds
- 500 µg/day for those over 6 years

Note that most toothpaste is now fluoridated and this is credited with much of the reduction in caries incidence since the 1960s in western countries. If children swallow large amounts of fluoridated toothpaste and are given relatively high amounts of supplemental fluoride compared to the normal intake from food and drink, this does increase the likelihood of at least mild symptoms of fluorosis; that is, mottling of the teeth.

There does seem to be a strong case for ensuring that young children consume sufficient fluoride to help protect their teeth against decay. The difference between a therapeutic dose and the level at which early signs of fluoride overload (tooth mottling) appear is small and there may well be some individuals who are particularly fluoride sensitive. It is therefore important to get the dose correct and this is complicated by the variety of sources that can contribute to total fluoride intake:

- Fluoride from most foods contributes little to total intake, although seafood is a good source if the bones of the fish are eaten.
- Tea is a rich source of fluoride and is a major contributor to the total intake of tea drinkers.
- The fluoride naturally present in drinking water can vary from almost zero in soft-water areas to over 10 mg/L in some parts of the world, which is sufficient to cause widespread and marked dental fluorosis.
- Fluoride is added to over half of the drinking water in the USA, but only about 12% of that in the UK.
- Most toothpaste now has fluoride added to it and the amount children swallow from this source can be variable.
- Fluoride supplements can be given by individual parents to their children.

There has been vociferous opposition to general fluoridation of water in the UK, even though the benefits to the dental health of children were convincingly demonstrated 40 years ago (DHSS, 1969 and WHO, 1970). This resistance is partly based on the issue of 'freedom of choice' and partly on anxieties about the long-term safety of these fluoride additions. While it is almost impossible to prove the absolute safety of such additions, the levels used are well within the normal range of natural drinking water and fluoride safety has been the subject of intense scrutiny for several decades.

Iodine

The UK RNI for iodine is 140 μg/day and in the USA the RDA is 150 μg/day; the LRNI in the UK is 70 μg/day. Iodine is present in relatively large amounts in seafood and sea salt (it is also sometimes added to salt, as iodised salt). Kelp is a dietary supplement that is marketed as a good source of iodine (see Chapter 8). The concentration of iodine in other foods varies according to the amount of iodine present in the local soil. In industrialised countries, dairy products contain relatively large amounts of iodine because of iodine supplementation of animal feeds and because of the use of iodine-containing disinfectants in the dairy industry.

Certain foods contain substances called goitrogens that either impair the uptake of iodine by the thyroid gland or impair the synthesis of thyroid hormones. These goitrogens are present in foods such as the Brassica vegetables (e.g. cabbage) and in cassava. Intakes of goitrogens in most western countries are unlikely to have a significant impact on iodine requirements, but in countries where cassava is the dominant staple they may precipitate iodine deficiency if intakes of the mineral are marginal. It has been suggested that in such places, intakes of iodine should be doubled to compensate for the effect of these goitrogens.

The sole function of dietary iodine is as a component of the thyroid hormones thyroxin and tri-iodothyronine, which control metabolic rate and development in children. The first indication of iodine deficiency is a compensatory swelling of the thyroid gland known as goitre. These goitres vary from barely perceptible swellings, which are considered attractive in women in some cultures, to large, nodular masses that may obstruct the airway. The thyroid is able to extract iodine from blood very efficiently and concentrate it within the thyroid gland. The ability of the thyroid to concentrate a dose of radioactively labelled iodine is used as a diagnostic indicator of thyroid function and high doses of radioactive iodine can be used to ablate the thyroid selectively when surgery is contraindicated.

The other symptoms of iodine deficiency in adults include impaired mental functioning, low metabolic rate and poor cold tolerance, hypotension and weight gain, a condition known as myxoedema. In children, iodine deficiency leads to an irreversible impairment of physical and mental development termed cretinism. In areas where iodine deficiency is endemic, it also leads to high levels of spontaneous abortion, stillbirth and increased frequency of babies born with congenital abnormalities like deaf-mutism, spasticity and mental deficiency.

Overt iodine deficiency is rarely seen in developed countries nowadays, although in the past it was common in specific regions, for example the area around the Great Lakes in the USA, in Switzerland and in the Cotswold and Derbyshire regions of England (hence the term Derbyshire neck, sometimes used to describe goitre). In affluent countries, the use of foods grown in diverse regions, the consumption of seafood, the high iodine content of milk and the use of iodised preparations such as salt have combined to make this condition unlikely.

Average intakes of iodine in the UK are well above the RNI for men and significantly above it in women, although according to Henderson *et al.* (2003), 12% of women aged 19–24 years have unsatisfactory intakes of iodine. Data on iodine intakes that relies on food tables, like the NDNS data, may not be wholly reliable as an indicator of total iodine intake. In a review, Zimmerman and Delange (2004) suggested that two-thirds of people in western Europe live in countries that are iodine deficient. These authors go on to suggest that most women in Europe are iodine deficient during pregnancy and they recommend that all pregnant women should receive iodine-containing supplements (150 µg/day) during pregnancy.

According to the WHO, as many as 1.6 billion people in the world live in places where they are at risk of iodine deficiency. They rely on local food, grown in mountainous areas or frequently flooded river valleys, where the soil iodine content is very low, for example in the Andes, the Himalayas, the Ganges river valleys and the mountainous areas of China. It is further estimated that around 200 million people suffer from goitre and maybe 10% of these show signs of resultant mental deficits. More than 5 million people worldwide suffer from gross cretinism and severe mental retardation. Iodine deficiency is the most common preventable cause of mental subnormality in children.

The mean intake of iodine from food in the UK is 220 μg/day, with the highest consumers taking in around double this amount. It is estimated that in some parts of the UK drinking water may provide up to a maximum of a further 30 μg/day. Iodine is a component of many vitamin and mineral multinutrient supplements, is present in kelp or other products of marine origin, but it is rarely used as a single supplement in western countries; these supplements may provide up to 490 μg/day, making a total estimated maximum exposure of 950 μg/day (FSA, 2003).

Iodine is a component of a number of medicinal products used for topical application because of its antiseptic properties. Some people are allergic to iodine used in this way and occasional cases of acute poisoning have resulted from accidental consumption of these products or their use in, for example, wound irrigation.

High intakes of iodine can lead to disturbances in thyroid function. This usually manifests as toxic nodular goitres and hyperthyroidism, but can sometimes manifest as hypothyroidism, as would be expected in iodine deficiency. These symptoms occur in populations who have chronically high iodine intakes or where there has been active intervention to boost iodine intakes. In the recent past, high iodine intakes in the USA as a result of the high iodine content of milk were the cause for some concern. These peaked in 1974 at 800 μg/day, although they have since declined. Dunn (2006) suggests that iodine-induced hyperthyroidism usually occurs in populations who have adapted to low iodine intake and developed a goitre, and thus they may become temporarily hyperthyroid if iodine intakes are suddenly raised (this author also gives a detailed account of iodine in nutrition). FSA (2003) suggests that supplemental iodine intakes of up to 500 μg/day (just above the estimated UK maximum) should not have any adverse effects in adults.

Iron

The most available form of dietary iron is the organic haem iron in meat and fish; inorganic iron in cereals (bread and flour are fortified with iron in the UK), vegetables and fruit is much less well absorbed.

The iron content of the red cells that deteriorate and are removed from the circulation each day amounts to around 20 mg, but most of this iron is conserved and recycled into new red cells. Total daily losses of iron from a healthy adult male are only around 1 mg/day, which is lost as sloughed skin and gut cells, hair, nails and bodily fluids. In women and older girls, menstrual losses increase this average daily iron loss to around 1.8 mg/day, although in women who have heavy menstrual bleeding this may be 2.5 mg/day or even more. The RNI for an adult male in the UK is 8.7 mg/day (RDA in the USA is 8 mg/day). The extra iron losses associated with menstruation are reflected in substantially higher dietary standards for women; the RNI for older girls and pre-menopausal women is 14.8 mg/day in the UK (RDA in the USA is 18 mg/day).

The RNI for iron seem superficially to be very high in relation to the average daily losses, which are the amounts that need to be replaced each day in order to maintain iron balance in adults. Even in women with heavy menstrual losses, the RNI is around five times the estimated daily loss. This is because only a relatively small and variable proportion of the iron consumed is absorbed in the gut. The amount that is absorbed depends on several variables, listed below:

- The form of the dietary iron has a large effect on the efficiency of absorption. Organic haem iron in meat and fish is much better absorbed than inorganic iron in milk and vegetable foods. Most of the inorganic iron in food is in the ferric state, whereas the ferrous iron used in most supplements is generally better absorbed.
- A number of substances in food can promote or inhibit the absorption of the inorganic iron in food. Vitamin C and alcohol increase the absorption of inorganic iron by increasing the amount of inorganic iron in solution, either directly, or indirectly by increasing gastric acid production. Phytate from unleavened bread and tannin in tea inhibit inorganic iron absorption. Very high fibre intakes may also have some adverse effect on iron absorption.
- Iron absorption is physiologically regulated: iron-depleted individuals absorb iron two to three times more efficiently than those whose iron stores are high.
- During pregnancy when there is an increased physiological need for iron, there is also a substantial increase in the efficiency of iron absorption during the course of the pregnancy.

As a rough rule of thumb, it has been estimated that about 15% of dietary iron is absorbed from a mixed diet. There are no mechanisms for excreting excess iron once it has been absorbed, so regulation of absorption is the main mechanism for homeostatic control of iron balance. Individuals with certain medical conditions that require repeated blood transfusions (e.g. the inherited blood disorder thalassaemia or failure of bone marrow to generate red cells, aplastic anaemia) are at risk of iron poisoning because they cannot excrete the iron that is being infused in the transfused blood and so bypass the normal gut regulation of iron balance. Some drugs are available that chelate iron and facilitate its excretion and these may also be used in cases of accidental iron poisoning.

Iron is a key component of haemoglobin, the oxygen-carrying pigment in blood, and of a similar protein in muscle called myoglobin. Iron is also an important component of mitochondrial cytochromes and is a co-factor for several enzymes, although the amounts involved are very small in comparison to the amounts in haemoglobin and myoglobin. A well-nourished adult male has around 4 g of iron in his body, with two-thirds of this present in haemoglobin and myoglobin; most of the rest is present as a protein–iron complex called ferritin, which is the main storage form of iron in the body. During body-iron depletion, there is initially reduced amounts of iron stored as ferritin (measured by a decrease in serum ferritin) – iron deficiency. This is followed by a fall in blood haemoglobin concentration – iron deficiency anaemia.

Iron deficiency is the most common micronutrient deficiency in the world, with perhaps 700 million people worldwide suffering from iron deficiency anaemia and many more with depleted iron stores. Although it is much more common in developing countries, we saw in Chapter 2 that inadequate iron intakes are common among women, children and the elderly in Britain. Many Britons in these categories have haemoglobin levels that are indicative of iron deficiency anaemia and many more have low serum ferritin levels, indicating iron deficiency (see Chapter 2 for details). A number of factors such as those listed below are likely to increase the risk of iron deficiency and anaemia:

- Low intake of available iron, for which vegetarians (10% of adolescent girls) are an obvious high-risk group because they exclude organic haem iron from their diets.
- High intake of substances like phytate (unleavened bread) and tannin (tea) taken with meals will reduce the efficiency of inorganic iron absorption and, conversely, so will low intakes of promoters of inorganic iron with meals, especially vitamin C.
- Any condition that leads to chronic blood or other iron loss, such as persistently heavy periods, repeated pregnancies, bleeding ulcers, intestinal parasites, prolonged lactation etc.
- Certain conditions that lead to reduced gastric acid secretion, such as gastrectomy or simply age-related achlorhydria; gastric acid helps to make inorganic iron more soluble and thus easier to absorb.
- Athletes have been regarded as particularly at risk of developing anaemia because of the belief that endurance training increases the requirement for dietary iron. This perception is increased because endurance training has a haemodilution effect; that is, plasma volume increases by more than circulating red cell mass, leading to a fall in blood haemoglobin concentration even though the absolute amount of circulating haemoglobin increases (Maughan, 1994). This effect is also seen in pregnancy. True anaemia in athletes is usually due to low iron intake.

Iron deficiency anaemia is characterised by small red blood cells (microcytic anaemia). The symptoms include pallor, fatigue, breathlessness on exertion and headaches. These symptoms are attributed to the impaired ability of blood to supply the tissues with oxygen, due to the reduced oxygen-carrying capacity of blood as a result of the reduced circulating amounts of haemoglobin in the blood. Iron deficiency without anaemia also has some adverse consequences, like reduced work capacity and memory, learning and attention deficits in children. Iron deficiency anaemia has traditionally been defined by a low blood haemoglobin concentration – a figure of less than 120 g/L at sea level has been often used as a cut-off point in the past, although more recent sources use 110 g/L (e.g. Gregory *et al.*, 1990).

Serum/plasma ferritin concentration is a more sensitive indicator of iron status than blood haemoglobin concentration. Levels of less than 25 μg/L indicate suboptimal iron stores and less than 12 μg/L indicate frank iron depletion.

There are several possible strategies that may be employed to improve the iron status of a population:

- Promotion of dietary changes to increase the amount of available iron in the diet, such as eating more lean meat or fish; taking vitamin-C-rich foods like orange juice with meals to increase inorganic iron absorption; not drinking tea with meals to prevent the tannin hindering iron absorption.
- Fortifying key foods with iron: there is already mandatory fortification of white and brown flour with iron in the UK and many breakfast cereals also contain added iron.
- The selective use of iron-containing supplements.

Given the apparent scale of the problem of inadequate iron intakes and iron deficiency, the use of supplements may well be a necessary component of measures that have a realistic chance of making a major impact on this problem, at least in the short term. Eating more organic iron in the form of extra lean meat and fish may be unacceptable to substantial numbers of people who are vegetarian or have vegetarian leanings. It may be wrongly seen as incompatible with other dietary advice to reduce the consumption of saturated fats. Mandatory fortification of still more foods with iron is unlikely to occur within a reasonable time frame, especially given the already high intake (three times the RNI) of some men.

It is possible for public health campaigns to make an impact on iron deficiency anaemia. In Sweden, the prevalence of iron deficiency was reduced by around three-quarters between 1965 and 1975. This was achieved by increased levels of fortification of flour, increased vitamin C intakes and the widespread use of iron supplements; in 1974 sales of pharmaceutical iron preparations in Sweden amounted to around 6 mg per head per day (see Anon, 1980).

Acute iron poisoning usually occurs when children take iron-containing supplements intended for their parents; it is the most common cause of accidental poisoning in children. The lethal dose in infants is 200–300 mg/kg body weight. Somewhere around 100 g is a lethal dose in adults, although treatment can make this survivable. The first obvious side-effects of more moderate iron supplements are gastrointestinal because it is an irritant of the gut: symptoms like constipation or diarrhoea, nausea and vomiting. At high doses there is damage to organs, especially cirrhosis of the liver.

Chronic iron overload is usually caused by infusion of blood or therapeutic iron. It is rarely caused by oral supplements unless the individual has a genetic susceptibility to iron overload. If total body iron exceeds 10 g then iron overload is classed as severe; apart from gastrointestinal symptoms it will also result in organ and tissue damage, especially cirrhosis of the liver. A condition known as hereditary haemochromatosis makes people highly susceptible to iron overload; it is inherited by a recessive autosomal gene and affects around 1 in 250 of Caucasian populations.

Mean adult intake of dietary iron in the UK is 12 mg/day, with the highest consumers taking in more than double this amount; that is, around three times the adult male RNI. Supplements may provide a further 20 mg/day or even more in individuals with a particular condition, such as pregnancy. This makes estimated total maximum exposure 44 mg/day (FSA, 2003). The low incidence of iron poisoning from oral supplements is partly because absorption efficiency decreases once iron stores are full. Constipation or diarrhoea and perhaps nausea and/or vomiting are the most common side-effects of iron supplements. FSA (2003) suggested that supplements of up to 17 mg/day of iron should cause no adverse effects among the bulk of the population who are not genetically susceptible to iron overload, as are those with hereditary haemochromatosis and perhaps those who are heterozygous carriers of the gene for this condition. A safety factor of threefold was used in reaching this figure of 17 mg/day (i.e. a third of 50 mg/day) because of the paucity of relevant data about the long-term consequences of large iron supplements in people who are not iron deficient.

Magnesium

COMA (1991) set RNI for magnesium at 300 mg/day for men and 270 mg/day for women; corresponding RDA in the USA are 400 mg/day for men and 310 mg/day for women. Leafy vegetables, whole grains, nuts, seafood and legumes are good dietary sources of magnesium. Drinking water may contain up to 50 mg/L of magnesium in some hard-water areas. Magnesium is present in many multinutrient supplements and is also available as a single supplement or in combination with calcium and vitamin D. Low magnesium intakes were noted several times in the discussion of general micronutrient adequacy in Chapter 2, as summarised below:

- Average recorded intakes of UK young and middle-aged women were below the RNI.
- 13% of women and 9% of men had intakes of magnesium that were below the LRNI and so were classified as inadequate; the prevalence of inadequacy was highest in the younger age groups of adults.
- Substantial numbers of older children recorded inadequate magnesium intakes.
- Around a quarter of elderly Britons recorded intakes that were below the LRNI.

This would suggest that purely on the grounds of ensuring nutritional adequacy, there is a *prima facie* case for the use of magnesium-containing supplements by many adults and older children in the UK. Of course, this presupposes that the dietary standards are an accurate reflection of the real need for magnesium.

Hundreds of enzyme reactions in the cell are magnesium dependent for one of two reasons:

- Magnesium binds to the substrate and so increases its affinity for the enzyme, e.g. magnesium complexes with ATP that enables kinases to bind to the ATP.
- Magnesium binds directly to the enzyme to make it active, e.g. RNA and DNA polymerase.

Most major metabolic pathways have magnesium-dependent enzymes, including the glycolytic pathway, the citric acid cycle, gluconeogenesis, β-oxidation of fatty acids and the pentose phosphate pathway. Magnesium deficiency has been experimentally induced in both experimental animals and human volunteers. The consequences of induced magnesium deficiency include low blood levels of magnesium, potassium and calcium; muscle weakness; spasms; personality changes; nausea, vomiting and anorexia. These symptoms regress during magnesium repletion. Primary symptomatic dietary deficiency of magnesium is rarely reported, but it is a fairly common consequence of other acute and chronic conditions such as renal disease, uncontrolled diabetes mellitus, alcoholism and a range of gastrointestinal conditions; such conditions increase losses of magnesium or reduce the amount absorbed from the intestine. There is a rare congenital condition in which there is a specific defect in magnesium absorption from the gut: primary idiopathic hypomagnesaemia.

As noted earlier, suboptimal intake of magnesium seems to be a common occurrence and magnesium depletion is a secondary consequence of a range of common conditions. There are numerous claims that adverse long-term consequences are associated with low magnesium intake or that magnesium supplements may have beneficial effects, including those listed below:

- It has been suggested that low magnesium status may increase the risk of coronary heart disease and this is one of the explanations offered for the slightly lower incidence of coronary heart disease in hard-water areas. There is no substantial evidence to support this suggestion and COMA (1994) did not mention magnesium in its review of 'nutritional aspects of cardiovascular disease'.
- Magnesium supplements have been claimed to reduce blood pressure, although several double-blind, placebo-controlled trials have failed to find any effect of magnesium supplements on blood pressure in healthy subjects or those with moderate hypertension (e.g. Cappuccio *et al.*, 1985; Sacks *et al.*, 1998). In a meta-analysis of 12 trials, Dickinson *et al.* (2009) found that magnesium supplements given for 8–26 weeks did not reduce systolic blood pressure, but did have a small but statistically significant effect in lowering diastolic blood pressure. These authors noted that trial quality was often low and that there was heterogeneity between trials, which makes bias a likely reason for the apparent lowering of diastolic blood pressure.
- Magnesium supplements have been claimed to be beneficial in reducing migraine headaches and symptoms of the pre-menstrual syndrome and in enhancing athletic performance – there is no substantial or consistent evidence to support these claims.

In general, the evidence to support the beneficial effects of 'extra' magnesium in the form of supplements is weak or preliminary in nature. Rude and Shils (2006) give a detailed review of the nutritional and physiological aspects of magnesium.

Around 60% of the body's magnesium is located in bones and hypocalcaemia is a manifestation of magnesium deficiency. Magnesium is required for both the secretion of parathyroid hormone and its effects on target tissues; it is also required for the hydroxylation of vitamin D to 25-hydroxy-vitamin D in the liver. This has led to suggestions that there is a link between magnesium status and osteoporosis and thus that improving magnesium status might help to prevent this condition, although there is no substantial evidence to support this.

Dietary supplements may provide up to 750 mg/day of magnesium, but doses are usually in the range of 100–500 mg/day. While when administered orally magnesium is generally considered as having low toxic potential, FSA (2003) felt that it did not have sufficient data to enable it to set s safe upper level for magnesium consumption. FSA suggested that for guidance purposes only, supplements of 400 mg/day should not have any significant adverse effects in healthy people. The most common symptom of excessive magnesium consumption is diarrhoea; many laxatives and antacids contain magnesium salts and Epsom salt is magnesium sulphate.

Manganese

Manganese is classified as an essential nutrient that is required in trace amounts. COMA (1991) felt that there was insufficient data to set firm dietary standards for manganese, but it suggested a safe intake for adults of at least 1.4 mg/day (1.8 mg/day in the USA).

There are several important manganese-containing enzymes, including pyruvate carboxylase, which is important in gluconeogenesis, and mitochondrial superoxide dismutase, which is important in removing the damaging superoxide free radical (see Chapter 5). Large numbers of enzymes are activated by manganese, although many, but not all, of these are also activated by other metals, especially magnesium. Manganese deficiency has been experimentally induced in several animal species, although deficiency symptoms in humans that can unequivocally be attributed to manganese deficiency are extremely rare; even the few potential examples are restricted to individuals consuming manganese-deficient, semi-purified diets or receiving TPN containing no manganese.

Average intakes in the UK are estimated to be around 5 mg/day, with as much as half of this coming from tea; the highest UK consumers take in over 8 mg/day from their diet. Given the lack of any spontaneous examples of manganese deficiency and given that average intakes are more than three times the UK safe intake, there seems to be no need for supplemental manganese to 'prevent deficiency'. There are suggestions that manganese supplements may be useful in some cases of diabetes and arthritis, but there are only anecdotal observations to support these claims and there is insufficient evidence to support claims that it may be useful in maintaining bone health (COMA, 1998b).

In the UK, manganese is present in some multinutrient supplements and some mineral supplements at levels of up to 10 mg/day. COMA (1991) and Buchman (2006) conclude that orally consumed manganese has very low toxicity, although poisoning by inhalation of airborne manganese does sometimes occur in miners and industrial workers, in whom it produces neurological symptoms similar to those seen in Parkinson's disease.

FSA (2003) reviews several studies of people chronically consuming high amounts of manganese in drinking water or prolonged use of manganese supplements. It concludes that there is insufficient evidence to set safe upper levels for manganese, but it suggests that a total intake of 12 mg/day would be unlikely to have any adverse effects in most adults. Older people may be more sensitive to manganese toxicity and so it reduced this value to 8.7 mg/day in the elderly. People consuming average amounts of dietary manganese and the maximum supplement dose will consume considerably more than these admittedly tentative and conservative upper limits. Heavy tea consumers would also take in considerably more manganese than average, but whether this is bio-available or physiologically significant is unknown.

Molybdenum

Molybdenum is recognised as an essential micronutrient. COMA (1991) set a safe adult intake for molybdenum of 50–400 μg/day (WHO set 100–300 μg/day and in the USA the recommendation is 45 μg/day).

Experimental molybdenum deficiency syndromes have been described in animals and molybdenum-responsive dietary deficiency has been reported in a single patient receiving prolonged TPN that was molybdenum free. Molybdenum is an enzyme co-factor for several enzymes, including:

- Aldehyde oxidase, which oxidises and detoxifies various nucleotide bases produced from nucleic acid breakdown.
- Xanthine oxidase, which is involved in uric acid synthesis (a product of purine breakdown).
- Sulphite oxidase, which converts sulphite (from sulphur-containing amino acid metabolism) to sulphate.

In the one patient with established primary molybdenum deficiency there was low urinary excretion of sulphate and uric acid, but increased excretion of sulphite and xanthine.

In the UK average dietary intake of molybdenum is estimated at 110 μg/day, with the highest consumers taking in around double this amount. Food supplements in the UK may contain up to 330 μg/day, giving a total estimated maximum exposure of 550 μg/day. FSA (2003) felt that it had insufficient data to make any judgement about safe maximum intakes for molybdenum. COMA (1991) suggested that intakes of 10–15 mg/day may result in altered nucleotide metabolism and reduced copper availability.

Eckhert (2006) suggests that molybdenum is a relatively non-toxic element and that levels far in excess of current maxima from food and supplements are required to produce toxic symptoms. As molybdenum deficiency does not occur and there is no significant evidence for benefit from supplemental doses, there seems to be no justification for the use of molybdenum supplements, even though they are probably safe.

Potassium

COMA (1991) set an RNI for potassium of 3500 mg/day for all people over 15 years of age (4700 mg/day for adults in the USA); the LRNI is 2000 mg/day in the UK. The richest dietary sources of potassium are fruit and vegetables, although potassium is present in all animal and plant tissues and in milk. One of the suggested advantages of consuming diets high in fruit and vegetables is that they would also provide a good intake of potassium. In the UK, food supplements may contain up to 200 mg of potassium and some licensed medicines (e.g. oral rehydration preparations) may contain more. Potassium chloride is widely used in salt-replacement products. The contribution of drinking water to total potassium intake is small.

The body of a 70 kg man contains around 135 g of potassium and more than 95% of this potassium is intracellular. The amount of potassium in a healthy person's body is a function of their lean tissue mass and indeed, measures of total body potassium are used to estimate lean tissue mass and body composition. Potassium is the major cation in intracellular fluid and sodium is the major cation in extracellular fluid. This differential distribution of cations across the cell membrane is maintained by the constant use of energy in cellular pumps, which pump sodium out of cells in exchange for potassium into them. This differential distribution of cations is crucial to many cellular functions, including generation and conduction of action potentials, active transport processes and the maintenance of acid-base balance.

Given the ubiquitous presence of potassium in all types of foodstuffs, overt primary dietary deficiency is an unlikely occurrence. Nevertheless, in the overview of micronutrient adequacy in Chapter 2, it was noted several times that relatively large numbers of British people have recorded intakes that are below those set by the dietary standards panels in the UK and the USA.

- The average recorded potassium intakes of adults are below the RNI and in the case of women substantially below it.
- 19% of women and 9% of men have potassium intakes below the LRNI; this inadequacy was particularly concentrated in the younger age groups.
- Substantial numbers of older UK children recorded potassium intakes below the LRNI.
- Around a quarter of elderly Britons had potassium intakes that were less than the LRNI.

Even though this apparent deficiency is not overtly symptomatic, these figures do seem to provide a *prima facie* case for relatively widespread use of potassium-containing supplements; certainly it suggests that multinutrient supplements should contain potassium. Additionally, low blood potassium can result from a number of medical conditions, including prolonged diarrhoea, vomiting or laxative abuse, and excessive secretion of aldosterone or other hormones with mineralocorticoid activity. Low blood potassium leads to muscle weakness, changes in cardiac function, reduced gut motility, alkalosis, depression and confusion.

Low potassium intake is likely to be a marker for low consumption of fruit and vegetables and/or low recorded total food intake. Low potassium intake is just one of several adverse consequences of low fruit and vegetable intake and many would suggest one of the least significant; potassium supplements would not compensate for the other problems that accompany low fruit and vegetable intake. Encouraging increased fruit and vegetable consumption would be more productive than focusing on potassium *per se*.

High sodium intake is generally accepted as a major causative factor in essential hypertension and most dietary recommendations suggest a reduction in total salt intake in order to reduce the incidence and consequences of high blood pressure; for example COMA (1991, 1994). Sodium reduction, coupled with better weight control and alcohol moderation, is the main focus for reducing blood pressure via health promotion. There is nonetheless a substantial body of evidence to indicate that high potassium intake may have some effect in reducing average blood pressure and that potassium supplements may reduce blood pressure (Cappuccio and MacGregor, 1991; COMA, 1991, 1994). In its report on the nutritional aspects of cardiovascular disease, COMA (1994) recommended that potassium intake should be increased to a population average of 3.5 g/day by increasing consumption of fruit and vegetables. Dickinson *et al.* (2009) did a meta-analysis of six randomised controlled trials of potassium supplements in the treatment of high blood pressure. They did not find a statistically significant effect overall, but the trials were small, of short duration and there was a big disparity between the results of individual trials.

FSA (2003) estimated that total maximum potassium intake in the UK was around 5 g/day from all sources and that average food intake was around 2.8 g/day. It felt unable to set a safe upper level for potassium, but concluded that supplemental doses of 3.7 g/day appear to have no adverse effects.

Selenium

The RNI for selenium in the UK for men is 75 μg/day and for women is 60 μg/day; the corresponding American RDA is 55 μg/day for both men and women. Selenium is found in meat (particularly offal), fish, eggs and cereals and it is largely present as the selenium-containing amino acids selenocysteine and selenomethionine. Selenium has been widely used as a nutritional supplement both in general multinutrient supplements and more specific supplements, for example in combination with the antioxidant (ACE) vitamins. It is present in food supplements in the UK at doses up to 300 μg/day.

Selenium is present in variable amounts in soil and thus in plants. In humans, selenium is incorporated into the amino acid cysteine to give selenocysteine and this in turn is incorporated into a number of selenoproteins. Several of these selenoproteins are important in systems that prevent damage to tissues by oxygen free radicals, such as glutathione peroxidases. The topic of antioxidants and free radicals is discussed more fully in Chapter 5. Another selenoprotein is involved in the conversion of the thyroid hormone thyroxin to the more active hormone tri-iodothryronine.

Deficiency of selenium is believed to result in a condition called Keshan disease in which there is progressive degeneration of the heart muscle (cardiomyopathy). Details of the relationship of this and other conditions to selenium deficiency may be found in Burk and Levander (2006). It has been claimed that because of its established role in antioxidant systems, supplements of selenium may prevent tissue damage by free radicals and thus have cancer-preventing and other beneficial effects in conditions where damage by free radicals is implicated. The COMA report on Nutritional Aspects of Cancer did not find any substantial evidence to support these claims, however (COMA, 1998a).

The average intake from food in the UK is 39 µg/day, with the highest consumers taking in more than 100 µg/day from their food. The food table database for selenium is incomplete and this will affect the reliability of these estimates. Combined with the maximum of 300 µg/day from food supplements, this gives a total maximum exposure in the UK of around 400 µg/day. Chronic selenium poisoning occurs in areas where the total selenium intake is above 900 µg/day and so FSA (2003) set a safe upper level for daily lifetime consumption of 450 µg/day. The first signs of selenium poisoning (selenosis) in humans are skin lesions and changes to the hair and nails, followed by a range of neurological symptoms.

Zinc

Zinc is clearly established as an essential nutrient. In the UK the RNI for adult men is 9.5 mg/day and for women 7 mg/day; the equivalent RDA in the USA are 11 mg/day and 8 mg/day respectively. Meat, whole-grain cereals, pulses and shellfish are good dietary sources of zinc and the mineral is found in all living tissue, where it is concentrated in cell nuclei. It is best absorbed from meat and fish. Phytate present in cereals may inhibit zinc absorption, but this is destroyed in the leavening of bread with yeast.

Zinc is important in cell division and there are more than 200 zinc-containing enzymes, which are involved in DNA synthesis and in the synthesis and metabolic breakdown of the three macronutrients. Superoxide dismutase, one of the key enzymes involved in the disposal of oxygen free radicals, is a zinc-containing enzyme.

In experimental animals, feeding a zinc-deficient diet rapidly leads to anorexia, reduced food intake and a reduction in growth that is only partly explained by the reduction in food intake. In other micronutrient deficiency states, there is usually a marked decline in tissue levels (stores?) of the nutrient before other manifestations of deficiency become apparent. In the case of zinc, the reduced food intake and growth are regarded as a homeostatic response to conserve the tissue zinc for its essential metabolic functions.

In studies carried out in Colorado, USA it has been shown that mild zinc deficiency may be a contributory factor in the low growth rate of some children and that zinc supplements may have a significant impact on final height in children who have a low height for age. Healthy children who had low height for age were selected for a double-blind, placebo-controlled trial of zinc supplements on their growth. Small zinc supplements (5 mg/day) increased height significantly in these growth-retarded children as compared to children receiving a placebo. Parallel studies of zinc supplements in children who were randomly selected (i.e. not selected on the basis of height) did not show any impact of zinc supplements. Some trials have shown reduced morbidity and mortality from infections and neuropsychiatric benefits of zinc supplements in children whose growth is improved by zinc supplements (reviewed by King and Keen, 1999; King and Cousins, 2006). In a review, Brown *et al.* (2009) confirmed the potential benefits of zinc supplements on growth and infection rates in children over 12 months of age, but found no neuropsychiatric benefits, although there was very limited data on this latter aspect.

Other manifestations of experimental zinc deficiency include reduced immune function, slow healing, hypogonadism and delayed sexual maturation, skin lesions, hair loss and other lesions in epithelial tissues. Zinc deficiency in pregnant animals leads to increased numbers of fetal abnormalities, including cleft lip and palate and spina bifida.

Severe deficiency of zinc in humans has been experimentally induced, and occurs when zinc-free infusions have been used in total parenteral nutrition and also in a rare inherited condition called acrodermatitis enteropathica, in which there is impaired absorption of zinc. This latter condition can be controlled by oral zinc supplements. In the 1960s and 1970s many cases of zinc-responsive growth failure and hypogonadism were identified in parts of Egypt and rural Iran. Diets in these regions consisted largely of unleavened whole-grain bread and it is thought that the high phytic acid content of this bread was an important precipitating factor, because it impairs zinc absorption. Note that phytic acid is destroyed during the fermentation process when leavened bread is made.

Zinc was highlighted several times in the discussion in Chapter 2 on the micronutrient adequacy of different age groups within the UK. Recorded average intakes of zinc are only just above the RNI for young and middle-aged men and women and slightly below it in older adults. In the UK the RNI for zinc is not increased during pregnancy, although in the USA it is increased by around 40%. For lactating women the RNI for zinc is more than doubled; as food intake only increases by a quarter, this would suggest that average intakes are substantially below the RNI. Average zinc intakes of pre-school children in the UK are below the RNI and substantial numbers of older children have intakes that are below the LRNI. In elderly people, especially elderly men, there is evidence of widespread zinc insufficiency: 8% of free-living men have zinc intakes that are below the LRNI, rising to 13% in those living in institutions for the elderly, and 15% of the institutionalised elderly show biochemical evidence of zinc insufficiency.

Zinc supplements have been investigated for their potential value in the following conditions and circumstances:

- In treating some cases of anorexia nervosa, presumably because anorexia is an early symptom of zinc insufficiency.
- In the promotion of wound healing.

- In reducing the symptoms of the common cold and more generally in improving immune function.
- In treating male infertility, presumably because hypogonadism and infertility were reported along with severe growth retardation in areas of endemic zinc deficiency in Egypt and Iran.

Given the known effects of zinc insufficiency on wound healing and immune function, it would seem prudent to ensure that people with injuries, at high risk of infection or undergoing surgery have good nutritional status for zinc; small supplements might be the most convenient way of ensuring this. The interpretation of any studies indicating beneficial effects of zinc supplements on wound healing and infection risk would be dependent on assessing initial zinc status prior to supplementation; that is, is the supplement correcting a deficiency or an addition to the normal estimated need?

The average intake of zinc from food in the UK is 10 mg/day, with the highest consumers getting over 17 mg/day. Zinc intake from drinking water is normally very low, but occasionally it may contain up to a further 10 mg/day. Supplements of zinc are widely available both in the form of multinutrient supplements and in more specialised or even single supplements. In the UK supplements may provide up to a maximum of 50 mg/day, giving a total maximum exposure of 77 mg/day (FSA, 2003).

High doses of iron may also interfere with zinc absorption and probably vice versa. Zinc supplements can cause gastrointestinal symptoms, especially if they are taken without food. Excess zinc interferes with the absorption of copper and so excessive use of zinc may precipitate a secondary deficiency of copper; this copper deficiency unfavourably affects the blood lipoprotein profile, decreases glucose tolerance and may produce heart arrhythmia. Excess of zinc also causes a decrease in the activity of the enzyme superoxide dismutase in red blood cells, an enzyme involved in the disposal of free radicals; this effect may be detected with doses of over 50 mg/day.

FSA (2003) set a safe upper limit for lifetime consumption of supplemental zinc of 25 mg/day; that is, about half the current maximum level in supplements. It chose this dose by halving the dose above which the effects of zinc on copper uptake and erythrocyte superoxide dismutase activity start to become apparent.

5 Free Radicals and Antioxidants

Introduction

Antioxidants and antioxidant systems prevent acute damage to health by quenching the oxidative free radicals that can damage cellular components. It is also widely believed that chronic degenerative diseases like cancer, atherosclerosis and even ageing itself may be the result of cumulative oxidative damage to cellular components.

Several vitamins and minerals have established roles as antioxidants or as essential factors necessary for the proper functioning of antioxidant enzyme systems, for example vitamin C, vitamin E and selenium. Many other dietary antioxidants are not recognised as true essential nutrients. It is now widely believed that these other substances in food that are not strictly 'essential' but have antioxidant activity may contribute to optimal long-term health by also reducing oxidative damage to cell components.

Antioxidants are discussed generally in this chapter whether essential nutrients or not. Examples of non-nutrient antioxidants are given below:

- The carotenoid pigments found in most dark green, red or yellow fruits and vegetables. Some of these, like β-carotene, can be converted by humans to retinol and so have vitamin A activity, but many do not. Antioxidant activity is independent of vitamin A activity.
- The flavonoids and other phenols and polyphenols found in foods such as grapes, nuts, many other fruits, green tea, olive oil and red wine (see Chapter 8 for more details of the categories of plant phenols and polyphenols).

Many antioxidant compounds are concentrated in foods from the fruit and vegetable groups and there are active campaigns in several industrialised countries to encourage people to eat more fruits and vegetables, for example the 'eat five a day' campaign in the UK. One of the suggested explanations for why high fruit and vegetable consumption is consistently associated with reduced risk of cancer and heart disease is their varied and abundant antioxidant content. Many foods are now marketed on the basis of their antioxidant content, some almost entirely on the basis of their claims to improve health, and some are relatively recent additions to

Dietary Supplements and Functional Foods, 2nd Edition. Geoffrey P. Webb.
© 2011 Blackwell Publishing Ltd.

British supermarket shelves, for example certain exotic berries and fruit juices (see the brief discussion of 'superfoods' in Chapter 9). Many dietary supplements are also, at least partly, marketed on the basis of their potential antioxidant activity. A major British mail-order supplier claims antioxidant activity (justifiably) for all of the following, either alone or in various combinations:

- Various combinations of essential vitamins and minerals, especially the so-called ACE vitamins: vitamins A (as β-carotene), C and E and selenium.
- Co-enzyme Q_{10} or ubiquinone (see Chapter 7).
- Alpha lipoic acid, ALA (see Chapter 7).
- Acetyl-L-carnitine, ALC (see Chapter 7).
- Zinc.
- Carotenoids like lutein and lycopene.
- French pine bark extract, containing a variety of bioflavonoids.
- Bilberry extract.
- Goji berry extract.
- Green tea extract.
- Grape seed extract.
- Pomegranate extract.
- Turmeric extract.
- Acai berry extracts.

It is interesting to note how much some of these tablets contain. For example, standard bilberry extract pills contain the equivalent of 500 mg (0.5 g) of whole fruit and the high-strength tablets 5000 mg (5 g). The goji berry tablets contain the equivalent of 1.5 g of berries and the acai berry extract the equivalent of 2 g of whole berries. Two blueberries taken from my fridge weighed 3 g!

The free radical or oxidant theory of disease

Free radicals or reactive oxygen species are highly reactive chemical entities that are produced as byproducts of the normal oxidative processes in cells. They are unstable and highly reactive species because they have an unpaired electron, whereas in stable chemical species the electrons are arranged in pairs that orbit around the atomic nuclei in opposite directions. (Note that nitric oxide is also a highly reactive and abundant free radical that is produced by many cells and has a number of important signalling functions in many physiological processes.) Free radicals are capable of reacting with many of the cells' components, for example DNA, proteins and lipids, and in reacting with these cellular components they may change the normal functioning of these molecules and so initiate pathological changes. Some examples are listed below (see Thomas, 2006 for further chemical details of these processes):

- Free radicals can cause breaks in the DNA chain as well as base changes and these mutations might initiate carcinogenesis. Modified bases are found in DNA as a result of oxidative damage, for example 8-hydroxy guanine and thymine glycol. Estimation of the levels of modified bases in urine can be used to assess the amount of oxidative damage to DNA in animal experiments.

- Peroxidation of polyunsaturated fatty acid residues in membranes can lead to major impairment of membrane function. Peroxidation of these lipids in food (rancidity) will seriously impair its flavour and consumption of rancid fat may lead to the consumed peroxides being incorporated into membranes. Measurement of lipid peroxidation products in plasma, especially malondialdehyde, is used as a measure of 'oxidative stress'.
- Oxidation of polyunsaturated fatty acid residues in LDL-cholesterol (see Chapter 6) can increase its potential to induce arteriosclerosis and increase the risk of cardiovascular diseases.
- Hyaluronic acid is a complex polysaccharide found in connective tissue and synovial fluid. It is viscous and acts as a lubricant in joints. Free radicals can degrade hyaluronic acid and inflammation leads to reduced amounts of synovial fluid in joints, which it is suggested may be the result of free radicals produced by neutrophils at the site of inflammation.
- According to Thomas (2006), free radicals can damage proteins in one of three ways:
- By causing fragmentation of proteins at vulnerable points in the chain.
- By irreversible oxidative damage to sites where metal ions normally bind in the functioning protein.
- By oxidising sulfhydryl (S-H) groups on cysteine or sometimes methionine residues. In some cases these sites can be re-reduced and so this can be part of a protective mechanism to mop up free radicals. For example, glutathione is an abundant cellular tri-peptide (glutamate-cysteine-glycine) that can be oxidised by free radicals and then the reduced form can be regenerated by the enzyme glutathione reductase.

Reactions of free radicals involve them gaining or donating an electron and thus they may produce another unstable product with an unpaired electron, which is also highly reactive and thus they have the potential to initiate damaging chain reactions. For example, interaction between membrane polyunsaturated fatty acid residues and the hydroxyl radical produces a lipid peroxyl radical, which can then interact with another fatty acid residue to produce a stable lipid peroxide and another lipid peroxyl radical and so on. Unless this chain is broken and the free radical quenched, this can result in the oxidation of many polyunsaturated fatty acid residues and alteration of the membrane's function. Quenching would occur as a result of scavenging of the lipid free radical by vitamin E or by the interaction of two lipid radicals to convert the two fatty acids to aldehydes and release the product malondialdehyde, mentioned earlier as a marker of oxidative stress.

Long-term cumulative oxidative damage caused by free radicals has been suggested to be important in the causation of many chronic diseases, including cancer, arteriosclerosis, arthritis, cataract, age-related macular degeneration (degeneration of the central part of the retina leaving the sufferer with just peripheral vision) and so on. It is also suggested that cumulative free radical damage may be responsible for many of the degenerative changes associated with ageing.

Oxygen free radicals are continually being produced in healthy cells and their production is accelerated in injured, infected or inflamed tissues. They are produced, for example:

- As a by-product of the electron transport chain that generates most of the energy (ATP) in aerobic metabolism.
- The superoxide radical is produced during oxygen-haemoglobin dissociation.
- Neutrophil leukocytes that infiltrate any injured, infected or inflamed tissues generate large amounts of oxygen free radicals, which it is suggested are essential for killing ingested micro-organisms, and these leukocytes may also secrete them into surrounding tissues.

It is also widely held that a number of potentially harmful environmental factors exert their harmful effects by increasing the generation of these free radicals. The excess free radicals produced by exposure to these harmful environmental factors produce cellular damage and are ultimately responsible for at least some of the acute and chronic consequences of the exposure. Examples of these harmful environmental factors include exposure to cigarette smoke, environmental pollutants, ionising radiations (including sunlight), exposure to high oxygen tension and some chemicals.

This 'free radical theory of disease' has been increasingly accepted and promulgated since the 1970s. Not only are many foods and dietary supplements promoted on the basis of their potential to quench or reduce the formation of these free radicals, a number of drugs have also been developed to stop production of free radicals or enhance their removal. The belief that neutrophil leukocytes kill micro-organisms and other 'foreign bodies' by generating an oxidative pulse of free radicals has been a key piece of the supporting argument for this theory of oxidative damage producing chronic disease. In layperson's terms, if these free radicals are powerful enough to kill tough micro-organisms then they must have the potential to do serious harm to human cells and tissues.

Mechanisms for limiting free radical damage

As free radicals are normal but harmful byproducts of cellular processes, mechanisms have evolved that 'quench' them and limit the damage they can do to tissue components. Some of the body's antioxidant systems are listed below:

- The enzyme superoxide dismutase (SOD) reduces the superoxide radical to hydrogen peroxide. There are several variants of this enzyme: the SOD present in the cytoplasm is a copper–zinc-requiring enzyme, whereas that in mitochondria requires manganese.

- The enzyme glutathione peroxidase is a selenium-containing enzyme that reduces hydrogen peroxide (a powerful oxidising agent) to water and in this reaction glutathione is oxidised.
- The enzyme catalase is a haem-containing protein that converts hydrogen peroxide to water and oxygen.
- The enzyme glutathione reductase converts oxidised glutathione (back) to its reduced state, which is required for glutathione peroxidase to function.
- The essential nutrients selenium, zinc, copper, manganese and riboflavin can all have co-factor functions for one of the above enzymes.
- Vitamin E, the carotenoids and co-enzyme Q_{10} (ubiquinone) are lipid soluble antioxidants present in membranes, whereas vitamin C is a water-soluble antioxidant and is the first antioxidant in plasma to be depleted during oxidative stress.

It should be noted that vitamin C is used by food manufacturers as a water-soluble antioxidant; that is, a preservative that slows the oxidative spoilage of foods. Vitamin E is used as a lipid-soluble antioxidant to prevent fatty foods becoming rancid. This demonstrates the antioxidant potential of these vitamins. Details of the chemical mechanisms involved in the quenching of free radicals by vitamins and the carotenoids can be found in Ball (2004).

In addition to these antioxidant systems, there are also mechanisms that can repair the damage caused by these free radicals, for example:

- DNA repair enzymes
- selenium-containing enzymes that remove lipid peroxides

In the tissues of a healthy, well-nourished person, one would expect that these quenching and repair mechanisms would largely counteract the effects of free radicals. Under some circumstances the production of free radicals may exceed the capacity of the quenching and repair mechanisms and the surplus free radicals may cause tissue damage and so initiate degenerative changes and disease.

According to this scenario, all of the following circumstances might be expected to lead to increased free radical damage and thus to increased degenerative change, which may ultimately manifest as cancer, heart disease, retinopathy, arthritis or simply more rapid ageing:

- A diet that is low in one or more of the vitamins and minerals that are essential components of the physiological mechanisms for quenching free radicals, e.g. vitamin E, vitamin C, selenium or zinc.
- A diet that is low in the other plant chemicals that, while not recognised as essential nutrients, may nonetheless have innate and useful antioxidant activity, e.g. the carotenoids, flavonoids and other polyphenols.
- Some genetic defect in one of the physiological antioxidant or repair mechanisms or perhaps a genetic defect that leads to accelerated production of free radicals.

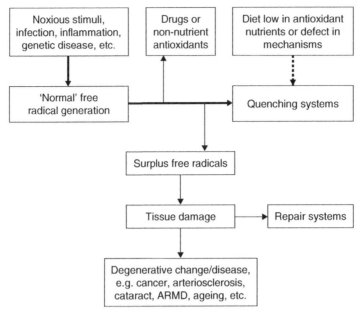

ARMD, age-related macular degeneration.

Figure 5.1   The 'free radical theory of disease' and some of the factors that may enhance or reduce free radical damage.

- Exposure to environmental factors that accelerate free radical production, such as excessive sunbathing or use of tanning lamps, cigarette smoking, certain chemical agents or exposure to other ionising radiation.
- Infection, injury or any noxious stimulus that leads to (chronic) inflammation and thus to increased generation of free radicals by the white cells that infiltrate the area in response to the inflammatory stimulus.

Conversely, certain circumstances like those listed below might be speculated to minimise the damage done by free radicals and thus to slow down the normal degenerative changes associated with ageing in tissues, and/or to ameliorate the effects of some of the influences listed above that might otherwise increase free radical damage and degenerative changes:

- Drugs that reduce free radical production or 'quench' them.
- Good intakes through food and/or supplements of antioxidants normally found in edible material.

Figure 5.1 summarises the sequence of events envisaged in the free radical theory of disease production and also summarises some of the environmental, dietary and physiological factors that can influence the amount of damage caused by free radicals and the chance of this leading to an increased risk of degenerative

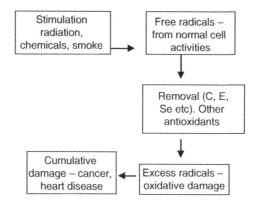

Figure 5.2   A highly simplified diagram to illustrate the free radical theory of disease (Webb, 2006).

disease. A much simplified version of the free radical theory of disease is shown in Figure 5.2.

For those dietary antioxidants that are known to be co-factors for antioxidant enzyme systems (e.g. selenium and zinc), one might expect the potential benefits to plateau once enough is available to maximise the activity of the relevant enzyme. That is, deficiency would compromise enzyme activity and increase free radical damage, but large surpluses would not be expected to offer additional benefits once the needs of the enzyme were satisfied. For those antioxidants that have innate antioxidant activity (like vitamins C and E, the carotenoids, flavonoids and other polyphenols), there seems to be no theoretical reason why there should be such a defined ceiling for their beneficial antioxidant potential.

This does not mean, of course, that very high doses of these antioxidants can only do more good and have no potential to do harm. For example, evidence will be discussed later in the chapter indicating that large supplements of β-carotene may cause long-term harmful effects under some circumstances. The COMA (1998a) report on the nutritional aspects of cancer development specifically counsels against the use of β-carotene supplements and generally encourages readers 'to exercise caution in the use of purified supplements of other micronutrients'.

Diets with plentiful supplies of (antioxidant-rich) fruits and vegetables are associated with a reduced risk of chronic diseases

The fruit and vegetable food group(s) are a major source of the essential nutrients and other plant chemicals with proposed antioxidant potential. There is overwhelming epidemiological evidence that diets with a plentiful supply of foods from the fruit and vegetable group(s) are associated with reduced risk of cancer, heart disease and the other degenerative diseases associated with ageing. It is generally assumed that this association is causal (i.e. that fruits and vegetables help prevent these diseases), hence the numerous officially sponsored health-promotion campaigns to encourage higher consumption (at least five portions a day) of fruits and vegetables. Note that possible alternative explanations for this association were mentioned in Chapter 1 (e.g. that high fruit and vegetable consumption may simply be an indicator of a generally healthy diet or perhaps even of a generally healthy lifestyle).

One widely promulgated explanation for this presumed causal association is that the high antioxidant content of fruits and vegetables is responsible for at least some of the reduced risk of chronic disease associated with eating good amounts of them. This argument, if correct, justifies the use of antioxidant supplements as being potentially able to reduce the risk of developing cancer, heart disease or any other degenerative condition that has been linked with free radical damage, such as age-related macular degeneration or even pre-eclampsia in pregnancy (see later in the chapter). A number of other observational studies also seem to support this hypothesis. There are numerous reports that high blood levels of antioxidants are associated with reduced risk of these diseases, for example:

- Gey *et al.* (1991) conducted a cohort study with 1600 middle-aged men from 16 European cities. They found an inverse relationship between blood levels of vitamin E and coronary heart disease mortality (i.e. an apparent protective effect of vitamin E).
- In a case-control study of 100 men with previously undiagnosed angina and 400 controls, Riemersma *et al.* (1991) found that blood levels of the antioxidant vitamins (β-carotene and vitamins C and E) were inversely related to risk of angina.
- Low blood levels of β-carotene and other carotenoids, especially lycopene, are associated with increased cancer risk (Ziegler, 1991).

Two large cohort studies have reported that high intake of vitamin E from supplements was associated with reduced rates of coronary heart disease, both in men (Rimm *et al.*, 1993) and in women (Stampfer *et al.*, 1993). There was no significant reduction in overall mortality in those taking supplements. Note that these were not randomised, controlled trials but epidemiological cohort studies, where the subjects using supplements were self-selecting. This means that there is the very real possibility of confounding variables being responsible for the apparent effects of the supplements, even though the authors will have tried as far as possible to correct for confounders. The supplement users were probably not representative of the total study populations in many respects; some of these differences would have been difficult for the authors to quantify and correct for.

What evidence is there that antioxidant supplements are beneficial or at least harmless?

Numerous trials with human subjects have been used to suggest that antioxidant supplements have beneficial effects. Many of these have had one or more of the following limitations:

- They have used small numbers of subjects.
- They have been of short duration.
- They have used reductionist outcome measures (e.g. a biochemical marker, a single symptom/disease).
- They have been poorly designed (e.g. not properly randomised and/or placebo-controlled).

Other studies have tested whether particular antioxidants can prevent the onset of chemically induced cancers in short-term studies with laboratory animals, or have looked at the effects on the growth of isolated human cancer cells in culture. Many studies have looked at the ability of these compounds to inhibit mutagenicity in bacteria, which is used as an indicator of anticancer potential. It must be said, however, that despite all these hundreds of studies spread over more than 30 years, there is still little direct holistic evidence that antioxidants, when take as supplements, afford any significant long-term protection against any major chronic disease or increase life expectancy in affluent, well-nourished populations.

COMA (1994), in its report on the nutritional aspects of cardiovascular disease, concluded that the evidence of a protective effect of the antioxidant vitamins E and C against cardiovascular disease was persuasive but not conclusive, and that it would be premature to make specific recommendations about increased intakes of these vitamins until several of the large controlled trials then underway (and now completed) were known. It warned that the use of pharmaceutical preparations containing high levels of vitamins cannot be assumed to be safe. It did, however, feel confident of recommending a diet rich in antioxidants; that is, rich in fruits and vegetables and containing nuts and seeds. Four years later, when some of the ongoing intervention trials referred to by COMA (1994) had been completed or terminated, the COMA (1998a) report on nutritional aspects of the development of cancer concluded that even though there is epidemiological evidence indicating that high intakes of the antioxidant vitamins (β-carotene, vitamin C and vitamin E) are associated with reduced cancer risk, most of the intervention trials conducted have failed to confirm a protective effect of these vitamins against cancer. They also recommend caution in the use of purified micronutrient supplements and counsel against the use of β-carotene supplements. They conclude also that there is insufficient evidence to reach any conclusions about the relationship between dietary selenium or zinc and cancer risk.

The Agency for Healthcare Research and Quality (AHRQ) commissioned a very extensive report into the efficacy and safety of supplemental antioxidants (vitamins C, E and coenzyme Q_{10}) for the prevention and treatment of cardiovascular disease (Shekelle *et al.*, 2003). The authors of this report sifted through well over 1000 articles that had addressed this topic and identified 144 clinical trials. Their conclusions after reviewing and reanalysing this information are summarised below:

- The evidence available in the literature does not support there being any benefit for supplements of vitamin E (either alone or in combination) on either cardiovascular or all-cause mortality.
- Likewise, there was no evidence of any harm caused by vitamin E supplements.
- More specific results gave no consistent evidential support for a beneficial effect on the incidence of fatal or non-fatal myocardial infarction.
- Vitamin E supplements do not appear to have any clinically or statistically significant effects on plasma lipids.
- Their conclusions for vitamin C were similar to those for vitamin E.
- For co-enzyme Q_{10} they found insufficient evidence to convincingly support or refute suggestions that supplements had any beneficial or harmful effects on cardiovascular outcomes. (Co-enzyme Q_{10} is discussed more specifically in Chapter 7.)

AHRQ also commissioned a similar report to investigate the effectiveness of these three antioxidants in the prevention and treatment of cancer (Coulter *et al.*, 2003). They also found no evidence to support the beneficial effects of vitamin E and/or vitamin C in the prevention of new tumours, the development of colonic polyps or in the treatment of patients with advanced cancer.

One often-cited intervention (experimental) study that did have an apparently positive outcome was conducted in the Linxian province of China. Using 30 000 middle-aged Chinese subjects, Blot *et al.* (1993) found that supplements containing β-carotene, selenium and vitamin E produced a substantial reduction in cancer incidence. However, people living in this area had low baseline intakes of micronutrients, and indeed micronutrient insufficiency was a suspected cause of the very high incidence of certain cancers in this region.

Over the last decade or so there have been several large, controlled trials that have found no indication of benefit afforded by various antioxidant supplements and even some indication that β-carotene supplements may be harmful under some circumstances. Several examples are briefly described below:

- In an Italian study of vitamin E and omega-3 polyunsaturated fatty acid supplements in 11 000 men who had had a previous myocardial infarction, there was no indication of any benefit from the vitamin E supplements after 3.5 years (GISSI, 1999). Note that this study did indicate beneficial effects of the fatty acid (fish oil) supplements and this is discussed in Chapter 6.
- A 12-year trial of β-carotene supplements in 22 000 American physicians found no benefits of these supplements on either cancer or heart disease incidence (Hennekens *et al.*, 1996).

- A study using male Finnish smokers found no evidence of benefit for either β-carotene or vitamin E. On the contrary, it reported significantly increased deaths from lung cancer, heart disease and strokes and increased total mortality in those taking β-carotene supplements (Group, 1994). Smokers were originally chosen as subjects for this study because it was perceived that they might have most to gain from antioxidant supplements.
- The CARET trial tested the effects of combined retinol and β-carotene supplements using 18 000 American men identified as being at high risk of lung cancer because of smoking or work exposure to asbestos. This study was terminated prematurely because rates of lung cancer were higher in the supplemented group than in the placebo group (Omenn *et al.*, 1996).
- Rapala *et al.* (1997) reported increased death rates from coronary heart disease in those subjects (smokers) given β-carotene supplements compared to those receiving either the placebo or vitamin E supplements.
- In a trial of vitamin E supplements in 2000 English men assessed from angiograms as being at high risk of having a heart attack, Stephens *et al.* (1996) reported that those taking the supplements had significantly fewer cardiac episodes, but cardiovascular death was not significantly reduced, in fact it was non-significantly higher.
- Lee *et al.* (2005) conducted a major randomised trial of vitamin E supplements compared to aspirin or a placebo in 40 000 healthy women aged over 45 years, with a follow-up time of over 10 years. They found no overall effect for vitamin E on major cardiovascular events, cancer, total mortality or mortality from either cardiovascular disease or cancer. They found no evidence to support healthy women being advised to take vitamin E supplements.

Vivekanathan *et al.* (2003) conducted a meta-analysis of seven large randomised trials of vitamin E supplements and eight trials of β-carotene supplements on long-term mortality and morbidity from cardiovascular disease. The vitamin E trials involved over 80 000 subjects and produced no evidence that these supplements reduced all-cause mortality, death from heart disease or from stroke. There was not even a non-significant trend supporting the use of vitamin E; the absolute death rate was very slightly, non-significantly higher in those receiving vitamin E supplements. There was also no evidence that vitamin E supplements conferred any benefits on patients who had already experienced a cardiovascular event. The analysis of the β-carotene trials suggested a small but statistically significant increase in all-cause mortality and cardiovascular deaths in those receiving supplements (doses were between 15 and 50 mg/day). Vivekanathan *et al.* (2003) conclude that these data provide no support for the routine use of vitamin E supplements and that they contra-indicate the use of supplements containing β-carotene. It was noted in Chapter 3 that in the light of such evidence about the potential for harm from β-carotene, FSA (2003) suggested a safe upper level for supplements of only 7 mg/day, compared to the 15–50 mg/day used in these studies.

A recent systematic review and meta-analysis of the effect of antioxidant supplements (β-carotene, vitamin A, vitamin C, vitamin E and selenium) on both healthy people (primary prevention trials) and those with a range of diseases (secondary prevention trials) has confirmed the lack of any demonstrable beneficial effect of taking these supplements (Bjelakovic *et al.*, 2008). These authors identified a total of 67 randomised trials involving about a quarter of a million participants; 21 of these trials included healthy people and 46 trials involved patients with a variety of different diseases. Overall the antioxidant supplements had no effect on mortality, but when the analysis was confined to the studies with low risk of bias, the supplements increased mortality by a small but statistically significant amount (relative risk 1.05 and 95% confidence intervals 1.02–1.08). The low-bias studies also found that vitamin A, β-carotene and vitamin E supplements increased mortality by small but statistically significant amounts, whereas vitamin C and selenium had no significant effect. There is now a substantial body of good-quality evidence to suggest that supplements of these nutrient antioxidants have no significant benefits on total, cardiovascular or cancer mortality, and that in some cases and under some circumstances these supplements are more likely to do harm than good.

As was also noted in Chapter 3, β-carotene has generally been regarded as non-toxic even in very high doses of 300 mg/day. There now seems to be disturbing evidence from intervention trials that chronic use of doses of supplements as low as 15 mg/day may lead to an increase in total mortality, heart disease mortality and, in particular, to an increased risk of lung cancer in those at high risk of this disease because of cigarette smoking or workplace exposure to asbestos. It is ironic that smokers and asbestos workers were initially chosen as subjects for these trials because it was thought that beneficial effects of antioxidants in general and β-carotene in particular might be more readily demonstrated in these high-risk subjects.

Several theories have been put forward to explain why β-carotene might increase the risk of lung cancer under some circumstances. Paolini *et al.* (1999) suggested that β-carotene might exert a co-carcinogenic effect by inducing enzymes that activate certain environmental carcinogens. This was based on short-term experiments with rats. This theory could reconcile the paradox that epidemiological studies are consistent with a protective effect of high β-carotene diets on cancer risk, whereas large supplements appear to increase lung cancer risk in those considered to be at high risk of developing this disease. Good intakes of antioxidants, including β-carotene, might prevent initial oxidative damage to DNA in the initiation of cancer, but high doses might activate carcinogens, including those from cigarette smoke, in those with high exposure to them.

Wang *et al.* (1999) used ferrets for some studies on the interaction between β-carotene and cigarette smoke, because they are thought to be a good animal model for humans in the way they absorb and metabolise β-carotene. They exposed groups of ferrets to either β-carotene supplements or cigarette smoke, both of these or neither of them. After six months of exposure the lungs of those receiving β-carotene supplements showed evidence of cell proliferation resembling the early stages of carcinogenesis. These changes were greater in those exposed to cigarette smoke and β-carotene, but were not seen in either the control group or the group exposed only to cigarette smoke.

Table 5.1 shows some of the individual chemicals and classes of chemicals found in edible material that are not classified as essential nutrients, but have nonetheless been claimed to have potentially beneficial antioxidant activity. The large number of potential antioxidants makes it highly improbable that a definitive demonstration of the benefit of any one of them in preventing chronic disease will be forthcoming in the medium term. Observational epidemiological methods can only provide evidence of association (not demonstrate cause and effect) and in any case would be largely unsuitable for pinpointing the likely long-term benefits (or harmful effects) of high consumption of any one of these. For example, an association between tomato consumption and some beneficial effect could be interpreted as evidence for a possible beneficial effect of lycopene, a powerful antioxidant carotenoid found in tomatoes. However, tomatoes also contain significant amounts of other carotenoids, vitamin C, vitamin E, folic acid, antioxidant minerals and so on. High tomato consumption may be a marker for a generally high consumption of fruits and vegetables, so it may be a marker for a generally 'healthy' diet and/or lifestyle.

Short-term human experiments can only show the effects that antioxidant supplements or increased antioxidant intake from food will have on acute conditions or acute markers of disease, such as, for example, biochemical indicators of oxidant stress. Chemical tests of antioxidant activity, *in vitro* tests of antimutagenic activity, tests of antioxidant activity with cultured cells or animal experiments may all be useful in generating hypotheses, but they cannot be relied on to predict the long-term response of human beings to high exposure to one or more of these chemicals.

The discussion in Chapter 8 on the potential health benefits of tea illustrates some of these difficulties. While there is a wealth of evidence from *in vitro* and animal studies that substances in tea, particularly green tea, have antioxidant activity and anticancer properties, there is almost no corroboration from human epidemiological studies. Evidence from *in vitro* and animal experiments alone is not sufficient to make holistic conclusions about the health effects of tea drinking or taking tea extracts as supplements.

Large, long-term controlled trials for all of the chemicals listed in Table 5.1 are clearly impractical except as a long-term aspiration. Indeed, the first such trials for even the key nutrient antioxidants have only recently been completed and even then the results of these trials have been challenged. For example, as noted earlier, major trials involving large supplements of vitamin E and β-carotene have found no indication that either protects well-nourished, affluent people from cancer or heart disease, and there are disturbing indications that β-carotene might actually increase risks slightly, at least for some types of people. Yet β-carotene supplements continue to be sold, some company spokespersons and others suggesting that the results are flawed because they have used pure β-carotene rather than 'balanced mixtures' of carotenoids. It has even been proposed that these unsuccessful studies have used insufficient doses! If β-carotene were a synthetic drug, it seems certain that it would fail to get regulatory approval as a cancer-preventing or cardio-protective agent, on the grounds that there is no convincing evidence of efficacy and positive evidence that its long-term toxicological safety is in doubt.

Table 5.1   Some of the potential antioxidants in food that are not recognised as essential nutrients

The carotenoids – around 600 of these. About 25% of the carotenoid content of the diet is β-carotene, which is one of around 50 carotenoids with vitamin A activity	
β-carotene	carrots, palm oil, green vegetables, red and yellow fruits and vegetables
α-carotene	palm oil, maize, carrots
lycopene	tomatoes, water melon, apricots, peaches
lutein/zeanthin	red peppers, green leafy vegetables, maize, tomatoes,
cryptoxanthin	oranges, mangoes
resveratrol	red wine, peanuts
The flavonoids – total US intake around 1000 mg/day (Birt *et al.*, 1999)	
quercetin	apples, red wine (white wine is much lower in antioxidants)
catechin	tea (green tea is richer in antioxidants than black tea)
gossypol	rice
hesperetin	oranges
Phenols and polyphenols – found in many herbs and spices, oranges and other fruits, tea, chocolate	
curcumin	turmeric
ferulic acid	many herbs
thymol	thyme
hydroxytyrosol	olive oil
Synthetic antioxidants – food additives used to prevent fats from going rancid	
butylated hydroxytoluene (BHT)	
butylated hydroxyanisole (BHA)	
Others	
ubiquinone (co-enzyme Q_{10})	meat, especially organ meats like liver and kidney, yeast extract
lipoic acid	dark green leafy vegetables
glutathione	yeast extract
glutamine	an amino acid that acts as a glutathione precursor
Many hundreds of mainly plant chemicals that fall into these and other categories	

Antioxidants and pre-eclampsia in pregnancy

Pre-eclampsia is a dangerous rise in blood pressure during pregnancy. There have been suggestions that oxidative stresses may be an important factor leading to pre-eclampsia. If true, this would mean that antioxidant supplements might be beneficial in preventing pre-eclampsia in women at increased risk of developing this condition during pregnancy. Poston *et al.* (2006) compared the effect of vitamin E and C supplements to a placebo in a randomised controlled trial involving 2400 women at high risk of developing pre-eclampsia. They found no benefit from these antioxidant vitamins and indeed, there was some suggestion that the onset of pre-eclampsia was slightly earlier in the antioxidant group and the incidence of low-birth-weight babies also slightly higher. A recent meta-analysis

(Rumbold *et al.*, 2008) confirmed the lack of benefit of vitamin C and E supplements on pre-eclampsia risk or any other serious complications of pregnancy. The only statistically significant effects of the supplements were adverse.

Vitamin E and dementia

Alzheimer's disease is an organic neurological disorder in which there is a progressive loss of memory and other neurological functions, which ultimately leads to death. The incidence of this condition rises sharply with age; it may be 20 times higher in those aged over 80 years as compared to those aged 60. Suggestions that damage by free radicals may contribute to the pathological changes associated with this condition have led to speculation that antioxidants and especially vitamin E may help to prevent this condition.

In a systematic review of trials of vitamin E in the treatment of Alzheimer's disease, Isaac *et al.* (2008) found only two randomised controlled trials that met their inclusion criteria. One trial of patients with existing moderate disease did find some indications that vitamin slowed the progression of the disease, but there was also an excess of falls in the supplemented group. The reviewers concluded that there was at present a lack of evidence to support the benefits of vitamin E supplements in either Alzheimer's disease or milder cognitive impairment.

Summing up the case for antioxidant supplements

There is convincing evidence that people who spontaneously consume large amounts of antioxidant-rich fruits and vegetables have a reduced risk of developing a chronic degenerative disease such as cancer or heart disease. It cannot be conclusively demonstrated that it is the high antioxidant content of this diet that confers these benefits, or even that it is due to the fruits and vegetables *per se*. Even if these apparent benefits are due to high antioxidant intake, will large, 'unbalanced' supplements of individual antioxidants or groups of antioxidants have the same effect as the broad increase in dozens of antioxidants that one would expect if fruit and vegetable consumption were increased? The free radical theory of disease causation is the theoretical basis for the use of antioxidant supplements. While this is widely accepted, it is nonetheless still a theory that this oxidative damage is a major cause of chronic disease rather than a proven fact. There are many perceived advantages to increasing fruit and vegetable consumption (see list below) and the available evidence certainly provides strong support for the safety of diets rich in fruits and vegetables.

Increased fruit and vegetable consumption would:

- Increase the intake of many essential nutrients.
- Increase the intake of many antioxidants: both nutrients and the hundreds of other non-essential compounds in food have antioxidant activity.
- Increase the intake of (soluble) dietary fibre.

- Lower the energy density of the diet (number of calories per unit weight of food) and so perhaps aid body-weight control.
- Probably displace some fat from the existing diet and so increase the carbohydrate-to-fat ratio in the diet.
- Perhaps displace some of the meat protein in the diet.
- Increase the intake of other phytochemicals that are not antioxidants but may have other beneficial effects (see Chapter 8 for a discussion of these other bio-active plant chemicals).

There are sound reasons for ensuring that people consume adequate amounts of all the essential nutrients, including those that are recognised as antioxidants. In order to ensure this, one might need to consider using targeted micronutrient supplements that include the antioxidant nutrients. Given this objective, the doses would be based on the dietary standards of adequacy. There is limited but persuasive evidence that supplements of antioxidant nutrients are beneficial in populations where micronutrient deficiencies are prevalent. There is no convincing evidence that large doses of antioxidants taken in the form of supplements confer any long-term holistic benefit in people who are already adequately nourished.

Given the evidence that there may be small but significant harmful consequences from consuming large supplements of β-carotene, and perhaps even some of the other antioxidant nutrients, it cannot be assumed that taking large doses of purified or semi-purified antioxidants is risk free. Given the lack of evidence for benefits from those antioxidants that have been rigorously tested, it also seems questionable whether the marketing and greatly increased intake of specific foods and drinks solely on the basis of their high antioxidant content are justified.

6 Natural Fats and Oils

The nature of fats, oils and other lipids

The principal component of dietary fats and oils is triacylglycerol (TAG), which is made up of three fatty acids attached by ester linkages to the simple three-carbon carbohydrate glycerol. These three fatty acids can be all the same (simple TAG) or different (mixed TAG). These fatty acids are composed of a hydrocarbon chain of variable length and a carboxyl (COOH) or acid group at one end (see Figure 6.1).

Palmitic acid (shown in Figure 6.1) is described as a saturated fatty acid because all of the carbons in the hydrocarbon chain are joined together by single bonds and all of the available valencies of the carbon atoms in this chain are 'saturated' with hydrogen. No more hydrogen atoms can be added into this hydrocarbon chain.

Fatty acids that have two or more of the carbons in the hydrocarbon chain joined by a double bond are termed unsaturated fatty acids. Under the right chemical conditions more hydrogen atoms can be added into this hydrocarbon chain; they are not saturated with hydrogen and two more hydrogen atoms can be added at the site of each double bond. Fatty acids with just one double bond in the hydrocarbon chain are termed monounsaturated (one point of unsaturation) and those with more than one are termed the polyunsaturated fatty acids. Oleic acid, illustrated in Figure 6.1, is an example of a monounsaturated fatty acid; and α-linoleic acid and eicosapentaenoic acids, also shown in Figure 6.1, are examples of polyunsaturated fatty acids.

Fatty acids with double bonds have lower melting points than the equivalent saturated fatty acid; the higher the number of double bonds, the lower is the melting point (see Table 6.1 for examples of melting points of saturated and unsaturated fatty acids). This means that many animal fats that are rich in saturated fatty acids (e.g. butter, lard, beef tallow) are solids at room temperature, while many vegetable and fish oils that are high in polyunsaturated fatty acids are liquids (e.g. sunflower oil, corn oil, cod liver oil). The double bonds cause the hydrocarbon chain of the fatty acid to bend back on itself in a U-shape, whereas in saturated fatty acids the chain is linear. Note that in most natural fatty acids, all of the double bonds are in the cis-isomeric configuration (i.e. both hydrogens are on the same side of the double bond), whereas in hydrogenated vegetable oils (e.g. some

Dietary Supplements and Functional Foods, 2nd Edition. Geoffrey P. Webb.
© 2011 Blackwell Publishing Ltd.

(a) Schematic representation of a triacylglycerol

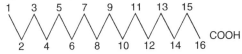

glycerol

(b) General chemical formula of a saturated fatty acid

(c) Diagrammatic representation of a saturated fatty acid (palmitic acid – 16:0)

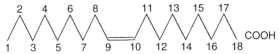

(d) Diagrammatic representation of a monounsaturated fatty acid (oleic acid – 18:1ω_9)

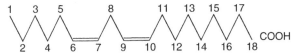

(e) Diagrammatic representation of linoleic acid (18:2ω_6)

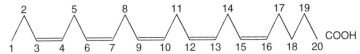

(f) Diagrammatic representation of eicosapentaenoic acid (EPA, 20:5ω_3)

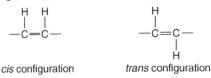

(g) Diagram to illustrate the *cis* and *trans* configurations of unsaturated fatty acids

cis configuration   *trans* configuration

Figure 6.1   The chemical nature of fat and the structure of fatty acids.
Source: G.P. Webb (2008) *Nutrition: A Health Promotion Approach*, 3rd edn. p. 264. Arnold, London.

margarines and vegetable shortening) relatively large amounts of trans fatty acids (i.e. the hydrogen atoms on opposite sides of the double bond) are produced during the hydrogenation process. Some natural fats like butter (4–8%) and other fat from ruminants also contain significant amounts of trans fatty acids.

The cis and trans configurations are also illustrated in Figure 6.1. Trans fatty acids have a more linear configuration than their cis equivalents and thus these fats with high levels of trans fatty acids have similar physical characteristics to satu-

Table 6.1 The melting points of some saturated and unsaturated fatty acids. The shorthand notation is fully explained later in the chapter, but the first number indicates the number of carbon atoms and the second one the number of double bonds (all double bonds are in the cis configuration except for elaidic acid).

	Melting point (°)
Lauric acid (12:0)	44
Palmitic acid (16:0)	63
Stearic acid (18:0)	70
Arachidic acid (20:0)	75
Oleic acid (18:1ω9)	13
Elaidic acid (trans oleic acid)	45
Linoleic acid (18:2ω6)	−5
Linolenic acid (18:3ω3)	−10
Arachidonic acid (20:4ω6)	−49°
Eicosapentaenoic acid (20:5ω3)	−54°

rated fats. They are regarded from a nutritional viewpoint as more akin to saturated fat than unsaturated fat and also have higher melting points than their cis equivalents (see oleic and elaidic acid in Table 6.1). Some margarine manufacturers have altered their manufacturing process so as to largely eliminate trans fatty acids from their products – a change in food for functional reasons, even if for something not usually regarded as a functional food.

Triacyglycerols belong to a family of chemical compounds known as the lipids, which are organic compounds characterised by their insolubility in water but solubility in organic solvents. Other substances that are covered by the term lipids are the phospholipids, glycolipids, sphingolipids, waxes and steroids (e.g. cholesterol). Glycolipids are substances found in plant tissue that have a sugar-derived unit replacing one of the fatty acids. Sphingolipids are derivatives of sphingosine, which is made from palmitic acid and the amino acid serine; these are important components of brain tissue.

Phospholipids are derived from phosphatidic acid, a compound where the third fatty acid in TAG is replaced by a phosphate group. A variety of other moieties can attach to this phosphate to give rise to a family of phospholipids. For example, if choline is attached to the phosphate this compound is called phosphotidyl choline (commonly called lecithin and discussed in Chapter 7).

Why are we preoccupied with the balance of our dietary fats?

As far back as the 1950s, studies with human volunteers were able to show convincingly that altering the balance between saturated and unsaturated fatty acids in the diet while keeping total fat intake constant could produce major changes in plasma cholesterol concentrations. These early studies suggested that high intakes of polyunsaturated fatty acids tended to lower plasma cholesterol levels, whereas saturated fatty acids tended to raise it. These studies had a profound impact on our perception of the healthiness of different fats because, of course, a high plasma cholesterol concentration is associated with increased atherosclerosis and increased risk of coronary heart disease.

At the time of these early studies, butter and animal cooking fats like lard and beef tallow, with their high levels of saturated and low levels of polyunsaturated fatty acids, were the predominant fats in British and American diets. Nowadays soft margarine, vegetable oil and low-fat spreads, with their high polyunsaturated, low saturated profiles, have displaced much of the butter and lard from our diets. In these early studies, dietary cholesterol *per se* was generally regarded as a relatively minor influence on plasma cholesterol, although some people are genetically susceptible to the plasma cholesterol-raising effects of cholesterol. Monounsaturated fatty acids were regarded as neutral in their effects on plasma cholesterol in these early studies, but are now thought to be more like polyunsaturated fatty acids and so oils rich in monounsaturates, like olive oil and rape seed oil (canola), currently have a very favourable health image.

In more recent years our perception of the relationship between plasma cholesterol concentration and atherosclerosis has become more sophisticated, or at least more complicated. Lipids, including cholesterol, are by definition insoluble in water and they are thus transported in water-based plasma as soluble protein-lipid complexes or lipoproteins. Most dietary fat after absorption in the intestine enters the bloodstream in the form of protein-coated droplets called chylomicrons that are rapidly removed from plasma and assimilated in the immediate post-prandial period. Three major classes remain in plasma once chylomicrons have been cleared and these can be separated according to their density by centrifugation techniques; their nomenclature reflects this usual method of separation: high-density lipoproteins (HDL), low-density lipoproteins (LDL) and very low-density lipoproteins (VLDL).

Low-density lipoprotein (LDL) is a cholesterol-rich lipoprotein fraction that accounts for around 70% of the total plasma cholesterol. Its main function is to transport cholesterol between tissues, where it can act as a component of membranes and serve as a precursor for steroid hormones and so on. When cells have adequate amounts of cholesterol, they reduce the number of receptors for LDL on their surface, which means that cholesterol tends to remain in the blood rather than being taking up by tissues. As blood levels of LDL cholesterol rise, so it tends to be deposited in artery walls to form atheroma, which can lead to scarring and fibrosis of arteries (atherosclerosis) and increased risk of thrombosis, which in turn predisposes to angina, coronary thrombosis, strokes and other cardiovascular diseases. An elevated plasma LDL cholesterol is thus predictive of an increased risk of coronary disease and it is this link that is responsible for the link between total plasma cholesterol and coronary disease.

More recent evidence suggests that the initial atheroma deposition is a relatively innocuous process *per se*, but that the serious and permanent damage to the artery wall occurs when this LDL cholesterol is oxidised. Antioxidants (see Chapter 5), it has been argued, may help to reduce this oxidation of LDL cholesterol and thus ameliorate some of the consequences of having an elevated plasma LDL cholesterol. Smoking, on the other hand, may help to increase levels of oxidative free radicals and thus increase the adverse consequences of having an elevated LDL cholesterol. Some people are genetically prone to having an elevated plasma LDL cholesterol concentration because one of their LDL-receptor genes does not produce functional receptor protein. These people have an elevated plasma LDL cholesterol concentration (familial hypercholesteraemia) and are very prone to premature heart disease, especially if they are male.

The cholesterol present in LDL is the sometimes referred to as the 'bad cholesterol' for the reasons outlined above. HDL cholesterol is, conversely, often referred to as the 'good cholesterol'. HDL cholesterol concentration is negatively correlated with risk of coronary disease; that is, HDL is apparently protective. Its role is to clear excess cholesterol and return it to the liver. Ideally, therefore, one might seek to increase the HDL concentration in blood while reducing the LDL concentration. It is principally by changing levels of LDL cholesterol that the manipulations of dietary fats referred to earlier produce their effects on total plasma cholesterol. Regular exercise and moderate intakes of alcohol are two factors that tend to raise the HDL concentration in plasma.

Very low-density lipoprotein (VLDL) is a triacylglycerol-rich lipoprotein fraction that is the main vehicle for exporting endogenously produced triacylglycerol from the liver to adipose tissue. In healthy people, the VLDL level in fasting blood is low. A high VLDL is found in several conditions (e.g. diabetes and obesity) that are associated with an increased risk of coronary disease, but it is not thought that a high VLDL concentration directly contributes to atherosclerosis and coronary disease, although it does have other adverse consequences.

Why are some fatty acids called 'essential'?

Essential fatty acids are polyunsaturated fatty acids that have one or two double bonds within the first seven carbon atoms of the hydrocarbon chain, counting from the methyl end of the molecule (note that throughout this discussion carbon atoms in fatty acids have been numbered from the methyl end of the molecule). While human beings do have the capacity to make fatty acids with double bonds, they do not have the ability to insert double bonds between these first few carbon atoms. This means that they can only be obtained by consuming fatty acids that already have these early double bonds present. There are two families of these essential fatty acids: the ω(omega)-3 (or n-3) and the ω(omega)-6 (or n-6) series. Throughout this book the ω (omega) notation is used but n and omega can be interchanged. In the omega-3 series the first double bond is between carbons 3 and 4 and in the omega-6 series it is between carbons 6 and 7. As the double bonds in natural fatty acids tend to run in sequence separated by a single saturated carbon (CH_2 group), the position of these first double bonds defines the position of the other double bonds as well. It is possible to define the structure of a natural fatty acid using a

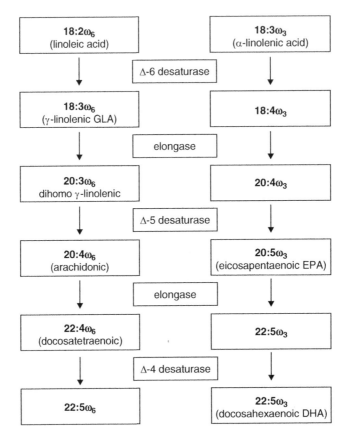

Figure 6.2   The production of other members of the omega-6 and omega-3 series of fatty acids from linoleic acid (18:2ω6) and α-linolenic (18:3ω3).

simple notation that gives the number of carbon atoms, the number of double bonds and the position of the first of these double bonds:

- Thus linoleic acid has 18 carbon atoms and 2 double bonds and the first double bond is between carbons 6 and 7, so its notation is 18:2ω6.
- Eicosapentaenoic acid (EPA) has 20 carbons and 5 double bonds and the first is between carbons 3 and 4, hence its notation is 20:5ω3. The position of the other four double bonds is implicit because there is a single saturated carbon separating them; that is, they are between 6 and 7, 9 and 10, 12 and 13 and 15 and 16 (counting from the methyl end).

Linoleic acid (18:2ω6) is the parent compound for the omega-6 series of polyunsaturated fatty acids and α-linolenic acid (18:3ω3) is the parent compound for the omega-3 series. Human beings can theoretically make the other five members of each series from the parent compound, as shown in Figure 6.2, but it is not possible for mammals to interconvert these two series. This means that if one has a dietary supply of linoleic acid, one can theoretically make all of the other fatty acids of the omega-6 series and likewise α(alpha)-linolenic acid and the omega-3 series (although this may only occur to a limited extent in humans). A dietary supply of any member of the omega-3 or omega-6 series enables us to synthesise the subsequent fatty acids of the series. Some limited manufacture of earlier fatty acids is also possible from the long-chain end products.

It was first shown in the 1920s that certain dietary fats are essential for the well-being of laboratory rats. Prolonged feeding of a fat-free diet induced a deficiency disease that could be cured by provision of small amounts of omega-6 polyunsaturated fatty acids and partially alleviated with omega-3 fatty acids. These rats did not grow properly, developed a scaly dermatitis, were infertile, had depressed inflammatory responses and had increased skin permeability and cutaneous water losses. It has thus been known for many decades that, at least in rats, there is an absolute but small requirement for some dietary omega-6 polyunsaturated fatty acids and that omega-3 fatty acids were partially effective as a substitute for these. It took a long time to shown unequivocally that this was also true in people; even six-month deprivation studies did not produce overt symptoms of deficiency in volunteer subjects. This is because:

- The requirement to prevent overt deficiency is very small: the minimum requirement for omega-6 fatty acids may be as little as 1% of total calories (current US and UK intakes c. 7% of total calories).
- A healthy adult has substantial stores of these acids in their body fat.
- It is difficult to eliminate them totally from the diet, because even certain vegetable foods categorised as essentially fat free do contain small amounts of essential fatty acids.

The best evidence for their absolute essentiality in humans comes from early attempts at maintaining patients for long periods solely by intravenous feeding (total parenteral nutrition, TPN). Symptoms developed relatively rapidly when the infusion did not contain fat but used carbohydrate as the sole energy source. Indeed, it was the development of the ability to infuse a source of fat safely that allowed the successful long-term nutrition of patients using TPN.

It is now generally accepted that small amounts of omega-3 polyunsaturated fatty acids are also essential in their own right for normal physiological functioning. While omega-6 fatty acids predominate in the membranes of liver cells and platelets, there are high and fairly stable concentrations of long-chain omega-3 fatty acids in brain and retinal membrane phospholipids in most mammals. It is not possible to set a minimum requirement for omega-3, but the above observations suggest that it is required in its own right and not merely as a partial substitute for omega-6 polyunsaturates; this issue is addressed again later in this section. Long-chain omega-3 polyunsaturated fatty acids may be particularly important during childhood for brain and retinal development.

While overt symptomatic deficiency of essential fatty acids is rarely, if ever, seen in industrialised countries, one biochemical indicator of essential fatty acid deficiency is the replacement of the normal long-chain omega-3 and omega-6 fatty acids in tissues with long-chain omega-9 fatty acids that can be made within the body; that is, fatty acids with the first double bond between carbons 9 and 10 made from ubiquitous oleic acid ($C18:1\omega_9$).

The functions of the essential fatty acids can be divided into two broad categories:

- The longer-chain members of these families are key structural components of membrane phospholipids and the presence of the multiple double bonds enhances the fluidity of membranes.
- Several important families of regulatory molecules – the prostaglandins, leukotrienes and thromboxanes – are synthesised from some of the fatty acid intermediates on the pathways in Figure 6.2. These are collectively termed the eicosanoids.

It is a common feature of synthetic pathways like those in Figure 6.2 that the first enzyme of the pathway (in this case the Δ-6 desaturase) is the slowest and thus the rate-limiting step. This enzyme's activity is inhibited by high levels of the end product(s) of the pathway (end product inhibition). The enzymes shown in Figure 6.2 are common to both pathways, so the Δ-6 desaturase is the rate-limiting enzyme for both pathways and is inhibited by the end products of either or both pathways. The two parent compounds, linoleic acid and α-linolenic acid, also compete for this enzyme, so that high levels of either will slow down the metabolism of the other. High intakes/production of the long-chain products of either pathway will also inhibit the production of the longer-chain products of the other pathway.

All dietary fats contain a mixture of saturated, monounsaturated and polyunsaturated fatty acids, but the relative proportions vary enormously. Fats from milk, farmed meat and tropical oils like coconut and palm oil tend to be rich in saturates and monounsaturates but low in polyunsaturated fatty acids; fat from ruminating animals is particularly low in polyunsaturated acids. Most commonly used vegetable oils like sunflower oil, corn oil and safflower oil tend to be rich in the linoleic acid and the omega-6 series of polyunsaturated fatty acids, while fish and other marine oils tend to be rich in the omega-3 series and are the only substantial dietary source of the longer-chain members of this family, such as eicosapentaenoic acid, EPA and docosahexaenoic acid, DHA. A few common vegetable oils such as rapeseed oil and soya oil do have comparatively high omega-3 to omega-6 ratios, while olive oil and rapeseed oil have particularly high levels of monounsaturated fatty acids.

Modern diets tend to have a much higher ratio of omega-6 to omega-3 fatty acids than has been found in the past. Historically, when diets were high in fat it tended to come either from animal sources or the traditional vegetable oils like palm oil and olive oil, none of which are rich in omega-6 polyunsaturated fatty acids. Modern omega-6 rich diets would be expected to lead to reduced production of the long-chain omega-3 fatty acids like EPA and DHA and thus to a reduced prevalence of these in membrane phospholipids. Sanders *et al.* (1984) showed that rat diets that were very rich in omega-6 polyunsaturated fatty acids could lead to reduced levels of brain and retinal EPA and DHA, despite the presence of significant amounts of the parent compound of the omega-3 series of fatty acids (α-linolenic acid, 18:3ω3) in their diets.

Feeding primates diets with very high omega-6 to omega-3 ratios (by using safflower oil) resulted in abnormal electroretinograms (Neuringer *et al.*, 1986). Individual case studies of children parenterally 'fed' with feeds that contained very high omega-6 to omega-3 ratios have also been reported to lead to visual and neurological disturbances. The growth in the use of vegetable oils and soft margarine has greatly increased the ratio of omega-6 to omega-3 polyunsaturated fatty acids in average US and UK diets; the current ratios are well over 10 and perhaps as high as 30 in some instances. The ratios in the diets of hunter-gatherers would probably be between 2 and 4. Most authorities agree that current ratios are too high. Estimates of what is optimal vary widely, but should be less than 10 (see Jones and Kubow, 2006). An optimal ratio of 4–5:1 has been suggested, although this is tentative. This discussion supports the essentiality of omega-3 polyunsaturated fatty acids or at least the desirability of a minimum intake for optimal health.

A number of dietary supplements, such as those listed below, are marketed because of their high concentration of particular fatty acids within the sequences shown in Figure 6.2 (usually ω3 fatty acids or γ-linolenic acid – $18:3\omega_6$).

- Evening primrose oil, starflower/borage oil and blackcurrant seed oil are rich in γ-linolenic acid GLA ($18:3\omega_6$). This bypasses the Δ-6 desaturase step in the metabolism of omega-6 fatty acids, the rate-limiting step in essential fatty acid metabolism. It increases the availability of dihomo γ-linolenic acid (20:3ω6), which as shown in Figure 6.3 is a potential source of eicosanoids.
- Fish oils and fish liver oils are the only rich dietary source of the long-chain omega-3 fatty acids eicosapentaenoic acid EPA ($20:5\omega_3$) and docosahexaenoic acid DHA ($22:6\omega_3$).
- Flaxseed/linseed oil is a rich source of omega-3 fatty acids, principally α-linolenic acid (18:3ω3), and is marketed as a source of these fatty acids that is suitable for vegetarians.
- Algal extracts of DHA (22:6ω3) are marketed as the only supplements providing good amounts of DHA that are acceptable to non-fish-eating vegetarians. Note that if these vegetarian supplements are marketed in capsule form, they must be in gelatine-free capsules to be acceptable to vegetarians.

Essential fatty acids and eicosanoid production

Eicosanoids are short-duration regulatory molecules that exert their effects very close to their site of production and are then rapidly inactivated. They are sometimes called locally acting hormones and they frequently regulate the cells that produce them. The name 'eicosanoids' originates because the prefix *eico* is derived from the Greek for 20 and they are made from polyunsaturated fatty acids that have 20 carbon atoms (by cyclooxygenase and lipoxygenase pathways). The origins of

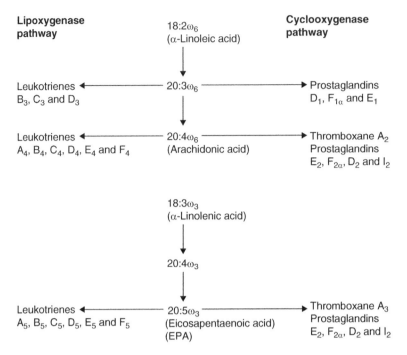

Figure 6.3 Production of eicosanoids from 'essential' omega-6 and omega-3 polyunsaturated fatty acids.

three categories of these eicosanoids, the thromboxanes, leukotrienes and prostaglandins, are illustrated in Figure 6.3. These eicosanoids regulate secretory processes, inflammatory and immune responses, reproductive function, cardiovascular and respiratory functions.

Arachidonic acid ($20:4\omega6$) is the precursor of the major group of eicsanoids, but some are also produced from dihomo-γ-linoleic acid ($20:3\omega6$) and from eicosapentaenoic acid, EPA ($20:5\omega3$). In general, the eicosanoids produced from arachidonic acid are more potent than those produced from the other two precursors.

It was noted earlier that there is competition for common enzymes for the metabolism of the omega-6 and omega-3 polyunsaturated fatty acids, and that there is the possibility of cross-regulation of these pathways. These eicosanoid precursors also compete for the enzymes of the lipoxygenase and cyclooxygenase pathways (see Figure 6.3). This means that altering the availability of omega-6 and omega-3 polyunsaturated fatty acid precursors by dietary manipulation or by the use of supplements can change the balance of eicosanoid production. In general, high intakes of omega-3 fatty acids will generally favour the production of eicosanoids made from eicosapentaenoic acid, while high intakes of omega-6 fatty acids will favour those produced from omega-6 precursors. More specifically, high intakes of γ(gamma)-linolenic acid, GLA ($18:3\omega6$) from supplements of evening primrose oil, starflower oil or one of the other plant oils rich in it will bypass the rate-limiting step in omega-6 polyunsaturated fatty acid metabolism, and especially increase production of those fatty acids produced from dihomo-γ-linoleic acid (20–3ω6). This is because many diets already contain substantial amounts of pre-formed arachidonic acid and high intakes of long-chain omega-6 or omega-3 fatty acids can reduce the activity of the omega-6 desaturase and thus the production of GLA and dihomo-γ-linolenic acid (see Figure 6.2). High intakes of fish oils that are rich in eicosapentaenoic acid, EPA (20:5ω3) and docosahexaenoic acid, DHA (22:6ω3) will especially reduce production of eicosanoids from arachidonic acid, with a corresponding increase in production of those for which EPA is the precursor.

Fish oil supplements

These may be consumed as fish liver oil or fish body oil. The former is usually cod liver oil, but may also come from halibut or shark liver, while the latter come from the bodies of oily fish such as herring, sardines or anchovies. Traditionally, fish liver oil was taken in liquid form, but because many people find it distasteful, fish oils and other oily supplements are now often marketed as oil-filled capsules. Fish and other animals store vitamins A and D in their livers and so fish liver oil is very rich in these vitamins and was traditionally taken solely as a supplementary source of them.

It was seen in Chapter 2 that significant numbers of people in various age groups have marginal or unsatisfactory intakes of vitamin A. Large numbers of elderly people who are largely housebound and so not regularly exposed to summer sunlight show biochemical evidence of poor vitamin D status. Poor vitamin D status is also prevalent among other sectors of the adult population, and there is increasing concern about its re-emergence as a problem for UK children, with small numbers of cases of overt clinical rickets being reported. Evidence was discussed in Chapter 3 that poor vitamin D may be associated with increased risk of a number of autoimmune diseases (like multiple sclerosis and type 1 diabetes) and with increased risk of hypertension and some cardiovascular problems. Fish liver oils would be useful as an additional source of these vitamins for such individuals and there is growing evidence that this would be an important preventive measure against the risk of osteoporosis in housebound elderly people.

Both fish liver and body oil are also the only rich sources of long-chain omega-3 polyunsaturated fatty acids in the diet and this has become a major reason for their use. The high levels of vitamins A and D in fish liver oil may even be seen as a disadvantage in these circumstances, because these vitamins are toxic in excess and so this limits the amount of fish liver oil that can regularly be taken with safety. A 10 ml dose of cod liver oil contains up to 1.5 times the adult RNI for vitamin A and up to the RNI of vitamin D for adults who are not regularly exposed to summer sunlight. Halibut and shark liver oil have even higher levels of these vitamins and the vitamin concentration is also usually higher in capsules than in liquid fish liver oil. The manufacturer's recommended dose of fish liver oil should not be exceeded and, because of the teratogenic effects of retinol, pregnant women probably should avoid fish liver oil supplements unless these have been approved by their physician.

There are no such safety concerns about fish body oil. The American Food and Drug Administration (FDA) suggested that daily doses of long-chain omega-3 polyunsaturated fatty acids equivalent to 10–20 fish body oil capsules could be 'generally regarded as safe'. There is a possibility that fish oil may exacerbate clotting disorders or enhance the effect of anticoagulant drugs. Both fish oil and fish liver oil naturally contain vitamin E and additional quantities are normally added to supplements to reduce the rate of oxidative deterioration.

In 1994, a group of UK experts (COMA, 1994) recommended that the average population intake of long-chain omega-3 polyunsaturated fatty acids (EPA and DHA) should be increased from around 100 mg/day to around 200 mg/day. This amounts to a recommendation to eat more fish and this committee recommended that people should eat two portions of fish per week, of which at least one should be oily fish. An alternative way of achieving the increased intake of these long-chain omega-3 polyunsaturated fatty acids is to take a daily supplement of fish (liver) oil in liquid or more usually capsule form. One capsule of fish (liver) oil should contain at least 100 mg of EPA and DHA and, depending on size and concentration, may contain over 400 mg (the amounts claimed to be in any particular brand should be stated on the packaging).

The American Heart Association (Kris-Etherton *et al.*, 2003), after a detailed review of the evidence, also made recommendations similar to those above from COMA (1994). It recommended that everyone should eat a variety of fish (preferably oily) twice a week and that patients with existing heart disease should consume 1 g/day of long-chain omega-3 fatty acids, preferably from oily fish but also perhaps from supplements. Considerably larger amounts as supplements were recommended to be used under clinical supervision for patients with excessively high plasma triglyceride levels.

One daily fish (liver) oil capsule will thus provide 1–3 g of EPA/DHA per week. This compares with:

- 25 mg in a 100 g serving of cod
- 1.31 g in 100 g of herring
- 1.93 g in 100 g of mackerel
- 1.67 g in 100 g of canned sardines in tomato sauce
- 1.5–3 g in a 10 ml dose of liquid cod liver oil

What are the suggested benefits of taking fish (liver) oil supplements?

Some people will take fish liver oils or give them to their children for the traditional reason, because they are a rich source of vitamins A and D. This will not be discussed further here, but should be seen in the light of the discussions in Chapters 2 and 3 on the prevalence of inadequacy of these vitamins and the benefits and risks of supplements of them. It is worth reiterating that the manufacturer's recommended dose of fish liver oil should not be exceeded because of the potential toxic effects of these vitamins. Pregnant women should seek advice from their doctor before taking supplements that contain vitamin A (retinol), because it is a known teratogen at high doses. When considering the safe dose of fish liver oil, one should factor in any other supplements that contain either of these vitamins and also the high concentration in animal liver, if this is eaten regularly.

Over the last two to three decades, the long-chain omega-3 polyunsaturated fatty acids (PUFA) found abundantly in fish oil have become a major motivation for taking fish (liver) oil supplements. Where this is the motivation for taking these oils and where there is any cause for concern about excessive intakes of vitamins A and D, fish body oil supplements should be used. These long-chain omega-3 PUFA in fish oil are claimed to reduce the risk of diseases linked to atherosclerosis, thrombosis and excessive inflammatory responses. Fish oils are claimed to have antithrombotic, anti-inflammatory and possibly antiatherosclerosis effects. One proposed mechanism by which fish oil supplements may exert these effects is by their effects on eicosanoid production. High concentrations of EPA and DHA would reduce the production of (see Figure 6.3):

- LTB-4 (a leukotriene that promotes inflammation)
- TXA-2 (a thromboxane that promotes platelet aggregation)
- PGI-2 (a prostaglandin with antiaggregating effects on platelets)

These would be partly replaced by eicosanoids produced from EPA:

- LTB-5 (a leukotriene with low activity)
- TXA-2 (a thromboxane with low activity)
- PGI-3 (a prostaglandin with antiaggregating effects on platelets)

Fish oils also reduce fasting and post-prandial TAG levels in plasma and may reduce irregular electrical activity (arrhythmia) within the heart (see Buttriss, 1999).

Several studies published in the 1970s and 1980s suggested that traditional Greenland Eskimos had low rates of heart disease even in comparison to their nearest geographical neighbours, the Danes (e.g. Dyerberg and Bang, 1979). The Greenland Eskimos in these studies ate a diet that was high in animal fat, but much of that fat came from marine animals rather than from farmed land animals, largely from fish and marine mammals like seals and whales. These Eskimos, and other populations consuming large amounts of fish like the Japanese, tend to have low mortality from heart disease, a relatively long clotting time and extended bleeding times; they also tend to have reduced incidence of conditions like arthritis that are linked to an excessive inflammatory response. It was thus suggested that the high intakes of long-chain omega-3 PUFA might help to prevent or treat coronary heart disease, and that they might be beneficial in the treatment or prevention of some inflammatory conditions by dampening the inflammatory response, rather like non-steroidal anti-inflammatory drugs (e.g. aspirin).

Evidence was discussed earlier (reviewed by Jones and Kubow, 2006) that DHA is a normal component of brain and retinal membranes, and that animals or children deprived of omega-3 fatty acids *in utero* and during early life show visual, learning and neurological impairments. These studies indicate that omega-3 fatty acids are essential for brain development in early life and probably necessary for optimal brain functioning throughout life. This has led to suggestions that fish oils may be useful in treatment of several overlapping behavioural problems in children, such as attention deficit and hyperactivity disorder (ADHD), dyslexia and developmental coordination disorder (DCD). A lot of publicity has also been given in the UK to claims that normal schoolchildren given dietary supplements containing fish oil show improved behaviour, attention span and examination performance. It has also been suggested that fish oils may help in the treatment of depression and in slowing the progression and or ameliorating the effects of Alzheimer's disease.

Fish oil supplements and heart disease: Evidence of effectiveness

It would be fair to say that apart from the studies with Eskimos, there is little support for a cardio-protective effect of fish oil from cross-population descriptive epidemiological studies. When the relationship between fish consumption and coronary heart disease mortality is compared across populations, there is either no correlation or at best only a weak negative association that is very dependent on the presence of the Japanese in the sample for any statistical significance. In the famous Seven Countries Study, some populations with negligible fish consumption (e.g. in inland former Yugoslavia) had very low mortality from coronary heart disease, whereas some populations with high fish consumption (like areas of Finland) had among the highest rates of coronary heart disease mortality (reviewed by Kromhout, 1990 and Buttriss, 1999). At least two factors make this an unsurprising finding:

- Fish consumption is a relatively crude indicator of omega-3 PUFA consumption.
- The very strong and positive cross-population relationship between saturated fatty acid consumption and coronary heart disease may mask any cardio-protective effects of omega-3 PUFA.

Buttriss (1999) reviewed several cohort studies that related reported fish consumption to risk of heart disease, and the majority of these do report a reduced risk of CHD as fish consumption increases. In one 20-year cohort study using 850 Dutch male subjects, it was found that the risk of death from CHD was negatively associated with level of fish consumption, and that in men who ate the equivalent of two portions (c. 200g) of fish per week, CHD mortality was about 50% lower than in those who ate no fish.

The most persuasive evidence to support the beneficial effects of fish oil on heart disease mortality risk comes from secondary intervention trials, where the effects of increased oily fish or fish oil supplements were tested in men in the years immediately after they had experienced a first myocardial infarction (heart attack). In the diet and reinfarction trial (DART), Burr *et al.* (1991) tested the effects of three dietary interventions (listed below) in 2000 men recovering from a myocardial infarction. This trial had a large impact, leading to increased awareness among the British public of the possible benefits of fish oil and also increasing scientific interest in this area. The men in this study were randomly allocated to receive or not receive each of the three interventions and the allocations to receive or not receive each intervention was independent of the other two. Thus four groups of the total of eight groups (i.e. c. 1000 of the c. 2000 men) received each of the three interventions:

- Advice to increase intake of cereal fibre.
- Advice to reduce total fat intake.
- Advice to eat two portions of oily fish each week, or take fish oil capsules for men who did not like fish.

Neither of the first two interventions produced any significant benefit, but the men advised to consume oily fish had significantly reduced total mortality over the two years of the study; that is, significantly more of them survived for two years after their first heart attack. It is very unusual in an intervention study of this type to get a statistically significant decrease in total mortality. There was no significant reduction in the number of myocardial infarctions in the fish oil men, but these heart attacks were less likely to have a fatal outcome.

A very large, multicentre Italian study (GISSI, 1999) confirmed the beneficial effects of fish oil for men who had experienced a heart attack; in this study there were significant reductions in both the total mortality and the number of non-fatal heart attacks in those men who took large supplements of omega-3 PUFA. These two studies provide very strong support for the notion that regularly eating oily fish or taking fish oil supplements has holistic benefits for men those who have had a first heart attack. They also provide support to the recommendation made by COMA (1994) to eat more oily fish, and therefore to the wider use of moderate fish oil supplements by those who do not eat much oily fish.

A major review of the effects of omega-3 fatty acids on cardiovascular diseases was commissioned by the Agency for Healthcare Research and Quality, AHRQ (Wang *et al.*, 2004). This review generally confirmed the above conclusions, that omega-3 fatty acids from fish or fish oil supplements reduces all-cause mortality and various cardiovascular outcomes. Almost all of the randomised controlled trials included in this review had used subjects who already had diagnosed cardiovascular disease; that is, secondary trials. These consistently suggested that fish oil reduced all-cause mortality and other cardiovascular events in this type of subject, although it did not reduce the risk of stroke. With one exception, the studies that had addressed the possible primary preventive role of fish oil in subjects with no previous clinical history of cardiovascular disease were epidemiological cohort or case-control studies. Those three cohort studies that had specifically estimated fish oil intake (rather than just fish consumption) all reported a significant reduction in all-cause mortality, cardiovascular deaths and myocardial infarction associated with high fish oil consumption (average follow-up duration of 10 years).

A slightly more recent review (Breslow, 2006) also concluded that fish oil supplements or increased consumption of oily fish reduced mortality in secondary intervention trials of people who had already experienced a heart attack. They concluded that this effect was probably due to a reduced occurrence of fatal arrhythmias. In a meta-analysis of 11 cohort studies relating fish consumption to relative risk of death from coronary heart disease, He *et al.* (2004) found a significant dose-dependent reduction in CHD mortality with increasing frequency of fish consumption. These studies had well over 200 000 subjects and the average follow-up time was almost 12 years. A systematic review by Wang *et al.* (2006) also generally supported the beneficial effects of fish oil supplements, especially in secondary studies. These authors found that omega-3 fatty acids consumed as alpha-linolenic acid (18:3ω3) from vegetable oils like flaxseed oil were not effective.

Evidence relating fish oils to inflammatory conditions such as arthritis

The observation (noted above) that traditional Eskimo populations also have relatively low prevalence of arthritic conditions led to the suggestion that regular fish (liver) oil might be of benefit in preventing or ameliorating arthritis and perhaps other inflammatory conditions. Kremer *et al.* (1985) reported that high intakes of EPA improved the clinical features of rheumatoid arthritis and reduced the levels of the inflammatory mediator LTB-4. Subsequent studies have found that high intakes of omega-3 PUFA provide symptomatic relief and reduce the doses of anti-inflammatory drugs need to control the disease symptoms (Kremer, 2000). It should be noted that there are several studies reporting substantial reductions in symptoms such as morning stiffness and joint pain, but the doses used in these studies are much higher than most people get either from eating oily fish or taking one or two capsules of fish oil per day; benefits also take several months to materialise after fish oil consumption has commenced.

Despite the widespread use of fish oil supplements by patients with rheumatoid arthritis and a prevalent view that they are effective, a more recent review (MacLean *et al.*, 2004) has found only limited evidence to support their use. This review was commissioned by AHRQ and looked at the effects of fish oils in a wide range of conditions, including type 2 diabetes, metabolic syndrome, and several inflammatory conditions like inflammatory bowel disease and rheumatoid arthritis. They reported that there was no significant beneficial effect of fish oils on any individual symptoms of rheumatoid arthritis as assessed by patients or on erythrocyte sedimentation rate (ESR), a more objective outcome measure. Six of the seven studies that assessed the requirement for anti-inflammatory drugs did record a reduced requirement for these drugs in those receiving fish oils. If a clinically significant reduction in use of these drugs as a result of fish oils were confirmed, it would be an important benefit in its own right, as these drugs have significant side-effects. The reduced use of these drugs in the test group would also have a potential confounding effect; that is, if patients had the same level of symptoms with fewer drugs, this could be masking a true effect of the fish oils.

Rosell *et al.* (2009) addressed the slightly different issue of whether oily fish might help in preventing the onset of rheumatoid arthritis in a very large case-control study involving almost 1900 people with rheumatoid arthritis and a larger number of matched controls. They found a very slight indication that regular oily fish consumption was associated with a decreased risk of developing rheumatoid arthritis. Such an observation should be viewed very cautiously as merely a basis for justifying further investigation.

Rheumatoid arthritis is an autoimmune condition that may be triggered by an infection. The symptoms and disability may develop in young people and may progress rapidly. Osteoarthritis is a much more frequent condition that has common symptoms to rheumatoid arthritis; it is regarded as a degenerative condition of ageing and affects two-thirds of elderly people to some extent. Stresses on joints lead to cumulative damage and erosion, which result in increasing pain and disability. There is little evidence about the impact of chronic consumption of modest amounts of dietary or supplemental fish oil on the progress of this condition, although there is a reasonable theoretical basis for it having an effect, and the evidence about the beneficial impact of large doses of fish oil in rheumatoid arthritis when taken for a few months is encouraging.

Many people take fish oils in the belief that they do have therapeutic or preventive benefits against joint pain, stiffness and osteoarthritis. Curtis *et al.* (2002) review some *in vitro* studies suggesting that supplementation with the omega-3 fatty acids found in fish oils can reduce the inflammation and erosion of cartilage that occurs in inflammatory joint diseases. In this review, almost all of the clinical evidence for beneficial effects of fish oils on arthritic disease that the authors refer to is from studies of rheumatoid arthritis; that is, evidence for benefits in rheumatoid arthritis is used to support its having benefits in osteoarthritis. One double-blind, placebo-controlled trial of the efficacy of cod liver oil as a supplement to non-steroidal anti-inflammatory drugs found that 10 ml of cod liver oil daily for 24 weeks did not produce any additional benefits to the drugs (Stammers *et al.*, 1992).

In a more general review of the role of nutraceuticals in the management of arthritis, Curtis *et al.* (2004) suggest that that the efficacy of fish oils 'has been demonstrated in several clinical trials, animal feeding experiments and in vitro models that mimic cartilage destruction in arthritic disease'. They do not, however, reference studies that have convincingly and specifically demonstrated holistic clinical benefits for patients with osteoarthritis. When I entered the terms 'fish oil supplements' and 'osteoarthritis' into an academic search engine (PubMed) in November 2009, I recorded only six hits and none of these was a controlled trial.

Fish oils, brain and behaviour

Some studies have looked at the possible use of fish oils in childhood development disorders such as ADHD, DCD and dyslexia, as noted earlier in the chapter. Children with ADHD present with lower levels of DHA and total omega-3 fatty acids in their red blood cell membranes than matched control children. The abnormal fatty acid profile is not explained by differences in intake and can be observed in different age groups of children (e.g. Colter *et al.*, 2008). These observations have led some authors to suggest that changes in endogenous production or metabolism of long-chain polyunsaturated fatty acids may be a factor (Burgess *et al.*, 2000). However, in a systematic review, Raz and Gobis (2009) found no evidence to support the use of essential fatty acid supplements to treat ADHD.

One controlled study (Richardson and Montgomery, 2005) in children with development coordination disorder (DCD, a syndrome with some features of both dyslexia and ADHD) found some evidence of benefits from taking supplements containing both fish oil (80%) and evening primrose oil (20%); that is, rich in long-chain omega-3 polyunsaturates and gamma-linolenic acid (GLA), $18:3\omega6$. Half of the 120 children were given active supplements for three months and half given a placebo. After three months the active supplement group showed no improvement in motor skills, but did show significant improvements in reading, spelling and behaviour. After three months the placebo group were also given the active supplement and they then showed similar improvements.

There have been several reports in the popular media of 'trials' of fish oils in normal schoolchildren, which have claimed that they lead to improved behaviour, attention span and examination performance. These have been uncontrolled trials that have had severe deficiencies of design from a scientific viewpoint and the results of these 'trials' have not appeared in peer-reviewed scientific journals. These studies are so poorly conducted that they cannot in themselves be taken as scientific evidence and, indeed, the dissemination of results from poorly conducted studies may be seen as hindering proper scientific evaluation of this hypothesis.

There is some epidemiological evidence to support the view that elderly people who consume good amounts of oily fish have better cognitive function and may be at reduced risk of developing dementia. Dangour *et al.* (2009), in an analysis of the relationship between fish consumption and tests of cognitive function in a sample of over 800 British people in their 70s, found a positive association between fish consumption and measures of cognitive function. However, when they corrected for confounding variables like age, sex, level of educational attainment and psychological well-being (e.g. depression), this association decreased and became statistically insignificant. Lim *et al.* (2006) were able to find no controlled trials of the effects of fish oil supplements on rate of cognitive decline in healthy elderly people that met their criteria for inclusion in a meta-analysis. As yet there is no evidence that fish oil as food or supplements can reduce cognitive decline in elderly people or lower the risk of developing Alzheimer's disease.

Fish oil supplements have also been suggested as being of potential benefit in depressive conditions, but there is as yet too little published data to assess this claim.

Evening primrose oil and other sources of GLA

Evening primrose, Oenothera biennis, is a plant that is native to North America, although it is now cultivated in many parts of the world. The leaves, shoots and roots of the plant were widely eaten by Native Americans and it has been cultivated in Europe for culinary purposes. The oil is extracted from its seeds. Evening primrose oil (EPO), starflower oil and several other plant oils mentioned earlier in the chapter are marketed as rich sources of gamma-linolenic acid (GLA), which is the second fatty acid on the omega-6 pathway in Figure 6.2. Evening primrose oil contains 8–11% GLA, starflower oil 20–25% GLA and blackcurrant oil 15–25% GLA. It is suggested that high intakes of GLA will increase production of the series of eicosanoids produced from dihomo gamma-linoleic acid (see Figure 6.3). There will be limited endogenous production of GLA in most human diets because they are usually abundant in arachidonic acid and so the Δ-6 desaturase activity is reduced by end product inhibition.

As mentioned in Chapter 1, two EPO preparations were licensed as medicines in the UK until 2002. They were prescribed for the treatment of breast pain (mastalgia) and less frequently for the treatment of atopic eczema. Both of these products had their product licences withdrawn because the evidence for their efficacy was considered to be insufficient to meet current standards for medicines. The licensing authorities stressed that withdrawal of licensing was not prompted by any concerns about their safety. EPO supplements continue to be widely available and used as dietary supplements.

The most common use of EPO and other GLA-containing oils is for the relief of pre-menstrual symptoms, especially breast pain, for which it was prescribed in the past. A systematic review of EPO for the relief of pre-menstrual syndrome (Budeiri *et al.*, 1996) identified seven placebo-controlled trials of EPO for this purpose. It concluded that the best controlled of these trials failed to show any benefits for EPO. While the small size of the studies meant that the authors could not rule out some modest beneficial effect, they concluded that the then available evidence suggested that EPO is of little value in the management of pre-menstrual syndrome. More recently, Srivastava *et al.* (2007) performed a meta-analysis of several treatments used for mastalgia and they concluded that EPO did not offer any advantage over a placebo.

In a systematic review of treatments for atopic eczema, Hoare *et al.* (2000) found insufficient evidence to make any recommendation on the use of EPO. Van Gool *et al.* (2004) similarly found no evidence from a meta-analysis of clinical trials to support the use of any GLA source (starflower oil, EPO or blackcurrant oil) to treat atopic eczema.

EPO is also taken for menopausal symptoms and for symptomatic relief of arthritis, although there is little substantial evidence to support these uses.

One of the most vociferous and influential advocates of the clinical uses of EPO was the late David Horrobin, and one of the companies that he founded sponsored many of the early clinical trials of EPO. A meta-analysis authored by Horrobin and colleagues representing his company (Morse *et al.*, 1989) was published in the *British Journal of Dermatology*. This review was influential in encouraging the belief that a preparation of EPO was effective in treating atopic eczema and had a striking beneficial effect on itching. As noted in Chapter 1, Williams (2003), in an editorial in the *British Medical Journal*, was critical of this meta-analysis because seven small trials (of nine included in the analysis) were sponsored by the authors' company and not published in peer-reviewed papers, and also because one relatively large independent study was excluded on what Williams implies were dubious grounds.

In 2003, the *British Medical Journal* published a highly critical obituary of Horrobin and his work on EPO (Richmond, 2003). This prompted well over 100 responses, which is close to the most for any article, let alone an obituary (these may be found on the journal's website. www.bmj.com). Richmond notes that one of the clinicians working on early clinical trials of EPO was found guilty of research fraud by the General Medical Council. She goes on to suggest that EPO 'may go down in history as the remedy for which there is no disease' and that Horrobin 'may prove to be the greatest snake oil salesman of his age'. It is only fair to add that a number of replies to this obituary were supportive of Horrobin and his work.

EPO is usually taken as capsules that contain 500 mg or 1000 mg of the oil. The GLA content of different EPO preparations varies, but typically GLA makes up about 10% of the total dose of EPO.

Flaxseed oil

Flaxseed oil is derived from the seeds of the flax plant, Linum usitatissimum, which originated in the Middle East where it was cultivated to make linen. The oil extracted from flax seeds is often called linseed oil and it has been widely used for non-culinary purposes, for example as a wood preserver and in paints and varnishes. The oil can also be used for cooking.

Flaxseed oil is marketed as a dietary supplement largely on the basis of its high content of alpha-linolenic acid, the parent compound of the omega-3 series of fatty acids. Over half of the fatty acid in flax seed is alpha-linolenic acid and the omega-3 to omega-6 ratio is over three. It has been suggested that as the parent compound of the omega-3 series of fatty acids, the alpha-linolenic acid in flaxseed oil can act as a source of EPA and DHA and thus be a vegetarian alternative to fish oil. It is now clear, however, that there is only limited conversion of alpha-linolenic acid to EPA in humans (slightly more in women than men) and very little conversion to DHA (Burdge, 2004). Flaxseed oil cannot therefore be regarded as a good source of long-chain omega-3 polyunsaturates, although one controlled study did find that very high doses of flaxseed oil (3 g/day) taken for 12 weeks did increase levels of EPA in serum by 60%, although it had no effect on levels of DHA (Harper *et al.*, 2006). Wang *et al.* (2004), in their commissioned review of the effects of omega-3 fatty acids on cardiovascular disease, found insufficient evidence to make firm conclusions about the independent effect of alpha-linolenic acid. There is currently no evidence that flaxseed oil has any beneficial effects on rheumatoid arthritis.

Flax seeds also contain a group of compounds called lignans, diphenolic compounds that are converted by colonic bacteria to active phyto-oestrogens enterolactone and enterodiol. Very little of these would be present in commercial preparations of flaxseed oil, but they would be found in less refined flaxseed products. Most of the research on phyto-oestrogens has been done using soya products, which contain isoflavones with weak oestrogenic activity; this is discussed at length in Chapter 9. Lignans are present in small amounts in most fibre-rich foods and so the total consumption in vegetarian-based diets may make them an important source of dietary phyto-oestrogens. Although there is little work specifically on the effects of lignans as phyto-oestrogens, theoretically one might expect that they would have similar potential effects to those discussed in Chapter 9 for phyto-oestrogens.

Conjugated linoleic acid (CLA)

Conjugated linoleic acid (CLA) is the collective name given to a group of isomers of linoleic acid, the parent compound of the omega-6 group of essential fatty acids. Isomers are substances that have the same chemical formula, but where the precise three-dimensional arrangement of the atoms is different. In linoleic acid, as seen earlier, the two double bonds of the hydrocarbon chain link carbons 6 and 7 and carbons 9 and 10, counting from the methyl end of the molecule; they are thus separated by a methylene (CH_2) group. Both double bonds in linoleic acid are in the cis configuration; that is, the hydrogens at either end of the double bond are on the same side of the double bond. In CLA, the double bonds are not separated by a methylene group but are contiguous, and they may be in the cis- or trans-isomeric configuration (see Figure 6.1 for illustration of cis and trans configurations). In the two largest components of CLA that usually make up 80–90% of the total, the double bonds are between carbons 6 and 7 and 8 and 9, or between 7 and 8 and 9 and 10, counting from the methyl end of the molecule. Both of these fatty acids have one double bond in the cis and one in the trans configuration. The structures of linoleic acid and these two most prevalent isomers in CLA are illustrated in Figure 6.4. (Note that it is more usual to designate the position of the double bonds from the carboxyl or Δ end of the molecule; see Figure 6.4). In this short account, no attempt has been made to differentiate between the different components of CLA, although it seems almost inevitable that they will differ in their effects and potency.

CLA is present in the human diet in small amounts and the principal dietary sources are dairy fat (from milk, cheese and butter) and meat fat, especially that from ruminant animals like cattle and sheep. Plant oils and fish contain very little CLA, although the CLA used in supplements is produced from vegetable oils like sunflower oil and safflower oil that are rich in linoleic acid. CLA is produced naturally in the rumen of cattle by the action of bacteria on dietary linoleic acid. The way in which cattle are fed markedly affects the CLA content of their meat and milk; those that graze on pasture have more CLA than those that are fed on grain and commercial cattle foods. It is possible to manipulate the CLA content of milk fat by changing the diet of cows (reviewed by Lawson *et al.*, 2001). In some non-ruminant species CLA precursors can be produced by their gut bacteria and these are converted into CLA after absorption.

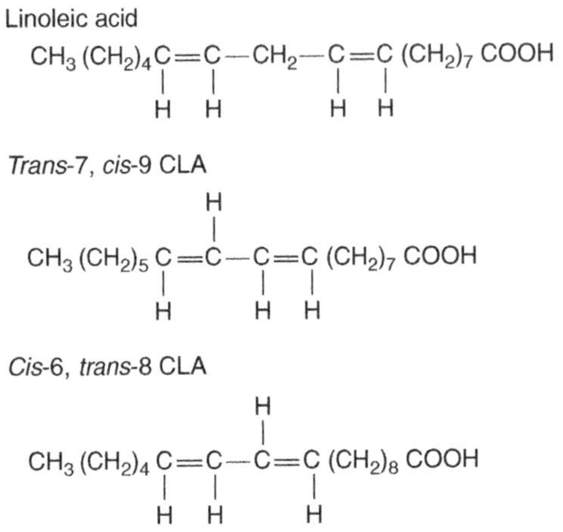

Linoleic acid

$$CH_3(CH_2)_4\underset{\underset{H}{|}}{C}=\underset{\underset{H}{|}}{C}-CH_2-\underset{\underset{H}{|}}{C}=\underset{\underset{H}{|}}{C}(CH_2)_7 COOH$$

Trans-7, *cis*-9 CLA

$$CH_3(CH_2)_5\underset{\underset{H}{|}}{C}=\overset{\overset{H}{|}}{C}-\underset{\underset{H}{|}}{C}=\underset{\underset{H}{|}}{C}(CH_2)_7 COOH$$

Cis-6, *trans*-8 CLA

$$CH_3(CH_2)_4\underset{\underset{H}{|}}{C}=\underset{\underset{H}{|}}{C}-\overset{\overset{H}{|}}{C}=\underset{\underset{H}{|}}{C}(CH_2)_8 COOH$$

Note that in the numbering of the positions of the double bonds in CLA the carbons have been counted from the methyl end of the molecule. Although in nutrition and biochemistry it is usual to refer to the omega-6 and omega-3 fatty acids (or n-6 and n-3) it is also usual to designate the position of double bonds from the carboxyl or Δ end of the molecule. Using this standard nomenclature the above isomers of CLA are more usually designated cis-9, trans-11 CLA and *trans*-10, *cis*-11 CLA respectively.

Figure 6.4 The structure of linoleic acid and the two major components of CLA.

In general, it is thought that human beings cannot synthesise CLA and feeding high levels of linoleic acid, for example, does not increase tissue levels of CLA. Human milk from women who eat no foods of ruminant origin is largely devoid of CLA. It is possible that there is some capability for endogenous synthesis from specific fatty acid precursors of dietary and gut bacterial origin (see Roche *et al.*, 2001).

The average intake of CLA by an omnivorous man in the UK was estimated to be around 150 mg/day in 1995, with two-thirds of this coming from dairy fat (milk, cheese and butter) and the rest coming from meat fat, especially ruminant meat (see Lawson *et al.*, 2001). Given the substantial reduction in the consumption of butter and whole milk in the last 15 years, it is likely that current estimates, using the same food composition assumptions, would be significantly lower than this.

Promotional material for CLA supplements sometimes suggests that CLA intakes in Britain and America have dropped markedly in recent decades because of changes in dietary and animal husbandry practices. This is used as an argument to support the widespread use of supplements of CLA that may contain several grams of CLA; that is, much more than 10 times current average dietary intakes. While the first statement is probably factually correct, this is not in itself a justification for taking large supplements of CLA. CLA is not an essential nutrient; many people manage to lead healthy lives with almost no CLA in their diet. CLA is not normally synthesised by human beings. This means that huge numbers of people worldwide manage with almost no CLA from either their diet or from endogenous synthesis. People with the highest intakes of CLA will be those consuming large amounts of dairy fat and fat from ruminant animals; this is the most saturated source of fat in the diet and consumption of saturated fat is generally seen as an unhealthy dietary characteristic.

Given that the normal range of intakes of CLA probably does not go much beyond 250 mg/day, the effects of gram quantities of it should be seen as pharmacological rather than physiological. These large supplements cannot be seen as compensating for some inadequacy in the diet. For completeness, the results of studies using large supplements of CLA are briefly overviewed, but these should be seen as pharmacological uses. One worrying aspect of these studies is that even where there is some evidence of benefit in animal studies, there is no clear explanation or rationale for these effects. It is possible that some of the effects of CLA are exerted through effects on eicosanoid production, but this area is still poorly understood. CLA is a natural component of many human diets and so has been in human food for centuries; there are also no serious adverse effects reported from studies where very large supplements have been consumed over relatively short periods. Despite this, there have been no studies of the chronic safety of large doses of CLA, when several grams per day are consumed by large numbers of people over years or decades.

There have been many studies with animals and *in vitro* systems that have suggested that large supplemental doses of CLA may have a number of potentially beneficial effects. Some of these are listed below:

- It has antimutagenic effects in bacteria. These mutagenicity tests (like the Ames test) are used to screen compounds for carcinogenic potential. Mutagens are often carcinogens and so inhibitors of mutagenesis may have anticancer potential in animals and people.
- CLA has been shown to reduce the chemical induction of tumours at various sites in rats and mice. These chemically induced tumours are used as models of human cancer development. Kritchevsky (2000) has reviewed the anticancer and antimutagenic effects of CLA.
- CLA has been shown to exert beneficial effects on blood lipoprotein profiles and cardiovascular risk factors in many but not all animal studies. It tends to reduce plasma cholesterol and plasma triacylglycerol concentrations and may reduce cholesterol-induced atherosclerosis in rabbits (see Kritchevsky, 2000 and Roche *et al.*, 2001).
- *In vitro* and animal studies suggest that CLA can modulate the inflammatory response, and this might be useful in the treatment of chronic inflammatory diseases.
- CLA has been shown to reduce body fat content and increase lean body mass in several species. This is probably the effect that has attracted most attention, because it suggests that CLA supplements may have some potential in the treatment and/or prevention of human obesity.

Most of the animal studies discussed above have used large doses of CLA, often between 5 and 10 g/kg of diet. Even using a conservative method of scaling between species, this is equivalent to several grams of CLA per day in humans.

Roche *et al.* (2001) review several relatively short-term trials (up to eight weeks) of CLA on body weight, body composition and blood lipoprotein profiles in humans. These have generally failed to consistently find the sort of changes in humans that might be expected from the animal studies – that is, no significant changes in body weight or body composition – although there may perhaps be a beneficial effect on plasma triacylglycerol levels. Roche *et al.* (2001) suggest that the doses of CLA (c. 3 g/day) used in these human trials may not have been sufficient to reproduce the beneficial effects on body weight and body composition seen in animal studies. Most methods of measuring body composition in humans are relatively insensitive and small changes achieved in short-term studies might be missed.

One long-term trial of large CLA supplements in a relatively big sample of overweight people did report significant effects on body weight, body composition and lipoprotein profile (Gaullier *et al.*, 2004). This group used 180 mainly female subjects with body mass index (BMI) in the range 25–30 kg/m^2, so considered to be overweight but not clinically obese. This was a double-blind, placebo-controlled trial that used a dose of up to 4.5 g of CLA for a whole year – a total of over 1.5 kg of CLA! At the end of the year, the CLA groups had lost an average of about 2 kg of body weight over the year. The researchers measured body composition using a very sensitive method (dual-energy X-ray absorptiometry DEXA) and found that the subjects had lost about 8–9% of their initial fat mass, but had registered a small but significant increase in lean body mass. There were no significant changes in these parameters in the placebo group. No serious adverse effects of CLA were noted in this trial, although there were some changes in cardiovascular risk factors that could be regarded as adverse, such as small rises in LDL cholesterol, small falls in HDL cholesterol and increases in levels of lipoprotein A. Even taking the results of this trial at face value, there must be doubt about whether such modest gains merit the chronic use of such high doses of a substance where there has been no long-term study of its safety, especially as one of the main problems of obesity treatment is maintaining weight losses.

In a systematic review of clinical trials of CLA, Salas-Salvado *et al.* (2006) found that relatively few clinical trials had been published and that, taken together, there was not enough evidence to decide whether CLA had any effect on body weight or composition in humans. They did suggest that there was some evidence that it had adverse effects on blood lipoproteins (including a reduction in plasma HDL), glucose metabolism (including a decrease in insulin sensitivity), lipid oxidation, inflammation and endothelial function. They concluded that indiscriminate use of CLA could not be recommended until large studies of its safety and efficacy had been conducted. CLA is metabolised in a similar way to other unsaturated fatty acids, although it tends to be metabolised more slowly and it may affect the metabolism of other polyunsaturated fatty acids and thus affect eicosanoid production. If taken in large doses over a protracted period it will accumulate in adipose tissue.

β-sitosterol and the phytosterols

β-sitosterol is the most abundant sterol found in plant foods. It is structurally similar to cholesterol, just with an extra ethyl group attached to carbon 24 (see Figure 9.1 in Chapter 9). Phytosterols like β-sitosterol are, unlike cholesterol, poorly absorbed from the gut, although they can interfere with the absorption and reabsorption of cholesterol from the gut and thus have the potential to lower blood cholesterol. This cholesterol-lowering potential of the phytosterols and β-sitosterol in particular was recognised as early as the 1960s.

β-sitosterol is available as a dietary supplement. Interest in these phytosterols has been reawakened in recent years because they are present in several margarines and other foods that are marketed as functional foods that are able to lower blood cholesterol concentrations. This issue is discussed in Chapter 9 in the section on phytosterols.

β-sitosterol is also one of several plant-derived products that are claimed to be beneficial in the treatment of benign prostatic hyperplasia (BPH). A brief description of this condition is given in the section on saw palmetto in Chapter 8. There are no clear mechanisms proposed for any action of β-sitosterol in the treatment of this condition, however. Wilt *et al.* (1999) conducted a systematic review of the effectiveness of β-sitosterol in the treatment of BPH (this was edited but not changed in 2008). They identified four randomised placebo-controlled trials of β-sitosterol for the treatment of this condition, with a total sample size of 519 men. These trials did suggest that in trials lasting from one to six months, β-sitosterol did improve urinary scores and measures of urine flow. An electronic search of the literature after 1999 identified no further trials of β-sitosterol alone in the treatment of BPH.

7 Non-Essential 'Nutrients' that are Used as Dietary Supplements

General rationale

This chapter deals with those chemical compounds that are taken as dietary supplements but are not covered in one of the earlier chapters; that is, they are not classified as vitamins or essential minerals or lipids. Although they are mainly derived from carbohydrate or amino acid precursors, they are chemically quite a diverse group of substances. Most of them are normally present in the diet and are natural components of the human body that have well-established biological functions, for example:

- They may be important as co-factors for important biochemical reactions.
- They may be precursors in the synthesis of important biologically active or structural molecules.

Thus their functional roles are in many cases similar to those of the established vitamins. However, they are not classified as essential nutrients, usually because the expert panels that prescribe which nutrients are essential and set the dietary standards for essential nutrients have concluded that their endogenous synthesis is sufficient to meet physiological needs. Nevertheless, as we saw in Chapter 3, the existence of some mechanisms for endogenous synthesis does not necessarily preclude something being classified as an essential nutrient, such as in the two examples below:

- In healthy adults, most vitamin D is produced endogenously by the photochemical conversion of a steroid produced in the skin into vitamin D when the skin is exposed to summer sunlight. A dietary supply becomes essential when there is inadequate exposure of the skin to sunlight, as in the housebound elderly (see the discussion of conditional essentiality below).
- Niacin can be synthesised from the essential amino acid tryptophan, and niacin deficiency occurs only if dietary supplies of both pre-formed niacin and tryptophan are inadequate.

Dietary Supplements and Functional Foods, 2nd Edition. Geoffrey P. Webb.
© 2011 Blackwell Publishing Ltd.

It is also true that dietary deficiencies of some established vitamins rarely occur because the diet almost invariably contains sufficient of the vitamin, so lack of a well-known 'deficiency disease; is again not a bar to something being classified as an essential nutrient. For example, overt pathological deficiencies of pantothenic acid and biotin are rarely seen, even in countries where dietary insufficiencies are common.

Of course, the underlying logic of taking supplements of the substances covered in this chapter is that despite their failure to meet the expert panels' criteria for essential nutrients, the endogenous synthesis and/or usual dietary supply is suboptimal. It may be considered inadequate for optimal physiological functioning or it may be considered that under some circumstances or in certain pathological states, additional supplies of the compound can have beneficial effects. For example, extra supplies may enhance training or performance in athletes or may have beneficial effects on the symptoms and/or progression of a disease. Harper (1999) suggests that some nutrients may be conditionally essential, 'not ordinarily required in the diet but which must be supplied exogenously to specific populations that do not synthesise them in adequate amounts'. In order to satisfy this definition of conditional essentiality, there must be, in the population for whom it is essential:

- A decrease in the blood levels of the substance to below the normal range.
- This decrease in blood levels must result in some abnormalities of structure or function.
- This abnormality can be corrected by exogenous supply of the compound.

Listed below are a number of examples of substances that are conditionally essential in premature babies, in certain pathological states and in some people with genetic defects (after Harper 1999):

- The amino acids cysteine and tyrosine are essential for premature babies because the enzymes for their synthesis do not develop until late gestation. Similarly, the long-chain omega-3 and omega-6 polyunsaturated fatty acids may be essential, because the elongation and desaturation enzymes needed for their production from linoleic and linolenic acid are not developed (see Figure 6.2 in Chapter 6).
- Cysteine and tyrosine may also become essential in some patients with cirrhosis of the liver, because their ability to synthesise these amino acids in the liver may be reduced.
- The amino acid glutamine may become essential in severe illness or after serious traumatic injury.
- Genetic defects in the pathway for carnitine synthesis may make it essential and carnitine supplements correct the myopathies (muscle wasting) that are otherwise associated with these defects.
- In addition to such examples, it could be argued that vitamin D is a conditionally essential nutrient that is only required when there is inadequate exposure of the skin to sunlight.

As well as the possibility that a nutrient may be conditionally essential, there are also several examples of substances that are normally synthesised in the body being an accepted pharmacological treatment for a particular condition (note that the usual definition of a drug specifies that it does not occur naturally in the human body). The most obvious examples are where hormone preparations are given to those people with no endogenous production or in whom it is insufficient. Thyroxin is used to treat thyroid insufficiency and oestrogen supplements are frequently given to reduce the acute and possibly the long-term consequences of reduced endogenous oestrogen production at the menopause. The adrenal hormone cortisol and its analogues are widely used to suppress inflammation and allergic reactions in many pathological states. The substance L-dopa, which is a normal metabolic product of brain and other nervous tissue, is an important and well-established treatment for Parkinson's disease. Parkinson's disease is characterised by low levels of dopamine in the brain and L-dopa is metabolised to dopamine.

The purpose of the above discussion is to show that there are precedents for compounds that are normally synthesised in the body being widely and effectively used in the prevention or treatment of some pathological conditions. Neither the absence of a well-characterised deficiency disease nor the existence of an endogenous synthetic pathway for a substance necessarily means that the rate of production of that substance is or is always sufficient for optimal functioning. Note that even though substances can still be classified as essential nutrients despite the existence of a synthetic pathway, it is also true that overt deficiency of these nutrients only occurs when there is a combination of very particular circumstances. Both a dietary lack of the vitamin and lack of sunlight exposure are needed for vitamin D deficiency; lack of niacin and low availability of the amino acid tryptophan are both necessary to produce pellagra. Note also that synthetic pathways are usually regulated by the availability of the end product; that is, when there is a lot of the end product present, the synthetic pathway slows, and accelerates when there is low end product availability. Such regulation reduces wasteful overproduction by synthetic pathways. This means that dietary supply or supplements of any substance would be expected to reduce its endogenous synthesis. Of course, using large supplemental doses may increase the availability of the substance despite reduced endogenous synthesis, but is this really dietary supplementation or pharmacological use of the substance?

Glucosamine and chondroitin sulphate

Supplements of glucosamine and chondroitin sulphate are frequently taken either separately or in combination, in the belief that they may maintain joint health and/or have therapeutic benefits for those suffering from arthritic disease. These substances are compounds that are normally present and synthesised in the body and are concentrated in cartilage. It is suggested that they may be 'chondroprotective', reducing the breakdown of cartilage that is a feature of arthritic conditions; they may also have anti-inflammatory effects.

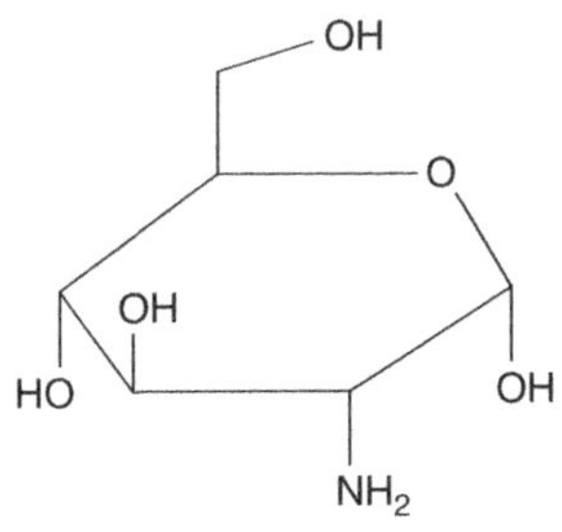

Figure 7.1   The structure of glucosamine.

Nature and functions of cartilage

Cartilage is a type of connective tissue that is more flexible than bone. The various types of cartilage have several important structural functions, such as:

- It covers the surface of bones where they meet to form joints.
- It provides the rigid support for structures like the larynx and trachea.
- It makes up the flexible material that connects the ribs to the sternum.
- It makes up the intervertebral disks.
- It makes up the flexible supporting tissue of the outer ear.

During uterine development, the fetal skeleton is largely composed of cartilage, but by the time of birth much of this has been calcified to form bone. When long bones grow, they grow at a cartilaginous area that connects the bone shaft with the epiphysis, the epiphyseal cartilage plate. New cartilage is produced in this plate and at the extremity of the plate this becomes calcified to form new bone. After adolescence, the shaft and epiphyses of the bone fuse (epiphyseal plate closure) and linear growth ceases.

Cartilage is rich in a group of substances, the proteoglycans, which contain some protein but are largely comprised of polysaccharides known as the glycosaminoglycans, which are important in determining the elastic properties and other physical characteristics of cartilage. Chondroitin sulphate is one of these glycosaminoglycans and it is made up of repeating disaccharide units; chondroitin, and all of the other glycosaminoglycans (dermatan sulphate, keratin sulphate, hyaluronate and heparin), contains a unit of glucosamine or galactosamine combined with glucuronic acid in their repeating disaccharide units. Glucosamine is synthesised by substituting an amine group from the amino acid glutamine onto position 2 of the glucose molecule (see Figure 7.1 for the structure of glucosamine).

Supplement forms and origins

The chondroitin sulphate used for supplements is derived from the cartilage of farm animals, such as pig or cattle trachea, or from the cartilage of cartilaginous fish like sharks. Glucosamine is produced by the acid hydrolysis of lobster, crab, shrimp or prawn shells and is marketed in a number of slightly different chemical forms, which partly depend on which acid is used for the hydrolysis of the shells:

- N-acetyl-D-glucosamine (the amino group of glucosamine is acetylated)
- D-glucosamine HCl
- D-glucosamine sulphate.2KCl
- D-glucosamine sulphate.2NaCl

These are all likely to be converted to glucosamine hydrochloride by the hydrochloric acid of the stomach.

Chondroitin sulphate is a large molecule that might not be expected to pass across the intestinal wall in its intact form. Chondroitin remains intact in the stomach and small intestine, but is degraded by bacteria in the large intestine. Ronca and Conte (1993) estimated that about 10% of chondroitin sulphate from shark cartilage (5000–10 000 molecular weight) is absorbed as large molecular weight moieties and a further 20% absorbed as low molecular weight breakdown products. Similarly, it has been shown that some chondroitin from farm animal cartilage is also absorbed; the amount of any given sample of chondroitin that is absorbed intact will depend on its molecular weight and other properties (Volpi, 2003). Volpi (2009) compared the quality of pharmaceutical-grade preparations prescribed by health practitioners in some continental European countries and some of those sold over the counter as dietary supplements in the USA, and concluded that many of the latter were of poor quality.

The maximum recommended dose of glucosamine is 1500 mg/day, which may be given in one more aliquots. No major adverse effects of taking glucosamine have been reported, apart from occasional incidences of usually transient, mild gastrointestinal discomfort. The usual maximum dose of chondroitin sulphate is around 1200 mg/day. Combinations of the two substances are also widely available and widely used.

Rationale for use and evidence of effectiveness

A continuous supply of glucosamine is required for the synthesis of the proteoglycans necessary for cartilage synthesis, which in turn is needed for the continual repair and remodelling of cartilaginous structures. One widely promulgated theory used by those marketing supplements of glucosamine is that the rate of endogenous production of glucosamine is slow, and is thus a rate-limiting factor in the production of proteoglycans in cartilage. Supplements of glucosamine would thus accelerate proteoglycan production in joints, and thus stimulate joint repair and reduce the erosion of cartilage seen in osteoarthritis. There are also suggestions that glucosamine may have anti-inflammatory effects, which contribute to its beneficial effects in arthritis (non-steroidal anti-inflammatory drugs are the main pharmacological treatment for osteoarthritis).

In vitro studies indicate that glucosamine can indeed increase the rate of proteoglycan production in cultured chondrocytes (Bassleer *et al.*, 1998). Glucosamine also inhibits the interleukin-1β-induced stimulation of some inflammatory mediators in isolated human chondrocytes (Shikhman *et al.*, 2001). The clinical significance of these *in vitro* findings is uncertain, because the concentrations needed to produce these effects in isolated chondrocytes are far higher than would be achieved in the cartilage of patients taking usual supplemental doses of glucosamine. Shikhman *et al.* (2001) suggest that high doses of glucose in the culture medium may compete with glucosamine for transporter molecules that facilitate glucose entry into the chondrocytes, and thus inflate the doses needed for these *in vitro* effects compared to the *in vivo* situation.

Clinical trials of the efficacy of glucosamine began more than 20 years ago. McAlindon *et al.* (2000) carried out a meta-analysis of trials of glucosamine and chondroitin for the treatment of osteoarthritis of the hip and knee that were of more than four weeks duration and that had been published before mid-1999. The initial analysis of all eligible studies suggested a moderate to large beneficial effect of both these substances in the treatment of osteoarthritis. However, they found that there was a high likelihood of publication bias; that is, negative findings were less likely to have been published than positive findings. Some studies had small sample sizes and there were also quality issues with some of the studies. The magnitude of the beneficial effects decreased when only the larger and higher-quality studies were used for the analysis. Many of the studies were funded by companies involved in the sale and manufacture of these supplements. Despite these flaws in the studies reviewed, however, these authors concluded that both compounds probably did have some efficacy in the treatment of osteoarthritis, although less than the crude aggregated data suggested. The analysis also indicated that periods in excess of a month may be required to get full efficacy.

Since this review by McAlindon *et al.*, several large and long-term controlled studies of glucosamine use have been published. Reginster *et al.* (2001) carried out a three year double-blind, placebo-controlled trial using a daily dose of 1500 mg of glucosamine. They randomised 212 patients with osteoarthritis of the knee to receive either the glucosamine or the placebo. In the placebo group, there was progressive narrowing of the knee joint space and a slight worsening of symptoms; whereas in the glucosamine group, there was no joint space narrowing and an improvement in the symptoms. A similar-sized study by Pavelka *et al.* (2002) reported qualitatively similar findings. Both groups of authors concluded that long-term treatment with glucosamine seemed to have a disease-modifying effect in osteoarthritis, positively affecting both symptoms and an objective measure of disease progression.

In 2003, the subject of the value of glucosamine in the treatment of osteoarthritis of the knee was debated at a major rheumatology centre in the UK. The report of that debate (Manson and Rahman, 2004) provides a readable summary of the case for and against glucosamine supplements. Much of the evidence quoted in this debate is summarised above and the assembled experts were split fairly evenly on whether glucosamine supplements were justified or not. Some of the key arguments put forward against the use of these supplements are listed below:

- The concentrations of glucosamine used in the *in vitro* studies are much higher than those that would be achieved *in vivo* with oral supplements (this issue was discussed earlier).
- The small size and dubious quality of many of the studies and the fact that most have been funded by the manufacturers.
- Doubts about whether narrowing of the joint space is a useful measure of the progression of the disease, as it does not seem to be correlated with symptoms.
- Several of the most recent positive studies had used patients with mild symptoms and had demonstrated only mild beneficial effects.
- One study that had used patients with a wider range of disease severity (Hughes and Carr, 2002) had not found evidence of a significant beneficial effect of glucosamine on symptoms or the primary outcome measure.

A systematic review first published in 2001 has been updated (Towheed *et al.*, 2005, also updated in 2009 with no change to conclusions) with a new search of the literature. This review covered 25 randomised controlled trials with almost 5000 patients in total. When all 25 studies were included, the results favoured a beneficial effect of glucosamine, with a significant reduction in pain after six months but no statistically significant effect on other parameters measured. When the analysis was restricted to just the higher-quality studies, there was no significant effect of glucosamine on pain. The authors suggested that there might be some difference in the results depending on whether a pharmaceutical-grade preparation or some other unregulated preparation was used in the trial, although the data was not clear. In general, the glucosamine preparations were seen to be safe and there were no more side-effects reported than for the placebo.

In a review of studies where glucosamine sulphate had been used for at least a year (and up to at least eight years), Black *et al.* (2009) found some evidence that it had modest effects on pain and resulted in a slight reduction in joint space loss (an objective measure of disease progression). There was less evidence to support beneficial effects of other glucosamine preparations or of preparations containing chondroitin. A major independent US study commissioned by the National Institute of Health (NCCAM, 2008) found no statistically significant reduction in pain from use of either glucosamine, chondroitin or a combination of both for patients with mild osteoarthritic pain. There was some preliminary evidence that patients with moderate to severe pain may have gained significant pain relief from the use of combined glucosamine and chondroitin preparations, although the sample sizes were small.

Given that even a group of clinical 'experts' in the field cannot come to a consensus on this topic, it is clear that the evidence is currently insufficient to make a firm recommendation as to the value of glucosamine supplements. The case for there being at least some small beneficial effect of glucosamine supplements in at least some patients looks slightly less convincing than it did when the first edition of this book was written. Those conducting trials of glucosamine have concluded that it is safe and with few adverse effects. Individual patients are left with the decision as to whether this probably small and not wholly certain benefit of taking glucosamine supplements justifies their cost.

The meta-analysis of McAlindon *et al.* (2000) came to essentially the same conclusions for chondroitin as those discussed for glucosamine. Another meta-analysis of seven controlled trials of long-term chondroitin supplements suggested that it significantly reduced symptoms as compared to the placebo (Leeb *et al.*, 2000). The more recent studies mentioned above (NCCAM, 2008; Black *et al.*, 2009) seem less positive than these older studies. The positive evidence that some large molecular weight components as well as smaller breakdown products of chondroitin are actually absorbed is clearly important in giving credibility to any claims about the benefits of oral supplements of chondroitin. Overall, the evidence for beneficial effects of chondroitin seems less than for glucosamine. Chondroitin supplements, especially those of marine origin, tend to be more expensive than glucosamine supplements; it is also common for combined chondroitin and glucosamine supplements to be taken.

s-Adenosyl-methionine (SAMe)

Nature and functions

s-Adenosyl-methionine (SAMe) is a natural component of the body that is synthesised from the sulphur-containing amino acid methionine; it is sometimes referred to as activated methionine. A healthy adult synthesises several grams of SAMe each day. The enzyme SAMe synthetase catalyses the addition of the adenosyl group (from adenosine triphosphate, ATP) to the sulphur atom of methionine.

The structure of SAMe is shown in Figure 7.2. It is the most important source of methyl (CH_3) groups for methyl transfer reactions that are catalysed by a variety of methyl transferase enzymes involved in many synthetic and other biochemical pathways.

Rationale for use and evidence of efficacy

Numerous claims have been made for the beneficial effects of SAMe supplements in several disease states, reflecting the involvement of SAMe in dozens of important

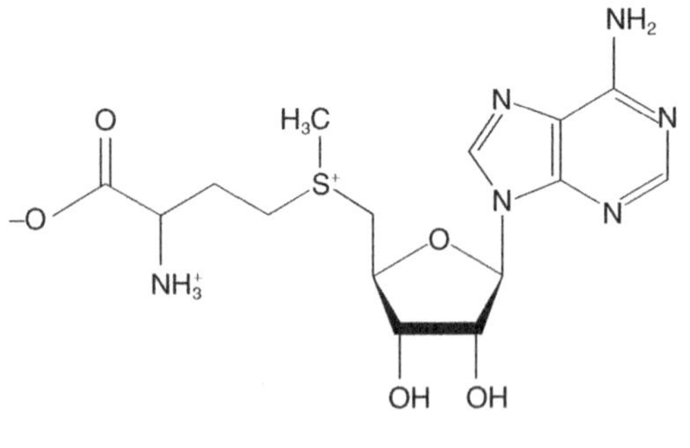

Figure 7.2 The structure of s-adenosyl methionine (SAMe).

biochemical pathways. It is, for example, essential for the synthesis of creatine, some neurotransmitters, glutathione, carnitine, phospholipids, proteins, DNA and RNA. The underlying hypothesis behind the use of SAMe in these disease states is that its endogenous synthesis and availability are rate limiting in one or more of these reactions, which produces adverse consequences and symptoms, and so provision of additional SAMe in the form of supplements should correct this. Three of the most persistent and researched claims are that it is beneficial in the treatment of arthritis, depression and liver disease.

Much of the information in this section up to 2002 is derived from a substantial review of the use of s-Adenosyl-methionine in the treatment of depression, osteoarthritis and liver disease, commissioned by the Agency for Healthcare Research and Quality (AHRQ) in the USA (Hardy *et al.*, 2002).

The structure of SAMe was elucidated in 1952 and a stable form that could be administered by intramuscular or intravenous injection was produced in 1974. However, it was not until the late 1990s that an enteric coated preparation of SAMe that could be administered orally was produced. It was only in 1999 that SAMe was introduced as a dietary supplement in the USA, but its popularity as a supplement grew rapidly, with US sales valued at around $40 million in 2001.

SAMe is present in various regions of the brain and is the main methyl donor in the central nervous system. SAMe-associated methylation is involved in the synthesis of several brain neurotransmitters and it may also affect membrane fluidity (and so nerve function) and receptor activity by its involvement in the methylation of phospholipids and other brain chemicals. Mind-altering (psychotropic) drugs are reported to increase the blood levels of SAMe and this led to it being tested early on as a possible treatment for schizophrenia. Suggestions that it might be useful in the treatment of depression arose as an observation from these early and unsuccessful trials. Levels of SAMe are low in the cerebrospinal fluid of people with depression and there have been reports that increased serum levels of SAMe have correlated with successful therapy for depression.

In a meta-analysis of 28 trials of the use of SAMe in the treatment of depression, Hardy *et al.* (2002) concluded that SAMe was significantly more effective than placebos and that this effect was clinically useful. When tested against conventional antidepressants, there was no statistically significant difference between outcomes for the treatments. Many of the studies reviewed were small scale and of variable quality; there was also the real possibility of publication bias (i.e. positive findings more likely to be published than negative ones). A very recent review in a major psychiatric journal (Papakostas, 2009) suggested that SAMe seemed to be more effective than a placebo and as effective as older tricyclic antidepressants in treating major depression when administered intravenously or intramuscularly, but that there is much less evidence of its effectiveness when given orally. Essentially this review suggests that there is not enough quality evidence available to judge the effectiveness of oral SAMe preparations or how well they are tolerated.

The suggestion that SAMe might be useful in the treatment of osteoarthritis arose as a side issue from trials of its use in treating depression. SAMe has been shown to have anti-inflammatory and analgesic properties when tested in animal models. Although the mechanism of these effects is unclear, it does act via a different mechanism to non-steroidal anti-inflammatory drugs (NSAIDs) like aspirin, which act by inhibiting prostaglandin synthesis. Orally administered SAMe does reach the synovial fluid and *in vitro* it stimulates cultured human chondrocytes and increases sulphate incorporation into proteoglycans. The process of sulphation in the synthesis of cartilage is known to involve SAMe derivatives.

A review of 10 trials of SAMe in the treatment of osteoarthritis suggested that it was more effective than placebos at reducing pain and that there was no significant difference when it was tested against traditional NSAIDs (Hardy *et al.*, 2002). A more recent systematic review (Rutjes *et al.*, 2009) found that the data on whether SAMe was effective in reducing pain and improving function in patients with osteoarthritis of the hip and knee was inconclusive, largely because many of the trials were small and of questionable quality. These authors concluded that while any effect of SAMe was likely to be small, it could be clinically significant and worthy of testing with larger, better-designed studies.

It has been reported that the activity of SAMe synthetase is decreased in cirrhotic livers. Alcohol-induced liver injury in baboons results in reduced levels of SAMe in their livers, and SAMe supplementation reduces the degree of liver injury (see Lieber, 2006). The adverse effects of SAMe depletion in experimental liver injury may be due to reduced availability of glutathione; SAMe is necessary for glutathione synthesis and glutathione is important in protecting the liver from free radical injury. SAMe may also prevent membrane damage induced by alcohol; SAMe-dependent phospholipid methylation is essential for optimal membrane function.

Hardy *et al.* (2002) identified 41 studies where SAMe had been used to treat a variety of liver conditions. There were sufficient studies to carry out meta-analyses of its effectiveness in treating the cholestasis (non-obstructive reduction in bile flow) of pregnancy and other causes of cholestasis. Cholestasis results in raised bilirubin levels in plasma, jaundice and severe itching. These pooled analyses suggested that SAMe was more effective than placebos in reducing the itching associated with cholestasis and in reducing bilirubin levels in the cholestasis of pregnancy. A 2001 Cochrane review of SAMe for the treatment of alcoholic liver disease did not find any significant effect of SAMe on mortality, liver transplantation rates or other complications of liver disease. Despite finding eight randomised controlled trials of SAMe use with patients with alcoholic liver disease, only one trial with 123 patients used adequate methodology and reported clearly on mortality and liver-transplantation rates. This review has been updated but with no change to the earlier conclusions (Rambaldi *et al.*, 2007).

Hardy *et al.* (2002) noted that few studies had looked at the responses to different oral doses of SAMe and so there was little information available to indicate a likely effective dose. Dosages recommended by manufacturers of the product vary between 200 and 1600 mg/day. Hardy *et al.* (2002) found no evidence from their review of clinical trials that there are any significant adverse effects associated with the use of SAMe. There has been speculation that SAMe might raise blood levels of homocysteine, which is an independent risk factor for heart disease. However, one

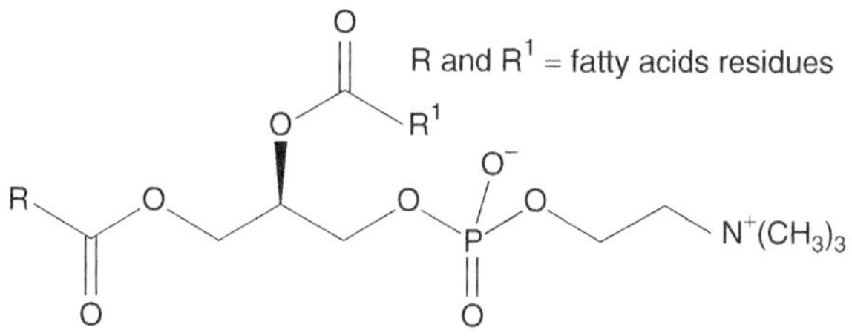

Figure 7.3   The structure of phosphatidylcholine (lecithin).

pharmacological study (Loehrer *et al.*, 1997) found that oral SAMe lowered blood levels of homocysteine and had no adverse effects on homocysteine metabolism.

Several other claims have been made for beneficial effects of SAMe, particularly for fibromyalgia (fibrositis), which is an arthritis-like condition affecting muscles and tendons rather than joints. Hardy *et al.* (2002) suggested that the data available for other conditions would almost certainly be less advanced than that for the conditions that they reviewed, depression, osteoarthritis and liver disease.

Lecithin and choline

Lecithin supplements contain a mixture of phospholipids that are usually extracted from soybean oil or, less commonly, from egg yolk. The principal phospholipid is phosphatidyl choline, with lesser amounts of phosphatidyl inositol and phosphatidyl ethanolamine. The terms phosphatidyl choline and lecithin are used as synonyms by biological scientists. Phosphatidyl choline is generally regarded as the 'active' ingredient in soy (or egg) lecithin supplements and it makes up a variable proportion of the total product. The structure of phosphatidyl choline is shown in Figure 7.3.

Choline is a component of commercial lecithin supplements and it has three main functions:

- It is a constituent of the key nerve transmitter acetylcholine.
- It is a component of the phospholipids in cell membranes and plasma lipoproteins.
- It acts as a methyl donor.

COMA (1991) did not include choline in its list of essential nutrients and in fact specifically decided not to include it as an essential nutrient (along with lecithin). There is an endogenous pathway for choline biosynthesis. However, it is not established that this pathway is capable of producing adequate amounts of choline at different stages of life. For this reason, in 1998 the US Food and Nutrition Board did add choline to its list of essential nutrients and set recommended intakes for individuals of all ages (425 mg/day for adult women and 550 mg/day for adult men).

Human choline deficiency does not normally occur, partly because of the endogenous synthesis and also because choline is present in many foods, such as soybeans, nuts, eggs, liver, meat, cauliflower, lettuce and many other foods. Lecithin is also used as a food additive because of its emulsifying properties, for instance in the production of margarine and low-fat spreads.

Choline deficiency has been experimentally induced in many non-ruminant animals, where it results in a wide variety of adverse consequences in the kidney, liver and pancreas as well as memory and growth disorders. Humans fed for three weeks on choline-deficient diets developed biochemical indications of choline deficiency. Fatty infiltration of the liver and liver damage have been reported several times in patients receiving total parenteral nutrition and this has been attributed to choline deficiency (Zeisel and Niculescu, 2006).

It has been suggested that lecithin and/or choline may be beneficial in dementia, based on the observation that there is low activity of the enzyme that synthesises acetylcholine in the brains of patients with Alzheimer's disease. A Cochrane review (Higgins and Flicker, first published in 2000 but recently updated with the same conclusions and no additional published data) found no evidence for any beneficial effect for lecithin in 12 controlled studies of its use in the treatment of Alzheimer's disease or other forms of dementia. The authors felt that there was so little evidence of any potential benefits that a large controlled trial was of low priority.

It has also been suggested that large doses of lecithin might lower serum cholesterol concentrations, but a properly controlled trial (Oosthuizen et al., 1998) concluded that phosphatidyl choline did not have independent effects on serum cholesterol. These authors attributed earlier positive findings to faults in the analysis or to the presence of polyunsaturated fatty acids in the preparations of lecithin.

The evidence for any beneficial effects from lecithin or choline supplements is thus generally very weak or non-existent.

L-carnitine

Nature and synthesis of L-carnitine

L-carnitine is another natural component of the human body that is synthesised, mainly in the liver and kidneys, from the essential amino acid lysine (the structure of L-carnitine and two of its esters are shown in Figure 7.4). Lysine is one of the so-called dibasic amino acids, which have a second amino group in their side chain. The synthesis of L-carnitine involves the transfer of three methyl groups to the nitrogen atom present in the side chain of lysine, while it is linked to other amino acids by peptide bonds within a protein (see Rebouche, 2006 for details of this synthetic pathway and general information about L-carnitine).

The synthetic pathway produces 11–34 mg/day of L-carnitine in a standard 70 kg adult and this endogenous synthesis is normally sufficient to meet the metabolic needs of adults and children, even those who are strict vegetarians (vegans) and obtain very little from their diet. Vegan adults do have blood levels of carnitine that are about 10% less than those in other adults; in vegan children they are about 30% less than those in matched omnivorous children. Meat, fish and milk

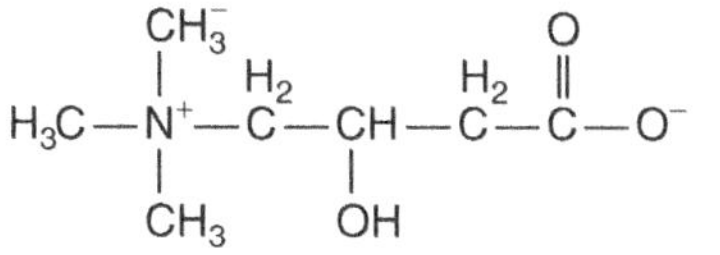

$$H_3C - \overset{\overset{\displaystyle CH_3^-}{|}}{\underset{\underset{\displaystyle CH_3}{|}}{N^+}} - \overset{H_2}{C} - \overset{\overset{}{|}}{\underset{\underset{\displaystyle OH}{|}}{CH}} - \overset{H_2}{C} - \overset{\overset{\displaystyle O}{\|}}{C} - C - O^-$$

Figure 7.4   The structure of L-carnitine. Acetyl-L-carnitine and propionyl-L-carnitine have acetyl of propionyl groups esterified to the OH group.

contain relatively large amounts of L-carnitine, whereas most vegetable foods contain very little. The diet of an omnivore probably contains 20–200 mg/day of L-carnitine, while that of a strict vegetarian might provide less than 1 mg/day. In normal healthy people there is efficient conservation and 95% of that filtered in the kidney is reabsorbed.

Up to 75% of the carnitine present in a normal diet is absorbed, whereas the absorption from supplements may be much lower (perhaps only 20% of a daily 2 g supplement). Oral supplements typically provide between 1 and 6 g/day of L-carnitine. In general, carnitine is regarded as relatively non-toxic, but doses in excess of 3 g/day can cause diarrhoea and a fishy body odour, caused by the organic breakdown products of carnitine. The body synthesises only the L-isomer of carnitine and this is also the only isomer present in normal food. Some supplements contain a mixture of D and L isomers (racemic mixture) and these should be avoided, because the D-isomer may interfere with the absorption and functioning of L-carnitine.

Functions of carnitine

Long-chain fatty acids with 16 or more carbon atoms can only enter the mitochondrion for oxidation and energy production when they are in the form of carnitine esters (acyl carnitine). Outside of the mitochondrion, coenzyme A derivatives of these fatty acids are esterified to acyl carnitine esters by the enzyme carnitine palmitoyl transferase I:

L-carnitine + acyl coenzyme A → Acyl carnitine ester (activated fatty acid) + reduced coenzyme A

A transporter protein called carnitine-acylcarnitine transferase facilitates the rapid entry of the acyl carnitine esters into the mitochondria. Once inside the mitochondrion, a carnitine palmitoyl transferase II reconverts the acyl carnitine ester back to acyl coenzyme A, which can then undergo β-oxidation within the mitochondrion to produce metabolic energy for the cell.

The coenzyme A or CoA moiety is derived from the vitamin pantothenic acid and CoA-activated compounds are key intermediaries in several biochemical pathways. If there is low availability of free reduced coenzyme A within the cell, this will have a limiting effect on any CoA dependent reaction. For example, both the β-oxidation of fatty acids and the oxidation of pyruvate in carbohydrate metabolism yield acetyl CoA. High rates of production of acetyl CoA from the β-oxidation of fatty acids would tend to inhibit the oxidation of pyruvate and thus block carbohydrate metabolism, because of the limited availability of coenzyme A. However, the enzyme carnitine acetyl transferase transfers the acetyl moiety from acetyl CoA to carnitine, thus releasing the coenzyme A for other reactions:

$$\text{Carnitine + acetyl CoA} \rightarrow \text{acetyl carnitine + reduced coenzyme A}$$

Coenzyme A derivatives of other short-chain organic acids, particularly propionyl CoA, can undergo similar conversion to acyl carnitine esters and these act as a reservoir of activated acyl residues. In certain inherited disorders of fatty acid metabolism, this mechanism is essential to maintain cellular metabolism. For example, in patients with deficiency of the enzyme propionyl coenzyme A carboxylase, propionyl CoA is an end product that would rapidly soak up available coenzyme A and prevent cellular energy production. However, in this condition, the propionyl moiety of propionyl CoA is transferred to carnitine and large amounts of propionyl carnitine are excreted. This condition leads to more rapid excretion of carnitine and large supplemental doses of carnitine may be prescribed.

Circumstances that may increase carnitine requirements

There are several conditions and/or circumstances in which carnitine deficiency may occur or the body's need for carnitine may be increased, although most of these are rare conditions.

- Carnitine is added to infant formula, especially soy-based formula, which is essentially carnitine-free up to the level found in human milk. There is no evidence even when infants are fed on unsupplemented soy formula that their growth is affected or that they have any other outward manifestations of deficiency. However, their serum carnitine levels are lower than those fed supplemented formula and levels of free fatty acids in the blood are elevated. Thus while endogenous synthesis may be sufficient to maintain growth in infants, unless it is supplemented by exogenous carnitine from breast milk or formula, rapid postnatal growth leads to a state of carnitine depletion. Carnitine is thus widely regarded as conditionally essential for infants and perhaps especially for premature infants, who have around ten times less carnitine in their skeletal muscles than adults.
- Primary carnitine deficiency results from a genetic defect in the enzyme that transfers carnitine across the plasma membrane. This means that the kidney fails to reabsorb filtered carnitine and there is a depletion of carnitine, which results in an impaired ability to metabolise long-chain fatty acids. Symptoms of carnitine deficiency include severe hypoglycaemia, cardiomyopathy, muscle weakness and skeletal muscle wasting. The condition responds to pharmacological doses of L-carnitine.

- There are several rare genetic disorders of fatty acid metabolism that can lead to secondary deficiency of carnitine. The deficiency of propionyl CoA carboxylase referred to earlier is an example of one of these. Details of these conditions and the role of carnitine in their therapy are beyond the scope of this book, but further details may be found in Vockley and Renaud (2006).
- In haemodialysis there is increased urinary loss of carnitine and this may increase the requirement for carnitine. There may also be reduced renal synthesis of carnitine in renal failure.
- Certain drugs, such as the anticonvulsant valproic acid and pivalic acid that are conjugated to some antibiotics (e.g. pivampicillin) to improve their absorption, may increase carnitine requirements. These organic acids are excreted as conjugates of carnitine and patients undergoing long-term therapy with such drugs may be given carnitine supplements.

Note that Nasser *et al.* (2009) did not find any controlled clinical trials of the use of carnitine supplements in children or adults diagnosed with an inborn error of metabolism; indeed, such controlled trials might be ethically dubious in some of these life-threatening conditions. The use of carnitine supplements and the choice of dosing regime are based on clinical experience and judgement.

Use of carnitine supplements

In addition to the above special circumstances, it has been suggested that carnitine supplements may be beneficial in the treatment of various pathological conditions, including acute myocardial infarction (heart attack), angina, intermittent claudication, Alzheimer's disease and chronic fatigue syndrome. Largely because of its role in facilitating fatty acid metabolism and thus potentially sparing glycogen, it has been suggested that carnitine may have the potential to boost athletic performance. In a concise referenced review of the use of carnitine supplements, Higdon (2002) found no controlled human studies that supported speculative claims that carnitine might boost athletic performance. More recent controlled trials of carnitine supplements have also found no evidence of any effect on athletic performance (Broad *et al.*, 2005; Smith *et al.*, 2008).

Two small pilot studies published in the early 1990s did suggest that carnitine supplements might have some slowing effect on the deterioration in Alzheimer's patients. However, two more recent and relatively large studies did not show any significant benefits over a placebo when using doses of 3 g/day of the acetyl ester of carnitine for one year. Thal *et al.* (1996) used a sample of 431 Alzheimer's patients and Thal *et al.* (2000) used 229 patients with early-onset disease.

Below is a summary of the findings in a review by Higdon (2002) on the use of carnitine supplements in the treatment of three cardiovascular conditions:

- Several small trials have been conducted of the use of carnitine supplements immediately after a myocardial infarction and these have produced no clear indication of whether they improve the clinical outcome. Some of these studies have used intravenous infusions of carnitine rather than oral supplements and in general the use of carnitine as an adjunct to the clinical treatment of a serious, acute condition is beyond the scope of this book.

- In a randomised controlled trial of the propionyl ester of L-carnitine in 226 patients with heart failure for six months, there was no overall difference in exercise tolerance between the carnitine and placebo groups. Further analysis of the data did suggest that that there might be some benefits in patients with less severe symptoms at the start.
- Intermittent claudication is a peripheral vascular disease in which atherosclerosis of peripheral arteries leads to ischaemic pain (due to poor blood flow) in the legs when walking. Higdon (2002) reviews preliminary evidence suggesting that doses of 2 g/day of the propionyl ester of carnitine for 6–12 months may have some beneficial effects on the distance patients were capable of walking. The significant benefits seemed to be confined to those patients with the highest level of disability and no significant benefit could be found in those with less severe disability.

Carnitine supplements: Conclusions

Thus carnitine supplementation of infant formula is generally recommended, especially soy-based formulae that contain almost none. There are some rare inherited conditions of carnitine and fatty acid utilisation that do respond to pharmacological doses of carnitine. There is no substantial evidence that carnitine supplements affect the progress of Alzheimer's disease, however. Large carnitine supplements may have a role as an adjunct to the clinical management of certain cardiovascular conditions, but the evidence is only preliminary and would certainly not warrant recommending self-medication. There is little evidence that carnitine improves athletic performance and little to suggest that carnitine supplements are likely to benefit healthy adults or children. At usual doses (typically 1–6 g/day), L-carnitine supplements are regarded as safe.

Creatine

Nature and origins of body creatine

Creatine is an amino acid and a typical adult body contains 120–160 g of this amino acid, largely concentrated in muscles. The amount of creatine increases with increasing lean muscle mass. It can be synthesised from other amino acids in the diet and is not therefore classed as an essential nutrient, nor is it one of the 20 amino acids found in protein. In the kidney, a substance called guanadinoacetic acid is produced from the amino acids arginine and glycine; in the liver this is methylated to creatine by the transfer of a methyl group from s-adenosyl methionine. The creatine synthesised in the liver is then transported to the muscles. The structure of creatine is shown in Figure 7.5.

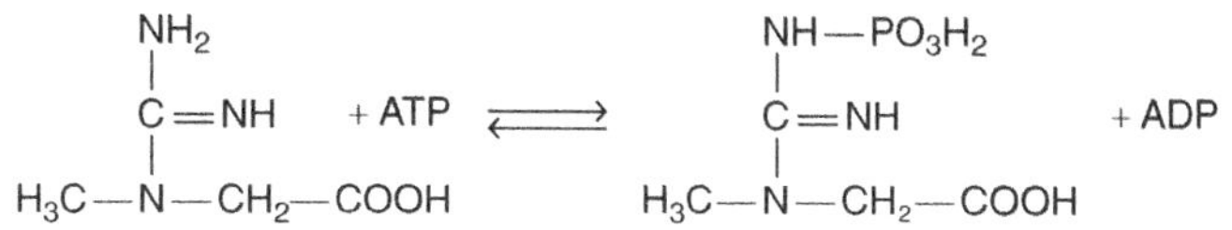

$$
\begin{array}{ccc}
\text{NH}_2 & & \text{NH}-\text{PO}_3\text{H}_2 \\
| & & | \\
\text{C}=\text{NH} \quad + \text{ATP} \; \rightleftharpoons & & \text{C}=\text{NH} \quad\quad + \text{ADP} \\
| & & | \\
\text{H}_3\text{C}-\text{N}-\text{CH}_2-\text{COOH} & & \text{H}_3\text{C}-\text{N}-\text{CH}_2-\text{COOH}
\end{array}
$$

Figure 7.5   The structure of creatine and creatine phosphate.

The daily synthesis of creatine is enough to maintain the body pool at 120–160 g without any dietary input. Daily synthesis depends on the amount present in the diet, as dietary input reduces endogenous synthesis. The amount present in the diet varies from almost nothing in vegetarian diets to around 2 g/day in omnivorous diets, where it is largely derived from meat and fish. Creatine is excreted in urine mainly as the metabolite creatinine and about 2 g/day is excreted in an average adult.

Functions of creatine

Within the muscles, creatine is phosphorylated to phosphocreatine or creatine phosphate by the transfer of a phosphate group from ATP and this is catalysed by the enzyme creatine kinase. This reaction is reversible and so stores of creatine phosphate within the muscle can be used to regenerate ATP for muscle work during short periods of intense activity.

$$\text{ATP} + \text{Creatine} \rightarrow \text{ADP} + \text{Creatine phosphate}$$

In effect, the creatine phosphate is acting as a short-term store of metabolic energy that can be used to directly rephosphorylate ATP during short periods of intense muscle activity. The ATP stores within muscles are limited and only sufficient for a couple of seconds of intense work; the creatine phosphate stores are ordinarily sufficient to maintain ATP levels for a few more seconds. If this level of exercise intensity is maintained, then ATP must be replenished by the anaerobic metabolism of glycogen and to a smaller extent by aerobic metabolism. Anaerobic metabolism leads to a build-up of lactic acid, which produces fatigue and this limits the duration of intense work in muscles. In endurance events the energy supply for the muscle largely comes from the aerobic metabolism of glucose, which is able to generate large amounts of ATP at a slower rate. There is an increasing contribution from the aerobic metabolism of fat, which cannot be metabolised anaerobically, the longer the exercise is maintained. In aerobic endurance events the work intensity in the muscle is at a level that is sustainable by aerobic metabolism.

Rationale and evidence for the use of creatine supplements

Creatine has been widely promoted and used as a legal performance enhancer or ergogenic aid by athletes. Given its role in replenishing ATP in the first few seconds of intense exercise, there are theoretical grounds for believing that increases in phosphocreatine levels in muscles might be useful in maintaining maximum work output in those activities that involve a single burst or multiple short bursts of intense activity. It was first shown by Harris *et al.* (1992) that creatine supplements could increase the phosphocreatine concentration in skeletal muscle. They used 20 g of creatine per day for five days and split this 20 g/day into four 5 g aliquots. This amount of creatine is well beyond that which could be obtained from boosting meat intake; Harris *et al.* (1992) suggest that a single 5 g supplement is equivalent to eating over a kilogram of raw steak. The average increase in muscle creatine recorded in this study amounted to around 20%, with the biggest increases seen in those who had the lowest initial levels; those with baseline levels towards the top of the maximum normal range showed less increase. Subsequent studies have shown that similar increases in muscle creatine levels can be brought about by smaller doses (say 3 g/day) of creatine administered for periods of up to a month.

There have been a number of small, controlled laboratory studies that supported the hypothesis that creatine loading can increase work output in single bouts of short-duration intense exercise or in intermittent bouts of intense activity separated by rest periods (see Hultman *et al.*, 1999). There are, however, almost as many other studies that have failed to report enhanced performance, especially when tested under field rather than laboratory conditions. These findings are generally consistent with the results of a meta-analysis of studies published up to 2003 (Branch, 2003). There is general agreement that creatine supplements do not enhance performance in endurance events and may even have a slight negative effect; in these events the extra muscle creatine phosphate would be expected to make an insignificant contribution. Creatine supplements do lead to a slight increase in body weight of around 1 kg and it probable that this is due to increased water content of muscles; this extra weight may be a net hindrance to performance in those events where there is no benefit from the extra muscle phosphocreatine. The role of creatine supplementation in skeletal muscle metabolism and performance has been reviewed by Casey and Greenhaff (2000).

Coenzyme Q_{10} (ubiquinone)

Nature and sources of coenzyme Q_{10}

Coenzyme Q_{10} is a lipid-soluble substance that is sometimes called ubiquinone because it is a 'quinone'-type compound that is ubiquitous in biological systems. It is made up of a benzoquinone component that has two carbonyl groups (C=O), which can be reduced to hydroxyl groups (C—OH) by the addition of two hydrogen atoms. Attached to this benzoquinone group are a variable number of so-called isoprene units; the most common mammalian form contains ten of these isoprene units, hence coenzyme Q_{10} (the structure of coenzyme Q_{10}

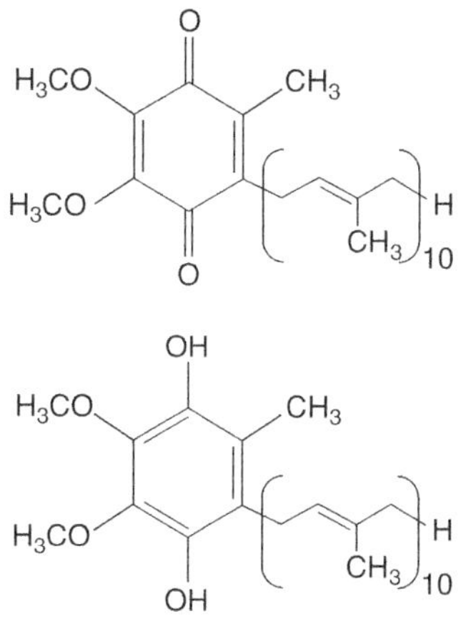

Figure 7.6   The structure of coenzyme Q_{10} (ubiquinone) and its reduced form ubiquinol.

is shown in Figure 7.6). Thus ubiquinone can be reduced to ubiquinol by the addition of two hydrogen atoms:

$$CoQ_{10} \text{ (ubiquinone)} + H_2 \leftrightarrow CoQ_{10}H_2 \text{ (ubiquinol)}$$

Coenzyme Q_{10} is synthesised in most human tissues. The benzoquinone part of the molecule is synthesised from the aromatic amino acids phenylalanine and tyrosine, and the isoprene side chain is synthesised from acetyl coenzyme A via a pathway that is partly common to cholesterol biosynthesis. The isoprene side chain is then coupled to the benzoquinone component to give coenzyme Q_{10}. The enzyme hydroxymethyl glutaryl CoA reductase (HMG CoA reductase) is an important regulatory point in both cholesterol biosynthesis and coenzyme Q_{10} synthesis.

The most important group of cholesterol-lowering drugs, the statins, work by inhibiting HMG CoA reductase. This raises the theoretical possibility that taking these drugs may reduce coenzyme Q_{10} production and thus increase the case for coenzyme Q_{10} supplements. In particular, it has been suggested that lower coenzyme Q_{10} production might be implicated in the myopathy that is occasionally associated with statin use. Marcoff and Thompson (2007) found that although statins reduced circulating Q_{10} levels, there was no evidence of their effect on intramuscular levels. They concluded that routine use of Q_{10} could not be routinely recommended for those receiving statin therapy, although there might be a case for testing its efficacy in patients with myopathy who do not respond to other treatments. While there are extremely rare genetic abnormalities of coenzyme Q_{10} biosynthesis that do respond to supplements, there is no general deficiency syndrome attributable to lack of coenzyme Q_{10} seen in the general population.

As its name suggests, ubiquinone is widely distributed in foods. Rich dietary sources are meat, fish, nuts, rapeseed oil and soya oil; it is also present in lesser amounts in fruits, vegetables, eggs and dairy products. There are few estimates of

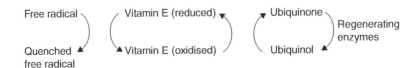

Figure 7.7 Ubiquinone (coenzyme Q_{10}) as an antioxidant.

usual dietary intake, but most diets probably contain less than 10 mg/day, with the average intake somewhere around half this figure. Endogenous synthesis is probably responsible for about three-quarters of the plasma coenzyme Q_{10}.

Functions of coenzyme Q_{10}

The best-known function of coenzyme Q_{10} is as a component of the electron transport system in the mitochondrion (oxidative phosphorylation). Reduced $NADH_2$ and $FADH_2$ generated by the oxidation of foodstuffs within the cell are reoxidised to NAD and FAD and the hydrogen eventually combined with oxygen to yield water. Most of the ATP produced by aerobic metabolism of fats and carbohydrates is generated during this electron transfer and reoxidation of these reduced coenzymes. $NADH_2$ transfers its hydrogen atoms to FMN (flavin mononucleotide) to give $FMNH_2$ and this $FMNH_2$ then transfers its hydrogen atoms to the oxidised form of Q_{10}, so converting it to the reduced form. $FADH_2$ transfers its hydrogen atoms directly to Q_{10}. The electrons of the hydrogen atoms of reduced Q_{10} are then transferred to a series of cytochromes and the protons (H^+) released into the intermembrane space of the mitochondrion, creating a proton gradient across the inner mitochondrial membrane. At the end of this sequence of cytochromes, protons, electrons and molecular oxygen combine to produce water; this reaction is 'driven' by the energy released when protons pass down the proton gradient that coenzyme Q_{10} has generated across the inner mitochondrial membrane. This means that coenzyme Q_{10} plays a pivotal role in the generation of the vast bulk of metabolic energy in the form of ATP.

Coenzyme Q_{10} is present in the lipid phase of almost all membranes in its quinol or reduced form, where it is believed to be an important antioxidant that, in combination with vitamin E, protects membranes from oxidative damage by free radicals. There are enzyme systems within membranes that can convert any oxidised CoQ_{10} (ubiquinone) that is generated back to the reduced $CoQ_{10}H_2$ (ubiquinol) form. When vitamin E quenches oxygen free radicals (ROS), it becomes oxidised and ubiquinol may then regenerate reduced vitamin E, while it itself is oxidised to the ubiquinone form. Any ubiquinone generated in this way is converted back to the reduced ubiquinol form by enzymes in the membrane (see Figure 7.7).

A third suggested role for CoQ_{10} is in lysosomes, where membranes have a relatively high concentration of coenzyme Q_{10}. Lysosomes are responsible for digesting cell debris and they have an acid pH, which is important in facilitating the activity of the digestive enzymes within them. Coenzyme Q_{10} may play a role in generating the protons necessary to maintain their acid pH.

Rationale and evidence for the use of coenzyme Q_{10} supplements

Oral supplementation with coenzyme Q_{10} does increase blood levels, but there is no evidence that it increases tissue levels in young healthy people or animals. Levels of coenzyme Q_{10} in some tissues does decline in old age and there is some evidence that supplements can increase some tissue levels in elderly animals or people. It is not clear whether this age-related decline in tissue levels should be regarded as an indication of deficiency, and thus whether there is any merit in trying to increase them by the use of supplements.

Listed below are some of the suggested uses for coenzyme Q_{10} and a brief assessment of their merits. A full list of references used for this summary may be found in a review of coenzyme Q_{10} supplementation by Higdon (2003a). Reference to the use of large, physician-prescribed supplements of Q_{10} as an adjunct to clinical therapy is included for completeness, but is beyond the scope of this book and patients are advised to avoid self-medication for these conditions without approval by their physician.

The age-related decline in tissue levels of coenzyme Q_{10} has prompted specula-tion that supplements might be beneficial in reducing the effects of ageing and perhaps in extending life expectancy. There is no evidence from animal studies that prolonged use of coenzyme Q_{10} supplements produces any measurable benefit on the rate of ageing (e.g. increased life expectancy), apart from the reported rise in tissue levels in elderly subjects referred to earlier.

The pivotal role of coenzyme Q_{10} in cellular energy production has prompted speculation that supplements might improve athletic performance. There is no sub-stantial evidence to support this proposal and no evidence that even prolonged use of large supplements causes any rise in muscle levels of coenzyme Q_{10} in healthy young animals or people.

Given its role as an antioxidant, according to the oxidant theory of disease (see Chapter 5) inadequate amounts of coenzyme Q_{10} would be expected to increase susceptibility to those diseases like cancer and cardiovascular disease that are believed to be promoted by oxidative damage to free radicals. For example, one might speculate that coenzyme Q_{10} might reduced the oxidation of LDL that is thought to be a key initiating step in atherosclerosis. At the moment, coenzyme Q_{10} is just one of many antioxidants that are postulated to help prevent these diseases, and there is no convincing and specific evidence that supplements of coenzyme Q_{10} have any protective effect. In their review of the role of antioxidants in the preven-tion and treatment of cardiovascular disease, Shekelle *et al.* (2003) concluded that there was no convincing evidence either to refute or to support the value of coen-zyme Q_{10} in cardiovascular disease. They found that there were only a few studies with over 60 patients and of at least six months' duration. They found one meta-analysis that had concluded that Q_{10} supplements were associated with a substantial improvement in measures of cardiac function (Soja and Mortensen, 1997; this review is discussed further in the next paragraph). However, several subsequent randomised controlled trials of sufficient size and duration to meet their inclusion criteria had not supported this conclusion, and those without substantial design or reporting flaws have found either no benefit from Q_{10} supplements or only clinically small improvements.

Large doses of coenzyme Q_{10} have been tested as possible adjuncts to other clinical treatments in the management of several types of cardiovascular disease, including angina pectoris, hypertension and congestive heart failure. It is also proposed that it might reduce myocardial damage if given immediately after a myocardial infarction (heart attack). Reperfusion and reoxygenation of heart muscle after an ischaemic attack may generate extra oxygen free radicals, and this may increase the amount of damage to the myocardium after the heart attack. Coenzyme Q_{10} might reduce this reperfusion injury because of its antioxidant activity. Most of the trials in this area have been small and preliminary studies and the results are as yet inconclusive. There has been a meta-analysis of eight trials that have used supplements of coenzyme Q_{10} in the treatment of congestive heart failure (Soja and Mortensen, 1997). This meta-analysis found that there were significant improvements in several measures of cardiac function in the Q_{10}-supplemented groups as compared to the placebo groups. In general, this possible role of coenzyme Q_{10} as an adjunct to the clinical management of established cardiovascular disease is outside the scope of this book. Ho *et al.* (2009), in a systematic review of the effects of coenzyme Q_{10} supplements in primary hypertension, found only four small trials, although these did suggest a beneficial effect. The poor design of some of these studies meant that they were unable to make any clear judgement on their effectiveness.

It is also suggested that because of its role as an antioxidant and its role in energy production in substantia negra (the affected area in Parkinson's disease) of the brain, coenzyme Q_{10} might slow down the progression of Parkinson's disease.

Over-the-counter supplements of coenzyme Q_{10} usually provide between 15 and 60 mg/day, although considerably higher doses have been used in some therapeutic trials. No serious adverse symptoms have been reported for coenzyme Q_{10} supplements except that it interferes with anticoagulant therapy (i.e. warfarin and other coumarin-type drugs).

Dietary supplements usually provide up to 60 mg of coenzyme Q_{10} in tablet form, but clinical trials done under medical supervision have used substantially higher doses than this. In general, there seems to be very little evidence that supplements of coenzyme Q_{10} offer any advantage to healthy young people, nor do they seem to improve athletic performance significantly. Indeed, supplements may not even raise tissue levels under these circumstances. Suggestions that coenzyme Q_{10} may play some role in reducing the effects of ageing are at present largely speculative. There seems to be no case for Q_{10} supplements to be recommended for the millions of people taking statins to reduce their blood cholesterol concentration. Supplements of coenzyme Q_{10} may have a role to play as adjuncts to the management of some cardiovascular diseases, but this research is still in its preliminary stages.

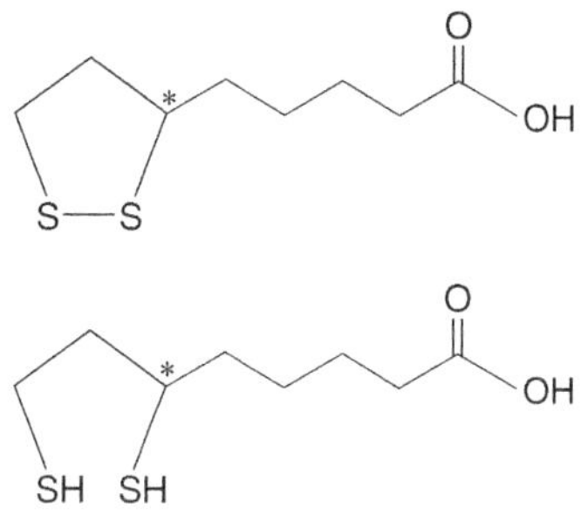

*Asymmetric carbon atom

Figure 7.8   The structure of α-lipoic acid and below its reduced form α-dihydrolipoic acid (DHLA).

Alpha(α)-lipoic acid

Nature and sources of body alpha-lipoic acid

Alpha-lipoic acid is a sulphur-containing compound that is synthesised by both plant and animal tissues and so is widely distributed in foods in small amounts, where it acts as an enzyme co-factor. It is both lipid and water soluble and the two sulphur atoms within the molecule can be reduced to give dihydrolipoic acid (DHLA); this is shown in Figure 7.8.

It can be seen in Figure 7.8 that α-lipoic acid has an asymmetric carbon atom and so two optical isomers of the compound can exist, the R and S isomers. All of the α-lipoic acid synthesised by plants and animals and thus all of that normally in the diet is present as the R isomer; only the R isomer can act as an enzyme co-factor. Chemical synthesis of α-lipoic acid yields a racemic mixture that contains equal quantities of both the R and S isomers. This means that most supplements also contain mixtures of the two isomers, although more expensive R-only preparations can be obtained; the S isomer must therefore be regarded as a chemical that is normally foreign to the body (xenobiotic). Note that the R and S terminology are alternatives to the D and L terminology used elsewhere in this book; for complex chemical reasons it is more convenient and usual to use the R and S terminology in this case.

There is no known deficiency syndrome associated with a lack of α-lipoic acid, so it is not classified as an essential nutrient because endogenous synthesis is deemed sufficient to meet normal physiological needs. It is widely distributed in foods, with meat (especially organ meat), spinach, broccoli and tomatoes being relatively rich sources; a list of the estimated lipoic acid content of some foods can be found in Higdon (2003b). Almost all of the lipoic acid present in food comes from enzymes that contain lipoamide (see below). Human digestive enzymes do not break the bond between lipoic acid and lysine, so it is thought that most dietary lipoic acid is absorbed in the form of lipolysine (lipoic acid — lysine). Unless supplements of pure lipoic acid are provided, no free lipoic acid can be detected in blood. While the amounts of lipoic acid ordinarily present in the diet are difficult to estimate, they are at least one order of magnitude lower than that provided by supplements, so supplements must be regarded as a pharmacological use of lipoic acid.

Functions of alpha-lipoic acid

Alpha-lipoic acid is a co-factor for several key enzymes in metabolism that catalyse oxidative reactions, including those listed below:

- The pyruvate dehydrogenase complex that converts pyruvate to acetyl CoA in carbohydrate metabolism.
- The α-ketoglutarate dehydrogenase complex that converts α-ketoglutarate to succinyl CoA in the Krebs cycle.
- Enzymes involved in the metabolism of the branched-chain amino acids leucine, isoleucine and valine.

The reduced form of lipoic acid, DHLA, also has the potential to act as an antioxidant. It can interact directly with oxygen free radicals and can be involved in the regeneration of the reduced form of other antioxidants that have become oxidised, such as vitamin C, vitamin E, glutathione and co-enzyme Q_{10}.

When alpha-lipoic acid acts as a co-factor for enzymes it is covalently bound to the enzyme; the carboxyl group (COOH) of lipoic acid binds to the free amino group in the side chain of one of the enzyme's lysine residues to form lipoamide. In the conversion of pyruvate to acetyl CoA by pyruvate dehydrogenase, this lipoamide is converted to acetyl lipoamide in a complex reaction that also involves the co-factor thiamin pyrophosphate, derived from vitamin B_1. In this acetyl lipoamide one of the sulphur atoms is reduced by the addition of hydrogen and the other is acetylated; that is, it has an acetyl group derived from pyruvate attached to it. This acetyl lipoamide then reacts with reduced coenzyme to give acetyl CoA and fully reduced dihydrolipoamide. This dihydrolipoamide is normally reoxidised by transfer of the hydrogen atoms attached to its sulphur atoms to NAD.

Rationale and evidence for the use of alpha-lipoic acid supplements

When supplements of pure alpha-lipoic acid are taken, it is rapidly absorbed from the gut (perhaps a third of the total oral dose) and rapidly taken up by cells. Within the cells alpha-lipoic acid is converted to the reduced form DHLA, which can act as an antioxidant, but this is rapidly removed from cells and metabolised. This suggests that any sustained antioxidant effect of lipoic acid would be more likely if the daily dose were split into several spaced aliquots.

Alpha-lipoic acid is available on prescription in Germany for the treatment of diabetic neuropathy (peripheral nerve damage associated with diabetes) and has been widely used for this purpose there. Diabetic neuropathy is one of a group of complications of diabetes that are associated with persistent hyperglycaemia, including diabetic retinopathy (retinal degeneration), diabetic nephropathy (progressive loss of renal function) and cataract. Better long-term glycaemic control is the primary focus of efforts to try to reduce these long-term complications (DCCT, 1993). Detailed discussion of the use of pharmacological doses for the treatment of diabetic neuropathy is beyond the scope of this book, but data from these trials do suggest that even very large doses administered over a period of years appear to be well tolerated and no serious adverse consequences have been recorded. This provides some reassurance about the use of smaller amounts as dietary supplements.

A review of the clinical trials of alpha-lipoic acid for this purpose does suggest that there is some preliminary evidential support for the belief that large supplements of alpha-lipoic acid (at least 600 mg/day) do have some beneficial effects on the acute symptoms and progression of diabetic neuropathy (Ziegler *et al.*, 1999; Singh and Jiala, 2008). Oxidative damage by free radicals is widely believed to contribute to these long-term degenerative changes seen in diabetics and so one possible mechanism of action for alpha-lipoic acid is via its antioxidant activity; there are also suggestions that it may increase insulin sensitivity and muscle glucose uptake.

Dietary supplements typically provide 50–300 mg/day of lipoic acid, although some clinical trials have used two to four times this maximum. There seems therefore to be little evidence to support the general use of alpha-lipoic acid as a dietary supplement. The size of the doses used in supplements far exceeds that which could be obtained from ordinary food and so any effects should be regarded as pharmacological. Doses used in clinical trials tend to be even higher than those used in supplements. There have been some preliminary reports that a combination of high doses of L-carnitine and alpha-lipoic acid have some beneficial effects on activity levels, short-term memory and measures of oxidative stress in ageing rats. Such animal studies are clearly an inadequate justification for the use of these supplements in people, although they have been used to promote such combinations in the advertising literature of some supplement suppliers.

Methylsulphonylmethane (MSM)

Nature and sources of MSM

Dimethylsulphonylmethane (MSM) $CH_3SO_2CH_3$ is an oxidation product of the organic solvent dimethyl sulphoxide CH_3SOCH_3. MSM is not an essential nutrient, but is found in small amounts in many foods, including fresh fruit and vegetables (1–4 mg/kg) and unpasteurised milk; because it is a volatile compound much of this is lost during cooking and prolonged storage. Adults excrete a few milligrams of MSM in their urine each day.

Dimethyl sulphoxide is an unpleasant-smelling liquid that has a strong, bitter taste. Despite intuitive expectations to the contrary, it has surprisingly low toxicity in both animals and people. Dimethyl sulphoxide has been used topically as an analgesic and anti-inflammatory agent. When taken systemically it imparts its unpleasant smell to the body odour of consumers, which, together with its unpleasant and persistent taste, means that it has not been widely used as a dietary supplement despite some claims for therapeutic benefits. Unlike dimethyl sulphoxide, MSM is an odourless compound and has been widely used as a dietary supplement.

MSM as a supplement

Extravagant claims about the health benefits and curative properties of MSM have been appearing in magazines, websites and advertising literature for well over 20 years. Many of these claims can be traced back to organisations and individuals involved in the production and marketing of MSM supplements. Indeed, claims that MSM has beneficial effects in the treatment of a host of medical conditions on one website prompted an official warning from the FDA in the USA that these claims were illegal for something marketed as a dietary supplement. These claims could only be used for drugs approved by the FDA. Details of the claims and rationale for taking MSM can be found on the 'official' website of the MSM – Medical Information Foundation (MSM, 2010). Despite over 20 years of promotion as a supplement, an electronic search of the medical and scientific literature produced only a handful of studies that have investigated the efficacy of MSM supplements, and these are mainly small-scale preliminary studies in laboratory animals.

The main rationale for using MSM as a dietary supplement in non-scientific sources seems to be as an organic source of sulphur for synthetic processes in the body. For example, because cartilage has a high sulphur content, it is argued that MSM as a potential source of sulphur could be useful in the management of conditions like osteoarthritis, where there is degeneration of cartilage. The sulphur-containing amino acids cysteine and methionine are found in most body proteins and nearly half of the body's sulphur is contained in muscular tissue; this has been used as a basis for promoting MSM use among athletes and body builders.

There is actually very little evidence that the body can utilise MSM as a source of sulphur for synthetic processes. Richmond (1986) found that small amounts of radioactively labelled sulphur from MSM administered orally to guinea pigs could be detected in their serum proteins, although most of the radioactivity was excreted in the urine. This report falls well short of demonstrating that mammals can make significant use of MSM as a source of sulphur for synthetic processes. Gut microorganisms may be responsible for any incorporation into animal protein that does occur.

The medical and scientific literature does not even provide promising preliminary evidence to support the use of MSM as a dietary supplement. A systematic review did find two small controlled trials of MSM (and four for dimethyl sulphoxide) for the treatment of osteoarthritis. While these trials did suggest that MSM had more effect than a placebo on arthritic pain, the methodology was said to be poor.

Suppliers and advocates of this supplement suggest daily doses of up to 2–5 g of MSM. No adverse effects were reported when rats were given 1.5 g/kg body weight for three months (Horvath et al., 2002). While very high doses appear to be well tolerated in acute and subacute trials, this is, of course, no guarantee that chronic mass consumption of these doses will not have adverse effects in some people.

8 Natural Products and Extracts

Scope of the chapter

Large numbers of plant preparations and extracts, as well as a few from animal sources, are currently marketed as dietary supplements. As was seen in Chapter 1, there are a number of advantages for companies in marketing such products as dietary supplements so that they are subject to regulations relating to foods rather than medicines. Dietary supplements can be sold over the counter in a range of outlets and the safety, quality and honest description provisions of food legislation are looser and applied liberally at the point of sale, rather than as a condition of being offered for sale.

The value of several 'dietary supplements' in the treatment of specific diseases is evaluated in this chapter. However, it should be remembered that in the UK no claims that a dietary supplement can cure or be beneficial as a treatment for or prevention of a disease can be made on the product packaging, advertising or sales literature unless the product has been licensed as a medicine. Similar restrictions apply to substances sold as traditional herbal medicines.

Some of the natural extracts marketed as supplements have authentic and widespread culinary uses, for example tea, garlic, ginger, turmeric and soybeans, and thus have a clear claim to be regarded as foods or dietary supplements. Many others have little or no culinary use, but do have a long history of use as folk or herbal medicines; these have been sold as food supplements partly to avoid the time and expense involved in obtaining a medicinal licence. Of course, in several cases it seems unlikely that, even given time and money, a credible case could be made that they are effective enough to get a licence as a conventional drug.

A 12-page list of herbal ingredients, with their botanical name, common names and recorded uses in food and medicine, as well as the parts of the plant used for these purposes, can be downloaded from the section of the MHRA website dealing with borderline products – those for which there is doubt about whether they should be regarded as food supplements or medicines: www.mhra.gov.uk/How weregulate/Medicines/Doesmyproductneedalicence/Borderlineproducts/index.htm. Kiple and Ornelas (2000) contains an extensive (c. 200-page) 'Historical Dictionary of the World's Plant Foods' and this is another authoritative source of information

Dietary Supplements and Functional Foods, 2nd Edition. Geoffrey P. Webb.
© 2011 Blackwell Publishing Ltd.

about the past and present use of plants as foods. These lists suggest that most of the plants used in supplements that would not normally be thought of as potential foods do have some reported history of food use, for example Echinacea, milk thistle, St John's wort and saw palmetto.

Extensive culinary use of a substance would be a positive criterion for inclusion in this chapter, but many big-selling 'food supplements' have little or no culinary use in the UK, even if there are some reports of the substance being eaten. This means that the decision about whether or not to include a substance in this chapter has been considered case by case and is consequently somewhat arbitrary. A few substances not normally regarded as potential foods in the UK but taken regularly over long periods with a view to improving risk factors for chronic disease have also been included. In general, I have not incorporated substances used for short periods as 'herbal medicines' to treat a disease or symptom, unless there are substantial direct over-the-counter sales of these substances as food/dietary supplements.

Note that from May 2011 four of the extracts discussed in this chapter (Agnus castus, Echinacea, milk thistle and St John's wort) will be classified as traditional herbal medicines within the EU, and those that are currently (2010) labelled 'food supplements' will gradually disappear from the shelves as existing stocks are sold. These products will continue to be freely available from authorised producers and will remain as 'dietary supplements' in the USA. This was discussed more fully in Chapter 1.

In Germany, there is a long history of use of herbal preparations by 'orthodox' medical practitioners. In 1978, the German government established a committee to determine the efficacy and safety of the many herbal preparations then being sold in the country. This Commission E has published a long series of monographs relating to the uses of a large number of herbal preparations. The Commission E list of approved herbal preparations amounts to almost 200 items. The size of this list illustrates the difficulty of deciding which of the many herbal extracts and preparations sold as dietary supplements should be included in this chapter. The Commission E list can be found on the website of the American Botanical Council (ABC, 2010) and there are links to short summaries about each of these preparations. These summaries include the drug's source and composition, its uses, indications and contraindications, side-effects, interactions, dosage, mode of administration and possible mechanisms of action.

Secondary plant metabolites

There is an overwhelming abundance of evidence to suggest that a diet that has a varied and plentiful supply of fruit and vegetables is associated with increased longevity and a reduced risk of developing a chronic age-related disorder like cancer or heart disease (e.g. Ziegler, 1991). This evidence has led to consumers throughout the industrialised world being advised to include fruit and vegetables in their diets. Consumers in the UK and the USA are urged to eat at least five 80 g portions of fruit and vegetables each day (in practice, only around a quarter of UK adults actually achieve this goal). Some of the benefits of a rich and varied intake of fruit and vegetables can be explained by conventional nutritional properties. For example, such a diet is also usually rich in vitamins and minerals, including those with antioxidant functions, has high levels of dietary fibre and is often relatively low in saturated fat. In recent years, other secondary metabolites found within plant foods have attracted attention as having protective potential; that is, even though they are not essential in the diet, their consumption may confer some benefits, such as the antioxidant properties of carotenoids that were discussed in Chapter 5.

Plants produce many thousands of so-called secondary metabolites, substances that are additional to those involved in the primary processes of respiration, photosynthesis, growth and development. 'Primary' metabolites are distributed throughout the plant kingdom and often throughout much of the animal kingdom as well. In contrast to the ubiquitous presence of primary metabolites, each plant produces its own complement of secondary metabolites that serve a variety of diverse functions, such as:

- Acting as attractants for insects and animals for pollination and seed dispersal.
- Discouraging consumption of the plant body by herbivores or insects, e.g. by imparting an unpleasant taste or causing adverse symptoms when consumed.
- Protecting against microbial infection.
- Protecting against damage by ultraviolet light.

Some of these compounds, like several of the carotenoids, are widespread in the plant kingdom, but many others may be confined to just a small number of plants. This is one reason why consumers are also advised to consume a variety of fruits and vegetables. Some of these secondary metabolites of plants have well-established medicinal properties, such as:

- The salicylates (aspirin-like substances) from willow bark.
- The cardiac glycosides (including digoxin) found in the purple foxglove, Digitalis purpurea, and used in the treatment of heart failure.
- The antimalarial drug quinine extracted from the bark of Cinchona succiruba.

Other secondary plant metabolites like the carotenoids have anti-oxidant effects and so may reduce tissue damage by oxygen free radicals. According to the 'oxidant theory of disease' (discussed in Chapter 5), free radicals are implicated in the cumulative damage to cellular components that helps to precipitate many of the age-related degenerative changes and diseases like cancer and heart disease.

Crozier (2003) classifies these secondary metabolites of plants into three major groupings based on their synthetic origins in plants rather than their dietary effects in animals and people. Details of the biosynthetic origins and chemical structures of these secondary plant metabolites may be found in this source. The three categories of Crozier's classification are:

- The terpenoids.
- The phenols and polyphenols.

- Sulphur-containing secondary metabolites and the nitrogen-containing alkaloids (note that these will be discussed under separate headings in this chapter).

Each of the groupings is briefly discussed below.

Despite the many tens of thousands of different substances that plants produce as secondary metabolites, this is not a random assortment of unrelated compounds. They can be logically classified into a small number of groups of compounds with common origins and overlapping properties.

Terpenoids

Terpenoids are a diverse group of over 25 000 different substances, which include the carotenoids and are classified according to the number of C5 isoprenoid units they contain. They are all derived from the precursor substance isopentenyl diphosphate:

$$CH_2 = C - CH_2 - CH_2 - O - P - P$$

$$|$$

CH_3 (isopententyl diphosphate)

Where P is a phosphate moiety.

The terpenoids are comprised of the subcategories listed below:

- The hemiterpenes with just one isoprenoid unit and thus with five carbon atoms (C5). The only one of these that is found widely in nature is the volatile compound isoprene, released by many plants.
- The monoterpenes with two isoprenoid units and ten carbon atoms (C10). These are components of the volatile oils that impart the characteristic odour to many plant oils and are widely used in flavouring and as perfumes, e.g. geranial in lemon oil, linalool in coriander oil, menthol in peppermint and thymol in thyme.
- The sesquiterpenes (C15), including zingiberene and λ-bisabolene, which are partly responsible for the characteristic smell of ginger.
- The diterpenes (C20) – gingkoglide A is a modified diterpene found in Ginkgo biloba extracts.
- The triterpenoids (C30) – two important plant sterols, stigmasterol and sitosterol, are triterpenes (see phytosterols and phytostanols in Chapter 9). Saponins are triterpenoid compounds that have surfactant properties; they form a stable foam when shaken in aqueous solution.
- The tetraterpenoids (C40), which are made up entirely of the carotenoids. The most prevalent carotenoids in human blood are β-carotene from, for example, carrots and tomato products, lutein from green leafy vegetables, red peppers and peas, lycopene from tomato products, α-carotene from carrots and oranges, β-cryptoxanthin from oranges. The pinkish colour of salmon and some

crustaceans is due to the presence of metabolites of plant carotenoids. Some of these carotenoids have vitamin A activity (see Chapter 3).

● Higher terpenoids (more than C40) – ubiquinone or coenzyme Q_{10} (see Chapter 7) is a derivative of a higher terpenoid.

Phenolic compounds (phenols and polyphenols)

Phenolic compounds have at least one aromatic ring with at least one hydroxyl (OH) group attached to it. More than 8000 phenolic secondary metabolites of plants have been identified, varying from simple molecules with a single aromatic ring to more complex polyphenols that have more than one ring. Some of the basic categories of phenols and polyphenols are listed below, but there are also polymeric and conjugated forms of these, which increases their diversity still further (the basic structures of the phenolic and polyphenolic compounds are shown in Table 8.1).

Table 8.1 The basic structure of plant phenolic and polyphenolic compounds

Carbon No.	Skeleton	Classification	Example	Basic structure
7	C_6-C_1	Phenolic acids	Gallic acid	
8	C_6-C_2	Acetophenones	Xanthoxylin	
8	C_6-C_2	Phenylacetic acid	p-Hydroxyphenyl-acetic acid	
9	C_6-C_3	Hydroxycinnamic acids	Caffeic acid	
9	C_6-C_3	Coumarins	Esculetin	
10	C_6-C_4	Naphthoquinones	Juglone	
13	$C_6-C_1-C_6$	Xanthones	Gentisin	
14	$C_6-C_2-C_6$	Stilbenes	Resveratrol	
15	$C_6-C_3-C_6$	Flavonoids	Quercetin	

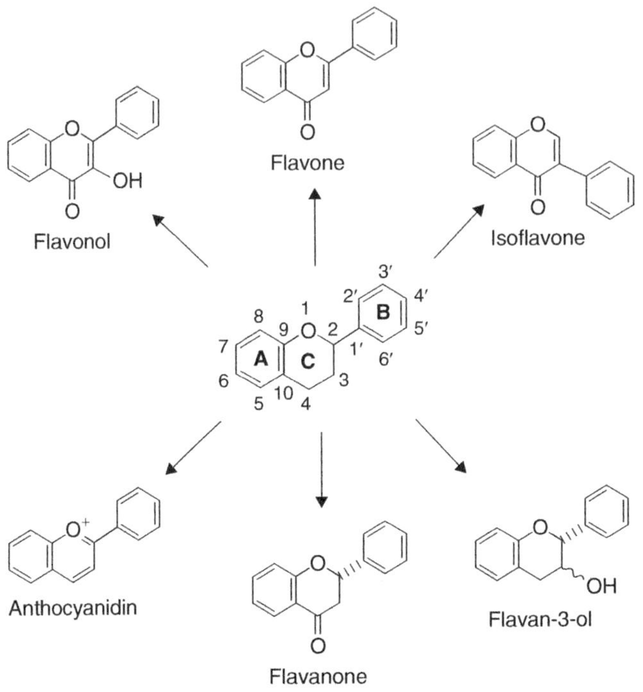

Figure 8.1   General structures of the major flavonoids.
Source: Reproduced from A. Crozier (2003) Classification and biosynthesis of secondary plant products: An overview. In: *Plants: Diet and Health. Report of the British Nutrition Task Force* (ed. G. Goldberg). p. 30. Blackwellm Oxford.

Phenolic acids are hydroxylated derivatives of benzoic acid and the principal component is gallic acid, so named because it is present in large amounts in plant galls.

Hydroxycinnamates have one aromatic ring and a three-carbon acidic side chain.

Stilbenes are polyphenols that have two aromatic rings connected by a two-carbon bridge; they are produced by plants in response to attack by microbial pathogens.

Flavonoids are polyphenols that have two aromatic rings linked together by a three-carbon bridge, a total of 15 carbon atoms (obviously polymeric forms have more than 15 carbon atoms). Prior (2006) has written a useful overview of the nutritional aspects of the flavonoids. They are the largest group of phenolic compounds and are often found in the epidermis of leaves and fruits, where they have roles such as pigmentation, protecting the plant from damage by ultraviolet light and conferring resistance to disease. The flavonoids (see Figure 8.1 for their general structures) are subdivided into:

- Flavonols such as quercetin, kaempferol, isorhamnetin, luteolin and myricetin are found in green vegetables, onions, apples, berry fruits, tea and red wine.

Around a quarter of the weight of Ginkgo biloba leaf extract is made up of flavonol glycosides (with an attached sugar residue), especially the first three on the list above.

- Flavones are not widely distributed in plants but are found in parsley, thyme and celery.
- Flavonols range from simple monomeric catechins, found in green tea, apples, and apricots, to more complex polymeric forms called proanthrocyanidins, found in apples, chocolate and red wine.
- Anthrocyanidins are pigments that are responsible for the red, blue or purple colouration of some fruits and flowers, like grapes and cherries. They protect against light damage and may help to attract insect pollinators to flowers.
- Flavonones are present in high concentrations in some citrus fruits.
- Isoflavones come mainly from soybeans and other legumes. Genistein and daidzein are known as phyto-oestrogens because they are able to bind to the mammalian oestrogen receptor and have slight oestrogenic activity; that is, they are partial agonists. It is the presence of these phyto-oestrogens in soy products that has led to them being widely used in an attempt to alleviate acute menopausal symptoms, and also to perhaps reduce the longer-term risk of osteoporosis and breast cancer (see phyto-oestrogens in Chapter 9).

Nitrogen-containing alkaloids

Alkaloids are a group of around 12 000 plant chemicals that contain at least one nitrogen atom. Most alkaloids are synthesised from amino acid precursors, but a few, like theobromine in cocoa and chocolate and caffeine in coffee, are synthesised from purine bases like adenine. In some alkaloids, the final product is combined with a steroid or terpenoid component.

Alkaloids were some of the earliest medicinal products derived from plants because they are relatively easy to extract. A number of well-known drugs and poisons are plant alkaloids (or derived from them), such as those listed below:

- Atropine from deadly nightshade (Atropa belladonna) binds with and blocks the acetylcholine receptor (antagonist) at parasympathetic nerve endings (muscarinic receptors) and so blocks the effects of the parasympathetic nervous system. Atropine is a CNS stimulant and has many clinical uses, including causing pupil dilation in some ophthalmic procedures; combating bradycardia and asystole (very slow or non-existent heart beat); inhibiting secretory processes like salivation. Atropine and other alkaloids from the nightshade family or Solenacae are sometimes referred to as the tropane alkaloids.
- Another tropane alkaloid is solanine, which is found in small amounts in potatoes (also a member of the nightshade family). On rare occasions, enough solanine can accumulate in green potatoes to cause nausea and vomiting and perhaps also respiratory symptoms.

- Nicotine present in tobacco is an alkaloid. It stimulates some acetylcholine receptors (known as nicotinic receptors), e.g. those at the autonomic ganglia, the neuromuscular junction and neurones within the central nervous system.
- Quinine is an alkaloid extracted from the bark of Cinchona succiruba and it was the first effective treatment for malaria.
- Curare is a poisonous extract of Chondrodendron tomentosum, a vine that grows in the canopy of South American rain forests. The main active constituent of curare is tubocurarine, an alkaloid that blocks the acetylcholine receptor at motor nerve endings and so causes muscle paralysis, including paralysis of the respiratory muscles. Native South Americans used curare as an arrow-tip poison for hunting. Curare-like compounds are used as muscle relaxants to reduce the anaesthetic dose needed in some abdominal surgical procedures and also to achieve muscle relaxation in some other clinical situations.
- Vincristine is an alkaloid extracted from the blue periwinkle plant Vinca rosea. It is widely used in the chemotherapy of several cancers, including acute childhood leukaemia, lymphoma, breast cancer and lung cancer.
- Codeine and morphine from the opium poppy are used as narcotic analgesics and morphine, together with a more potent chemically modified derivative, heroin, is used as an illegal recreational drug.
- Cocaine from the coca plant (Erythroxylon coca) was used as a local anaesthetic and was also present in early versions of cola drinks. It is a CNS stimulant producing short-lasting euphoric effects and it is widely used as an illegal recreational drug.
- Theobromine in chocolate (from the seeds of the plant Theobroma cacao) has recently attracted media attention as a possible cough remedy. It is a mild stimulant in humans but is toxic to dogs; a 200 g bar of plain chocolate contains enough to kill an average-size spaniel.
- Caffeine is present in coffee and is a mild CNS stimulant; it is derived from the roasted beans of the coffee tree Arabica coffea.
- Colchicine is an alkaloid from the autumn crocus, Colchicum autumnale, which is used in the treatment of gout. Colchicine prevents white cells from migrating to joints where uric acid has been deposited and so reduces the pain and inflammation provoked by white cell infiltration.

Sulphur-containing plant secondary metabolites

The two categories of sulphur-containing plant secondary metabolites are:

- The glucosinolates found in members of the cabbage or Brassica genus (in the family Cruciferae).
- The S-alkylcysteine sulphoxides found in members of the onion or Allium family, discussed later in this chapter in the section on garlic.

The Cruciferous plants include cabbage, broccoli, brussel sprouts, cauliflower, swede, turnip, mustard, radish, watercress, rocket, horseradish and rape, and these all produce glucosinolates. Breakdown products of glucosinolates called isothiocyanates, which are released when the plant is damaged by processing or chewing, are responsible for the hot and bitter flavours associated with foods like mustard and horseradish. The seeds of ordinary varieties of rape have a bitter taste due to the presence of a glucosinolate, but genetically modified varieties have been produced in which this compound does not accumulate, making it more palatable, for example as an animal feed.

A number of *in vitro* studies have shown that certain isothiocyanates derived from glucosinolates in dietary Brassicae have potential anticancer properties, although the WCRF/AICR report (2007) found that the evidence to support this was sparse. There is also some epidemiological evidence that high consumption of Brassica vegetables is associated with a low risk of lung and colorectal cancer (see Johnson, 2003 for more details and references).

How might these secondary metabolites reduce the risk of chronic disease?

Jackson (2003) has reviewed the potential mechanisms by which bioactive substances, including plant secondary metabolites, might act to reduce the risk of chronic degenerative diseases like cancer and heart disease. Some of the potential sites of action of plant secondary metabolites and other bio-active substances that Jackson (2003) discusses are listed below:

- Some potential environmental carcinogens are activated and made more damaging to DNA and other cellular components by the initial stages in the body's detoxification processes. So-called phase I enzymes convert environmental chemicals into more water-soluble metabolites to facilitate their excretion. This may amount to a metabolic activation of some potential carcinogens. It has been suggested that certain isothiocyanates derived from dietary glucosinolates (e.g. from Brassica vegetables) may inhibit this metabolic activation of potential carcinogens.
- The second stage in the detoxification of foreign chemicals involves their conversion by so-called phase II enzymes to harmless metabolites. Some plant chemicals may induce the formation of phase II enzymes and so accelerate the detoxification process. The sulphur-containing compounds found in the Allium (onion) family, as well as some isothiocyanates, may have such an effect. This has led to suggestions that garlic and broccoli, for example, may have anticancer properties. High doses of compounds exerting this effect may also increase the rate of metabolism of some prescription drugs and thus render them less effective. For example, Hypericum (St John's wort) extracts are believed to interfere with the actions of several prescription drugs in this way.
- Certain carcinogens may interact with DNA to cause alteration of bases like guanine and cytosine, for example by the addition of hydroxyl or alkyl groups. If these changes are not repaired by the cell's DNA repair mechanisms, they can

ultimately lead to potentially carcinogenic mutations. Many plant substances with antioxidant activity such as the antioxidant vitamins, carotenoids and many flavonoids may reduce this DNA damage.

- Once the production of potentially cancerous cells has been initiated by DNA damage, other substances may act as promoters that cause the abnormal cells to develop into tumours and spread to other sites. These promoter substances may not in themselves be carcinogenic. A number of environmental and dietary chemicals, as well as some hormones, are known to act as cancer promoters. Thus androgens (male sex steroids) promote prostate cancer and oestrogens promote many breast cancers. The phyto-oestrogens found, for example, in soy foods are postulated to have potential against breast cancer because they can be anti-oestrogenic (see Chapter 9).
- A high blood cholesterol concentration and, more specifically, an elevated level of LDL cholesterol in plasma is causally associated with an increased risk of atherosclerosis and coronary heart disease (see Chapter 6). Some plant chemicals may reduce plasma cholesterol concentration and thus exert a protective effect against those cardiovascular diseases that are precipitated by atherosclerosis. Some plant sterols (see phytosterols in Chapter 9) that are structurally similar to cholesterol may reduce blood cholesterol by inhibiting its absorption and reabsorption from the gut. Sulphur compounds in garlic and other members of the Allium family are also claimed to lower blood cholesterol levels in high doses.
- When LDL is oxidised it becomes much more damaging to arterial walls and thus more atherogenic. A number of plant chemicals with antioxidant potential may reduce LDL oxidation within the arterial wall and thus reduce the risk of cardiovascular disease. Such claims have been made for the antioxidant vitamins and minerals, the carotenoids and many flavonoids (see Chapter 5).
- The development of atherosclerotic lesions in arterial walls is a chronic process that may manifest itself symptomatically as angina or intermittent claudication: ischaemic (due to oxygen deprivation) pain in the legs when walking. However, atherosclerosis can also precipitate acute life-threatening thromboses: the formation of blood clots that may lodge in key arteries causing ischaemic damage in the tissues they supply. The result may be a myocardial infarction (heart attack), stroke or pulmonary embolism. Plant substances may reduce the risk of embolism by inhibiting the initial aggregation and activation of blood platelets or by affecting the blood clotting process *per se*. A number of plant substances inhibit platelet aggregation in some *in vitro* studies, for example certain polyphenols and salicylates (like aspirin). Some phyto-oestrogens may inhibit platelet aggregation and thrombin formation; thrombin is the key enzyme that, once activated, causes blood to clot.
- High levels of several carotenoids are found in parts of the human retina where they may protect it from light-induced free radical damage by virtue of their antioxidant effects. It has been suggested that carotenoids may help to reduce the degenerative changes in the retina seen in age-related macular degeneration. They may also protect other structures like skin from damage caused by

UV light and, indeed, one of their functions in plants is to protect the plant tissues from damage by UV radiation.

Jackson (2003) warns that many of the studies on which these theories are based have employed purified chemical products in short-term reductionist laboratory experiments using *in vitro* systems or animal models. Such studies can be very useful in generating testable hypotheses or possible explanations for epidemiological observations or the results of clinical trials. However, these studies cannot accurately predict the effects of long-term human consumption of crude plant extracts or even of the purified chemical; they cannot, in themselves, justify the long-term use of such products by healthy people. Just because a plant contains a substance or substances that can be shown to reduce DNA damage *in vitro* or to act as an antioxidant does not mean that eating the plant or taking extracts of it will reduce a person's risk of cancer or heart disease. Many of the claims about the cancer-preventing or heart disease-preventing properties of particular foods or supplements are also based on such studies. Evidence from these studies should be regarded with extreme scepticism unless the safety and efficacy of any supplement has been substantiated in large, well-designed clinical trials.

Natural extracts as a source of drugs

Several examples of drugs derived from plant extracts (especially alkaloids) have been noted in the preceding sections, illustrating the principle that many clinically important drugs are based on natural substances produced by plants or, less commonly, by animals. Many important medical drugs are based on herbal or traditional remedies. The short list of alkaloid-based drugs also reinforces the message that just because a substance or extract is 'natural' does not mean that it can be assumed to be harmless and safe to consume; several of the compounds listed are potent poisons. Many suppliers and advocates of herbal preparations suggest that because they are natural, even though they often contain an ill-defined mixture of chemical substances, they are somehow likely to be safer than purified chemicals; that is, medical drugs. If a substance has a long history of food use, this does offer considerable reassurance about its safety as a herbal remedy, but that becomes less so if:

- A highly concentrated extract is used and so the amounts of active chemical constituents consumed are much greater than would be eaten in food.
- A part of the plant that is not usually used in food is used to make the remedy or supplement.

It is easy to think of a large number of drugs that are natural compounds extracted from plants or occasionally from animal sources. Others are nature-related compounds that are based on naturally occurring plant or animal compounds, but that have been chemically modified to enhance their usefulness as a therapeutic drug, for instance to enhance a therapeutic effect, minimise a toxic effect or increase bio-availability. It is, however, more difficult to think of potent and widely used pharmaceutical drugs that have originated from a common food. Perhaps one reason for this is that many drugs are toxic when relatively small overdoses are taken or they may produce symptoms perceived as unpleasant. People living in areas where the plant grows will thus have learned to avoid eating the plant (or animal) regularly as food. One exception to this generality is the anti-ulcer drug carbenoxolone sodium, which is derived from a glycyrrhizic acid found in liquorice root. However, the natural substance is substantially modified to produce the drug and, according to Sircus (1972), its pharmacological actions are totally different from the natural starting material. Some fish oil preparations have also been given a medicinal licence for the treatment of hyperlipidaemia.

The individual plant and animal extracts

Agnus castus

Agnus castus is an aromatic tree or shrub (Vitex agnus-castus), also known as the chaste tree. The ancient Greeks used it to reduce libido, hence the name chaste tree; paradoxically, it also been said historically to have aphrodisiac qualities. According to Kiple and Ornelas (2000), the berries, which resemble peppercorns and smell and taste like pepper, have been used as a spice; its use by Christian monks is the origin of the alternative name 'monk's pepper'. The list of herbs and their uses on the HMRA website, referred to at the beginning of this chapter, does not list a food use for this herb, which suggests that any food use is historical or very limited.

Extracts of Agnus castus contain many substances in small amounts and it is unclear which are responsible for its biological activity. Casticin is a flavonol present in the lipophilic fraction of extracts and, since the pharmacological activity is also present in this fraction, extracts are often standardised to contain a set amount of this ingredient. To obtain the extract the crushed fruits are extracted with aqueous alcohol and 20 mg of this extract is the standard dose. Current use of Agnus castus is almost always to alleviate symptoms of pre-menstrual syndrome (PMS), which may be experienced to some extent by up to 50% of young women during the luteal phase (second half) of all or some of their menstrual cycles. It is characterised by:

- A range of psychological symptoms, including anxiety, aggression, irritability and depression.
- Fluid retention, a bloated feeling and weight gain.
- Breast tenderness.

In around 5% of women of reproductive age the symptoms may be severe enough to seriously disrupt their lives and their relationships and to meet the American Psychiatric Association's formal diagnostic criteria (DSM-IV) for pre-menstrual dysphoric disorder (PMDD). The causes of these pre-menstrual symptoms are unclear. One suggestion that has attracted much attention in recent years is that hypersecretion of the pituitary hormone prolactin may play a role. Prolactin may cause breast tenderness and may shorten the luteal phase of the menstrual cycle, leading to deficits of luteal hormones, especially progesterone. The major physiological regulator of prolactin release from the pituitary gland is the nerve transmitter dopamine, which in this context is also sometimes termed 'prolactin inhibitory factor'. Drugs that inhibit the release of prolactin by mimicking the actions of dopamine therefore may offer the potential for treating PMS.

Agnus castus extracts are now known to bind to dopamine receptors and to inhibit the release of prolactin *in vitro*, in animals and in women. Jarry *et al.* (1994) used an *in vitro* culture of rat pituitary cells to show that an active principle of Agnus castus was able to bind to dopamine receptors from these pituitary cells and selectively to inhibit prolactin release without affecting the secretion of other pituitary hormones. More recently, Meier *et al.* (2000) have confirmed a dopaminergic effect of Agnus castus extracts and have also suggested that it has effects on opioid receptors that may contribute to its pharmacological actions.

There are some clinical trials in the German literature (e.g. Milewicz *et al.* 1993) suggesting that Agnus castus may be of value in the treatment of pre-menstrual syndrome; on the basis of such trials the German Commission E approved its use for this purpose. A large and well-designed study (Schellenberg, 2001) published in English has also supported the efficacy of this herb. This group used 170 women who met formal diagnostic criteria for PMS, who were randomly assigned to receive either a placebo or 20 mg of Agnus caster extract. Using the women's own assessment of their condition and the physician's global clinical impression, the Agnus caster performed highly significantly better than the placebo. The researchers concluded that Agnus caster is a well-tolerated and effective treatment for pre-menstrual syndrome. A more recent trial conducted in Chinese women with moderate to severe PMS came to essentially the same conclusion (He *et al.*, 2009).

In a detailed and extensive review of the safety of Agnus caster, Daniele *et al.* (2005) found that the available evidence suggested that it was safe and that any occasional side-effects were mild and reversible, for example nausea and gastrointestinal symptoms, headache, menstrual disorders, acne, pruritis and rashes. They did suggest that it not be used during pregnancy or lactation.

This herb seems to be an effective and safe treatment for a specific medical condition and is approved for this use in some countries like Germany. Given its clear pharmacological activity, it would seem to be unsuitable for use as a general dietary supplement for people not suffering from this condition; that is, it should be regarded as a herbal medicine rather than a dietary supplement. The usual dose is 20 mg of extract, which in the pharmacological-grade preparation Ze440 is equivalent to 180 mg of the dried fruits. Its safety in pregnancy and lactation has not been established and it should be avoided in these conditions.

Aloe vera

Aloe vera is a gelatinous substance that is obtained from the thick leaves of the cactus-like Aloe vera plant. The most popular and most familiar use of this extract is for topical use in cosmetic preparations and after-sun lotions. Aloe vera is also used as an ingredient of ointments to treat skin conditions, because it is claimed to have anti-inflammatory, itch-relieving, pain-killing and healing properties. It has also been promoted more recently as an oral supplement, with claims that it may reduce blood lipid levels and blood glucose levels in type 2 diabetes. The leaves of this plant also exude a bitter yellow substance called aloe latex or aloe juice. This contains anthroquinone, which is a harsh laxative, and drying the juice yields dark brown granules that are approved by the FDA in America as an over-the-counter laxative.

Kiple and Ornelas (2000) give no dietary use for this plant and this is not surprising, given the bitter taste and laxative effects of aloe latex. Aloe vera gel for use as a dietary supplement should contain no juice and should not have laxative effects.

The aloe gel contains polysaccharides that would be classed as components of the soluble dietary fibre, as well as vitamins, minerals, saponins (triterpenoids with surfactant properties) and essential fatty acids. Despite the exaggerated claims made by suppliers and advocates of aloe vera supplements, there is very little evidence in the scientific literature to support the claims that these oral supplements have beneficial effects on blood lipoprotein profiles or are useful in the management of type 2 diabetes. One systematic review published in 1999 suggested that the clinical effectiveness of neither oral nor topical aloe vera was sufficiently defined at that time, and in fact very few controlled clinical trials of oral aloe vera were found (Vogler and Ernst, 1999). A more recent study (Yeh *et al.*, 2003) systematically reviewed the effects of a number of herbal and other dietary supplements in glycaemic control in diabetes. This study found only two non-randomised and single-blind clinical trials (published in 1996) and some animal studies on the use of aloe vera in the treatment of diabetes. While the clinical trials gave some evidence of a positive effect of aloe vera, this type of study must be regarded as very weak evidence of any beneficial effect.

In the UK, aloe vera is usually taken as tablets or capsules (one or two per day) that contain the concentrated aloe vera gel extract. There seems no significant evidence to justify the oral consumption of aloe vera supplements, although there is also no evidence of harmful effects of these supplements.

Bee products

Honey is the most used of the products derived from beekeeping, but because it is a normal food it is not discussed in this book. Three other byproducts of beekeeping – royal jelly, bee pollen and bee propolis – are used as dietary supplements. Detailed information about all products produced from beekeeping can be found in Krell (1996).

Royal jelly

Royal jelly is a substance secreted by young worker bees and used to feed the young larvae and the queen bee throughout her life. Royal jelly is not normally stored in the hive because it is fed directly to the larvae or queen as it is secreted. However, some accumulates around the larval queen in the 'queen cell' in the early stages of development. Krell (1996) explains that in order to produce royal jelly commercially, the hive must be stimulated to produce queens at inappropriate times, and that one hive has the potential to produce about 500 g of royal jelly during the course of a summer.

The observation that the royal jelly diet of the queen bee is associated with great fecundity and a much longer life than other female bees has probably led to suggestions that it may have similar beneficial effects in humans and that it is the 'queen of foods' for human beings.

Fresh royal jelly varies in composition, but a typical composition might be:

- 70% water
- 12% carbohydrate (mainly as glucose and fructose)
- 12% protein
- 5% lipids

Given that a typical daily dose in supplements is 250–500 mg, these amounts of macronutrients are nutritionally insignificant. Royal jelly is practically devoid of fat-soluble vitamins and vitamin C. It does contain B vitamins and several minerals, but the amounts present in a typical supplement dose are nutritionally insignificant and would probably not reach 1% of the RNI for any vitamin or mineral. Royal jelly also contains an assortment of other chemically diverse substances, which from a human perspective are present in minute amounts, for example free nucleotide bases, acetylcholine and two heterocyclic compounds, biopterine and neopterine.

There are huge numbers of claims for the beneficial effects of taking royal jelly supplements and some for its topical use; according to Krell (1996), however, there is almost no scientific substantiation for these claims. Prominent among these claims for royal jelly is that it acts as a general tonic, reducing fatigue, improving mental and physical performance and leading to a general health improvement. There are reports that *in vitro* it has antibacterial activity and that it has antitumour activity in animal studies, but their significance for human consumption is impossible to say.

There is one review of the effect of royal jelly on serum lipids in animals and humans (Vittek, 1995), which does suggest that previous studies have shown it to be effective in reducing blood cholesterol levels in animals and people. No other studies or reviews on the effects of royal jelly on blood lipids were found in the English-language literature, either before or after 1995, during an electronic literature search.

There are numerous case reports of people developing allergic reactions after consuming royal jelly. These allergic reactions can occasionally be severe and life threatening. People with asthma should avoid royal jelly because it may precipitate severe asthma attacks (see for example Thien *et al.*, 1996). Leung *et al.* (1997) suggested that in Hong Kong, where use of royal jelly supplements is very common, the risk of allergy to royal jelly was high and positively associated with other allergic conditions, including asthma.

Bee pollen

Bee pollen is a mixture of pollens collected by bees from flowers, which is mixed with nectar and regurgitated honey and so also contains digestive enzymes of the bees. It is collected from bees as they enter the hive by a wire mesh that brushes the pollen off into a collecting vessel. The exact composition of bee pollen will obviously depend on the types of flowers from which it has been collected. Typically, bee pollen contains about 20% protein and 30–40% carbohydrate, mainly in the form of simple sugars. It contains smaller amounts of lipids, including essential fatty acids. It does not contain fat-soluble vitamins, except carotenoids, but does contain water-soluble vitamins and essential minerals. As typical doses in supplements are in the range 0.5–1.5 g, this will make little contribution to the human requirements for either macro- or micronutrients.

Bee pollen contains flavonoids, carotenoids, free amino acids, nucleic acids and many enzymes (although these will be inactivated and digested in the human gut). Several of these constituents are known to have antioxidant activity and so bee pollen probably has some antioxidant activity, and is also claimed to have anti-inflammatory activity.

As with royal jelly, there are numerous claimed beneficial effects from taking bee pollen supplements, including a general increase in vitality, improved athletic performance, reduced atherosclerosis and a blood pressure-lowering effect. It is also claimed to be beneficial in the treatment of benign hypertrophy of the prostate gland in men, but no clinical trials were found in the English-language literature to support this. Some trials of its effects on athletic performance were carried out in the 1970s and 1980s (e.g. Maughan and Evans, 1982 in swimmers), but none of these found it to be effective.

Once again, there are several reports of allergic reactions to bee pollen, some of which have resulted in serious life-threatening anaphylaxis. Anyone with a known allergy to pollen should avoid bee pollen and it should probably be avoided by anyone with a history of atopic disease (eczema, asthma or allergic rhinitis). Claims that it may actually be helpful in curing allergies are based on false logic. Pure pollens collected directly from the plant to which a person is allergic can be used to desensitise him or her to particular pollens when injected in controlled doses. Eating bee pollen with its unpredictable content is likely to provoke allergic reactions rather than to desensitise. Given the risk of allergic reactions and the lack of any substantial evidence for benefit, bee pollen is not recommended as a dietary supplement.

Bee propolis

Bee propolis is a complex mixture of plant resin collected from plants, beeswax and bee secretions. The bees use it for various construction purposes in their hives, including sealing up brood cells. It has antibacterial, antifungal and perhaps even antiviral properties, which helps reduce microbial spoilage within the hive and presumably also infections in the bees. The caffeic acid esters found in bee propolis have been shown to have antitumour activity using *in vitro* human cancer cell lines and with animal models of cancer (e.g. Rao *et al.*, 1993). Propolis itself has also been shown to have anticancer activity *in vitro* (e.g. Aso *et al.*, 2004).

The exact composition of propolis will vary according to a number of factors, not least of these being the plant sources of the resin component; almost 200 individual components have been identified. Krell (1996) suggests that a typical composition might be:

- 50% plant resin, rich in flavonoids and phenols, including caffeic acid and other hydroxycinnamic acids
- 30% lipids, mainly beeswax but also some plant lipids
- 10% essential oils
- 5% pollen
- 5% other organic material and minerals

Much of the suggested benefit of bee propolis is based on extrapolation of its *in vitro* antimicrobial activity and its antitumour activity in human cancer cell lines and experimental animal models. No clinical trials of propolis were found in the English language in an electronic search of the literature.

Bee propolis or its extracts (usually ethanolic extracts) are sold for use as supplements in the form of tablets, capsules or liquids. The dose is not established, but manufacturers recommend the equivalent of 0.5–1 g of propolis. There are numerous case reports of contact dermatitis resulting from exposure to bee propolis as well as other reports of allergic reactions. There seems to be little basis for recommending bee propolis as a general dietary supplement.

Chitosan

Chitin is a very abundant, long, fibrous polymer of N-acetyl glucosamine that is found in many invertebrates and fungi. It is, for example, a major component of the shells of crustacean like crabs, lobsters and shrimps. Chitin can be partly deacetylated by treatment with sodium hydroxide to produce chitosan. Chitosan has been available for about 30 years, despite the current advertising claims of some suppliers that it is a new product that acts like a 'fat magnet' and will revolutionise weight control. The implication is that you can eat what you like and still lose weight with chitosan supplements.

The theory is that fat and cholesterol bind to ionised sites on the chitosan, which prevents its digestion and absorption. Claims of the fat-binding capacity of chitosan vary from four times its own weight up to more than double this. Such claims are not based on *in vivo* studies but on chemical laboratory experiments. There is technical evidence that chitosan can bind fat and that large doses may increase the fat content of faeces in some animal studies. Evidence that it has any significant effect on faecal fat losses in humans is not apparent in the scientific literature. Gades and Stern (2003) evaluated the effect of chitosan (4.5 g/day spread over five doses) on faecal fat content in 15 male subjects. They concluded that the extra daily fat loss in faeces associated with this large dose of chitosan amounted to only 1.1 g/day; that is, about 10 calories per day. This is a clinically insignificant effect. Guerciolini *et al.* (2001) compared the effects of chitosan and a prescription drug, orlistat, on faecal fat excretion using 12 adult subjects in a crossover study. Orlistat works by inhibiting the enzyme lipase, which is responsible for fat digestion in the gut, and in this study orlistat treatment resulted in an average 16 g/day increase in faecal fat content compared to the baseline values. In this study there was no statistically significant effect of chitosan.

Human trials of chitosan for weight control have generally been consistent with the negative findings for its effects on faecal fat excretion: it appears to be ineffective as an aid to human weight loss. Mhurchu *et al.* (2004) conducted a relatively large, controlled trial using 3 g/day of chitosan or a placebo in 250 overweight or obese adult subjects. The intervention period lasted for 24 weeks and the difference in average weight change between the control and placebo groups over this period was about half a kilogram. While the weight loss associated with chitosan was just statistically significantly more than that of the controls, it was not clinically significant. A small but clinically insignificant fall in circulating LDL cholesterol was also associated with the chitosan consumption in this study.

A study by Pittler *et al.* (1999) found no weight-reducing effects of chitosan in a smaller and shorter-duration study. Bokura and Kobayashi (2003) also found that chitosan produces a small but statistically significant cholesterol-lowering effect. Chitosan would thus seem to have little if any effects on faecal fat loss in humans, and no clinically significant weight-reducing effects even when taken in large doses for up to six months. It may have statistically significant effects in lowering plasma (LDL) cholesterol, but these are probably transient (they only last while the supplement is being taken) and of little clinical significance.

In a systematic review and meta-analysis of 15 published trials (1200 participants), Jull *et al.* (2008) found that when all trials were included, chitosan preparations did lead to a statistically significantly greater weight loss than a placebo and to a reduction in plasma cholesterol, but they were not able to find any significant effect on fat excretion. The quality of some of the trials was less than ideal and when only the better studies were considered, the effects of chitosan were substantially reduced. They concluded that in high-quality trials any effect of chitosan on body weight is minimal and unlikely to be of clinical significance.

Doses of chitosan recommended by suppliers vary from 1.5–3.5 g/day and this requires consumption of up to 10–15 tablets/capsules each day spread into several doses that precede meals. There are few reports of adverse effects of chitosan and these are minor, such as bloating. People with shellfish allergies should note that chitosan is obtained from the shells of crustaceans, usually shrimps. Theoretically, any substance that interferes with fat absorption could also impair the absorption of fat-soluble vitamins; this is certainly the case with orlistat and manufactured indigestible fats (olestra) used as dietary fat substitutes in the USA. However, given the insignificant effect of chitosan on human fat absorption, this is probably no more than a theoretical risk.

Echinacea

Echinacea purpurea is also sometimes called the purple coneflower. These are tall weeds with purple flowers that grow in the prairie regions of the USA. The plants have edible roots, leaves and seeds and were used by Native Americans mainly for medicinal purposes. Both the roots and above-ground parts of the plant are used in supplements and they contain a number of phenols that are derivatives of caffeic acid (e.g. cichoric acid and caftaric acid), which are in the category of phenols listed earlier as hydroxycinnamates. As with many herbal extracts, it is not known which (if any) of the many secondary metabolites are the 'active ingredients', although the phenol content is used to assess the quality of Echinacea preparations.

The main claims for Echinacea are that it is an immune stimulant and that it may be beneficial in preventing and/or treating upper respiratory tract infections (colds and flu). There have been numerous trials of the benefits of Echinacea for treating and preventing colds and flu, which have used a variety of different preparations and many of which have had major methodological flaws. Melchart et al. (2000) conducted a systematic Cochrane review of Echinacea and identified eight prevention trials and eight treatment trials. Their conclusions were that some Echinacea preparations may be better than placebos, although the data were not of sufficient homogeneity or quality to perform a quantitative meta-analysis. The authors concluded that the evidence then available was not sufficient to recommend Echinacea for the treatment or prevention of colds (Linde et al., 2006, discussed later, is an updated version of this review).

Since 2000 there have been several other trials of Echinacea, most of which have found it to be ineffective in preventing colds (Sperber et al., 2004) or in reducing the duration and severity of symptoms in adults (Barrett et al., 2002; Yale and Liu 2004) or in children (Taylor et al., 2003). One trial did report that subjects given Echinacea at the onset of an upper respiratory tract infection had significantly lower scores on a subjective 'severity of symptoms' scale than those receiving a placebo (Goel et al., 2004). The latter authors used a formulation made from freshly harvested Echinacea purpurea plants and suggest that perhaps the negative results obtained in many other trials may be attributable to the low level of active ingredients in the Echinacea preparations used. Even in this positive study, however, the apparent benefits of the Echinacea were modest.

In the most recent Cochrane review, Linde et al. (2006) found no evidence that Echinacea preparations are effective in preventing a cold, but some preparations of Echinacea purpurea might have some effect in reducing the severity of symptoms or duration of the cold in adults, although not in children. One trial did report rashes in some children receiving an Echinacea preparation. These authors commented on the great diversity of Echinacea preparations on the market at that time, with variation in exact species, parts of the plant used and the method of preparation of the extract, which would be likely to have major effects on the composition of the different extracts available and used in the trials.

There seem to be no grounds for the routine long-term use of Echinacea as a dietary supplement (it will no longer be classified as such within the EU from

May 2011); the evidence supporting its use as a short medication at the onset of an upper respiratory tract infection is also very weak. Echinacea is available in tablet or liquid form and special preparations for children are also sold. It is very difficult to specify a dose because of the variability in the content of the commercial preparations. One major UK supplier produces tablets containing concentrated extracts of the plant juice, which they say is the equivalent of just over 3 g of the fresh herb and is standardised to contain 3% of cichoric acid, one of the phenols that may be bioactive.

Garlic

Sulphur-containing secondary metabolites in the Allium (onion) family

Garlic is a member of the Allium family of plants, which also includes onions, leeks and chives. It has been widely used as a food flavouring and as a traditional medicine for centuries. Garlic has antibacterial properties *in vitro* and garlic preparations have been used topically for the treatment of skin infections and wounds, although their clinical potential is still being evaluated. Cutler and Wilson (2004) have produced a stable, aqueous extract of allicin (see later) from garlic that was able to kill 30 clinical isolates of methacillin-resistant staphylococcus aureus (MRSA), even those that were resistant to the topical antibiotic mupirocin.

All members of the Allium family contain compounds known as S-alkyl cysteine sulphoxides. These compounds are all derived from the sulphur-containing amino acid cysteine:

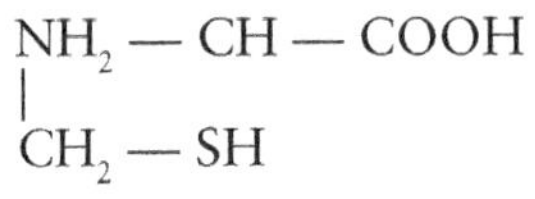

$$NH_2 - CH - COOH \qquad Cysteine$$
$$|$$
$$CH_2 - SH$$

In these S-alkyl cysteine sulphoxides, the normal side chain of cysteine ($-CH_2SH$) is oxidised and alkylated to give side chains with the following general formula:

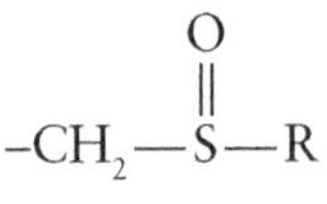

$$
\begin{array}{c}
O \\
\| \\
-CH_2 - S - R
\end{array}
$$

Where R is an alkyl or hydro carbon group
Below are examples of the side chains of some of the S-alkyl cysteine sulphoxides commonly found in members of the Allium family.

S-methyl cysteine sulphoxide, which is found in all or most Allium species:

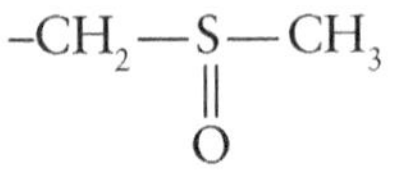

$$
\begin{array}{c}
-CH_2 - S - CH_3 \\
\| \\
O
\end{array}
$$

S-propyl cysteine sulphoxide, which predominates in chives:

$$-CH_2-S-CH_2-CH_2-CH_3$$
$$\overset{\|}{O}$$

S-propenyl cysteine sulphoxide, which predominates in onions – when onions are cut it is a metabolite of this compound that causes the eyes to water:

$$-CH_2-S-CH=CH-CH_3$$
$$\overset{\|}{O}$$

S-allyl cysteine sulphoxide, which predominates in garlic and is usually called alliin:

$$-CH_2-S-CH_2-CH=CH_3$$
$$\overset{\|}{O}$$

Fresh undamaged garlic cloves have little smell, but when they are cut or crushed, an enzyme called allinase cleaves off the side chain of alliin to give allyl sulphenic acid:

$$CH_2=CH-CH_2-S-OH \quad \text{(allyl sulphenic acid)}$$

Two molecules of allyl sulphenic acid then condense to produce allicin, which is responsible for the characteristic odour of crushed garlic and is also regarded as an important biologically active compound in garlic:

$$CH_2=CH-CH_2-S-S-CH_2-CH=CH_2 \text{ (allicin)}$$

Allicin is relatively unstable to heat and is degraded to a number of sulphur-containing compounds during cooking; it is also relatively unstable even when the crushed garlic is not cooked. One 2–4 g clove of fresh garlic has the potential to produce about 5–20 mg of allicin. To put this into context, the odourless garlic capsules marketed by one large company contain the extract from 1 g of fresh garlic and are claimed to contain 0.05 mg of allicin.

One major problem encountered in trying to study the effects of garlic, and indeed to interpret other studies, is that the exact nature and preparation of the garlic used will have a large effect on the amounts and make-up of the sulphur-containing compounds within it. Fresh raw garlic may contain more than 10 times as much allicin as some of the extracts used in supplements. Drying garlic preserves both the allicin potential and the allinase enzyme and so good amounts of allicin can be generated when this is rehydrated. There is not much hard evidence that it is actually allicin that is responsible for much of the supposed biological activity of garlic preparations, but this is widely assumed to be the case.

Rationale and evidence for the use of garlic supplements

The major benefits claimed for oral garlic supplements are listed below:

- Garlic supplements are claimed to lower blood cholesterol and perhaps to have other beneficial effects on the blood lipoprotein profile.
- They are claimed to have favourable (antithrombotic) effects on blood coagulation, such as reducing platelet aggregation.
- Garlic supplements have been claimed to lower blood pressure.
- It has been suggested that garlic may be of value in the management of type 2 diabetes.
- It is suggested that garlic may have anticancer properties.
- Garlic supplements are claimed not only to have topical and *in vitro* antibacterial effects, but also to have similar effects when administered systemically.

The effects of garlic on the cardiovascular system and on cancer have been the subject of a major review by the Agency for Healthcare Research and Quality in the USA (Mulrow *et al.*, 2000). The authors identified randomised controlled trials of garlic of at least four weeks' duration that had used a variety of cardiovascular measures and outcomes. Thirty-seven trials of garlic supplements on blood cholesterol that met their inclusion criteria were identified and these consistently reported a small but statistically significant reduction in plasma total cholesterol in the garlic group compared to the placebo at one month and three months. However, the few trials (eight) that reported the effects after six months found no statistically significant effect of the garlic supplements. Taken at face value, these findings suggest that garlic supplements do probably have a small but transient cholesterol-lowering effect. Such a small and transient effect would be of very limited clinical value, because it is the prolonged exposure to elevated cholesterol levels that is responsible for the increased risk of atherosclerosis and heart disease associated with an elevated blood cholesterol concentration. Another possibility is that the apparent differences in the short- and longer-term response to garlic supplements may be the result of methodological or other differences between the studies, rather than a true reflection of time differences in the response to garlic supplements.

A more recent meta-analysis of 13 RCTs of between 12 and 24 weeks' duration (Khoo and Aziz, 2009) found no evidence that garlic preparations had any useful effect on plasma total or LDL cholesterol concentration. They remarked that the quality of the studies was generally good, but they also noted that the results of different studies were quite variable. Even the best interpretation of these data suggests that garlic supplements are an inefficient way of achieving a clinically insignificant reduction in plasma cholesterol and thus that they have little if any clinical usefulness in this respect. Other natural products like the phytosterols (discussed in

Chapter 9) and drugs like the statins that inhibit cholesterol biosynthesis have clear and more substantial cholesterol-lowering effects.

Mulrow *et al.* (2000) identified 27 short-term studies testing the effect of garlic supplements on blood pressure. These studies reported mixed results, but none of them suggested that garlic supplements caused any substantial reduction in blood pressure. Most studies found no statistically significant effect of garlic on blood pressure, and even in the few that did report a significant effect it was only a small effect.

There was some evidence from 10 short-term randomised controlled trials that garlic supplements might have some useful effects in reducing platelet aggregation and thus perhaps also lowering the risk of thromboses.

Garlic has been suggested to be of value in the treatment of type 2 diabetes, which is also an important risk factor for cardiovascular disease. However, Mulrow *et al.* (2000) found no evidence from their review of published material that garlic supplements had any effects on blood glucose concentration or insulin sensitivity (reduced insulin sensitivity is the primary pathological change in type 2 diabetes).

There is little evidence in the scientific literature to support the proposition that garlic has anticancer properties. Most of the studies reviewed by Mulrow *et al.* (2000) were case-control studies and these found that garlic supplements used for up to between three and five years were not associated with reduced risk of breast, lung, gastric or colorectal cancer in any of the studies reviewed. Some individual case-control studies did find an association between garlic consumption and cancer at some sites, but evidence from this type of study must be regarded with great scepticism unless there is corroboration from studies that have used other more robust methodologies. Dorant *et al.* (1996) used a cohort of 120 000 Dutch people to evaluate prospectively the association between the consumption of several Allium species in food, the consumption of garlic supplements and risk of colorectal cancer over a period of 40 months. They found no suggestion that high consumption of Allium foods or garlic supplements had any protective effect against bowel cancer.

In a major review of the relationship between diet, physical activity and cancer, WCRF/AICR (2007) did find some evidence, mainly from case-control studies, to support a preventive effect of garlic and other Allium vegetables on colorectal cancer and perhaps stomach cancer. In the latter case they speculated that garlic might inhibit the growth of Helicobacter pylori in the stomach and that this might ultimately lead to a reduced stomach cancer risk. In stark contrast to this, however, Satia *et al.* (2009) specifically looked at the association between use of dietary supplements and risk of colorectal cancer, and found that use of garlic pills was associated with a significant increase in colorectal cancer risk. These findings were based on analysis of cancer cases over a 10-year period in around 77 000 people who had filled in a detailed questionnaire about their supplement use at the start of the period. Overall, there seems to be no evidential justification for taking garlic supplements in order to reduce the risk of developing cancer.

Lissiman *et al.* (2009), in a Cochrane review, found little evidence from the scientific literature that garlic was of any use in treating or preventing the common cold and that claims of its effectiveness seemed to be based on poor-quality evidence.

These authors only found only one trial (Josling, 2001) that met their inclusion criteria and they judged its quality to be reasonable. Josling did report that daily doses of 180 mg allicin for 12 weeks did reduce the frequency of colds and the total number of days of illness compared to the placebo, but that it did not have much effect on the duration of each cold. The very large dose of allicin used in this trial should be noted: the equivalent to 10–40 cloves of fresh garlic per day. This is the equivalent in terms of allicin content to several thousand of some odourless garlic capsules per day for some brands sold as food supplements.

Mulrow *et al.* (2000) also looked at the side-effects that were reported to be associated with high garlic use, which included:

- Unpleasant breath and body odour.
- A range of abdominal symptoms, including increased flatulence and abdominal pain.
- Dermatitis, rhinitis and asthma (typical symptoms of allergic reactions).
- Bleeding.
- A small number of cases of possible potentiation of anticoagulant drugs.

Apart from the effects on breath and body odour, it cannot be certain that these adverse symptoms were side-effects caused by the garlic supplements. Despite the lack of substantial evidence of a cause-and-effect relationship between garlic and these adverse effects, it would seem prudent for people taking anticoagulant medication to avoid garlic supplements, or at least to make their physician aware of their garlic use.

There is no clearly established dose for the use of garlic supplements, but many trials have used 400–1000 mg of dried garlic, which is equivalent to one or two cloves of fresh garlic per day (theoretically also providing 10–40 mg of allicin). Some preparations sold as food supplements may contain very small amounts of allicin and this may be particularly true of some odourless preparations.

Ginger

Ginger refers to the underground rhizome of the tropical flowering plant Zingiber officianale. The term *officianale* in the Latin name of a plant indicates that this was sold by apothecaries in past times and so that it has a long history of medicinal use. *Zingiber* means horn-shaped in Sanskrit and refers to the shape of the ginger rhizome. Ginger has a sharp, sweet flavour and is used to flavour foods and drinks. The oil of ginger root contains the sesquiterpenes zingiberene and λ-bisabolene, while the oleoresin contains a group of pungent phenolic compounds called gingerols and their degradation products. The gingerols are widely regarded as the components of ginger and ginger extracts that are responsible for any pharmacological actions. The gingerols are structurally related to capsaicin in chilli peppers and they bind to the same pain receptors (vanilloid receptor 1, VR1) that are abundant in the mouth and skin. Activation of VR1 receptors is responsible for the searing sensation of eating chilli peppers and also presumably for the pungency of ginger (Dedov *et al.*, 2002). The chemical structures of capsaicin and several gingerols may be found in Dedov *et al.* (2002). These same VR1 receptors may also be largely responsible for the chest pain experienced during a heart attack. Dedov *et al.* (2002) suggest that studies with gingerols and capsaicin may help in the development of substances that interact with and block the VR1 receptor (antagonists) and that this may offer a new approach to some types of pain control.

There are many historical claims for the medicinal usefulness of ginger, but the main focus of interest today is its potential to help with minor stomach upsets and, more particularly, for the control of certain types of nausea and vomiting:

- morning sickness in pregnancy
- post-operative sickness
- motion sickness
- sickness caused by cancer chemotherapy

It is also suggested on the basis of animal studies that gingerols may exert an anti-inflammatory and analgesic effect in conditions such as osteoarthritis by inhibiting prostaglandin and leukotriene biosynthesis (Kiuchi *et al.*, 1992).

Ernst and Pittler (2000) did a systematic review of clinical trials of the efficacy of ginger for controlling nausea and vomiting from a variety of causes. The found just one study each for sea sickness, morning sickness and chemotherapy-induced nausea that met their inclusion criteria. While these generally favoured ginger over placebo, it would be premature to draw any firm conclusions from single studies. Ernst and Pittler (2000) identified three trials in which ginger had been used for the control of post-operative nausea and vomiting. Even though two of these studies suggested a positive benefit for ginger use, when the data from the three studies was pooled the ginger was not found to be statistically more effective than the placebo. A more recent and relatively large trial with 180 patients (Eberhart *et al.*, 2003) reported that ginger did not reduce the incidence of post-operative nausea and vomiting any more than the placebo in patients after they had had gynaecological laparoscopy.

It has been proposed that ginger might exert an antinausea and vomiting effect in motion sickness by reducing the increase in gastric rhythmicity and the rise in antidiuretic hormone (ADH or vasopressin) that accompanies motion sickness. In a small trial, Lien *et al.* (2003) found that pre-treatment with 1 g or 2 g of ginger reduced the nausea, the increase in gastric activity and the rise in plasma ADH when subjects were put in a rotating chair to induce motion sickness. Two other trials using the rotating chair as a method of inducing motion sickness have not detected any beneficial effects of ginger over the placebo, however. Stewart *et al.* (1991) found that neither 500 mg nor 1 g of ginger provided any protection against motion sickness nor did it significantly affect gastric function during motion sickness; a standard motion sickness drug did register positive effects. A study to test the efficacy of several antisickness drugs for NASA found that three doses of ginger had no more effect than the placebo (Wood *et al.*, 1988). One study, in a more naturalistic setting, tested the effects of ginger on sea sickness in 80 naval cadets during a voyage. The ginger significantly reduced the tendency to vomit and reduced cold sweats, but the reduction in the symptoms of nausea and vertigo did not reach significance compared to the placebo (Grontved *et al.*, 1988).

White (2007), in an overview of the therapeutic uses of ginger, concluded that it was effective in reducing the nausea and vomiting in pregnancy and in post-operative patients, but that there is much less evidence that it is effective in controlling other causes of these symptoms, including motion sickness. Borrelli *et al.* (2005) published a systematic review of the effects of ginger on pregnancy-induced sickness. They found six trials that met their inclusion criteria; four of these suggested that ginger was more effective than a placebo, and the other two suggested that ginger was as effective as vitamin B_6, which is also prescribed for morning sickness. Chaiyakunapruk *et al.* (2006) did a meta-analysis of five randomised controlled trials (360 patients in total) on the effect of doses of at least 1 g of ginger on nausea and vomiting experienced in the first 24 hours after surgery. They did find evidential support for the effectiveness of ginger and the only side-effect reported was some abdominal discomfort.

Kiuchi *et al.* (1992) reported that gingerols inhibit the enzyme prostaglandin synthetase, which synthesises prostaglandins, and probably also inhibit the enzyme arachidonate 5-lipoxygenase, which is involved in the synthesis of leukotrienes (see Figure 6.3 in Chapter 6). As prostaglandins and leukotrienes are key mediators of the inflammatory response, these laboratory data suggest that gingerols might have anti-inflammatory and analgesic effects. They might therefore alleviate the pain and/or swelling associated with osteoarthritis by a similar mechanism to aspirin.

Bliddal *et al.* (2000) conducted a randomised, double-blind cross-over trial comparing the effects of ginger extracts, ibuprofen and a placebo in 56 patients with osteoarthritis of the hip or knee. Each patient spent three weeks on each of the three treatments in random order, with a one-week 'wash-out' period between each of the three treatments. While some preliminary analysis did suggest a possible beneficial effect of ginger compared to the placebo over the whole study, there was no statistically significant effect of ginger compared to the placebo and ginger was clearly less effective than ibuprofen. The authors noted that this study did not support the beneficial effects of ginger, but that a longer study with more potent extracts of ginger was warranted.

Ginger has a very long history of safe use as a foodstuff and there have been few adverse effects noted in trials of concentrated extracts, and these have not been serious. Most of the trials discussed above have used doses that are equivalent to at least 1 g of fresh ginger.

Ginkgo biloba

Ginkgo biloba is also known as the gingko nut or maidenhair tree. The gingko nut tree probably originated in China, where it has been grown for many thousands of years. It is sometimes called a 'living fossil', because the modern trees are almost unchanged from fossils found in China that are over 100 million years old. The ginkgo tree produces an inedible yellow fruit containing a hard-shelled nut or kernel, which has been used as a human food. Ginkgo nuts are still widely used in Asian cuisine in soups, appetisers and desserts. These nuts are also used in traditional Chinese medicine, but it is extracts of the leaves that are used to make modern western dietary supplements and herbal medicines. One well-defined extract, denoted EGb 761, has been one of the most widely prescribed medications in Germany and Ginkgo biloba is the most popular of the herbal supplements in western countries. Most clinical trials have used this extract and many of the trials have received funding from the producer company (Birks and Grimley-Evans, 2009). Another well-defined extract, LI 1370, has been used in some trials. Unlike many herbal preparations, high-quality standardised extracts of Ginkgo biloba have been widely available for many years.

The standardised Ginkgo leaf extract contains around 25% of flavonoid glycosides like quercetin, kaempferol and isorhamnetin and about 6% of terpenoid derivatives, including a series of so-called ginkgolides and bilobalide. These flavonoids and terpenoids are believed to be the active constituents of Ginkgo biloba leaf extracts.

Rationale and evidence for the use of Ginkgo biloba supplements

There are several claims about the beneficial effects of Ginkgo leaf extracts, and some of the most studied and most likely are listed below:

- It is said to improve memory in people with age-related cognitive deficiency.
- It may improve memory in healthy people.
- It may slow down the progression of Alzheimer's disease and other forms of dementia.
- It may be helpful for people with intermittent claudication (pain in the legs when walking).
- It may be beneficial for people suffering from chronic tinnitus (the perception of sound with no external auditory stimulus – 'ringing' in the ears).

The exact mechanism by which Ginkgo biloba extracts exert any physiological or clinical benefits is not established, but a number of pharmacological activities such as those listed below have been demonstrated, often using animal models (see Barnes, 2002a; Ahlemeyer and Krieglstein, 2003; and the Commission E monograph on Ginkgo biloba – ABC, 2010):

- It has free radical scavenging and antioxidant activity and, as discussed in Chapter 5, this could be helpful in preventing or slowing almost any 'degenerative change'. It might, for example, lead to a reduced rate of neuronal death in neurodegenerative conditions.
- It inhibits platelet aggregation by inhibiting platelet-activating factor. This might improve blood flow by reducing its viscosity.

- It improves both cerebral and peripheral blood flow by the effects on blood viscosity and also by relaxing vascular walls.
- It may affect neurotransmitter metabolism.
- It may increase neuronal regeneration in some experimental brain injury models in animals.

There have been dozens of clinical trials of Ginkgo biloba extracts for the clinical indications listed earlier and a few for other indications, and there have been a number of systematic reviews of these trials. Many of the early trials were not published in English but often in French or German. One of the earlier reviews published in English evaluated the literature relating to the effects of Ginkgo biloba on 'cerebral insufficiency' (Kleijnen and Knipschild, 1992). Cerebral insufficiency is a term that was used to describe a myriad of psychological symptoms, including poor concentration and memory, thought to result from an age-related reduction in cerebral blood flow. Kleijnen and Knipschild identified 40 controlled trials of Gingko biloba for 'cerebral insufficiency', but described only 8 of these as well performed. Despite their reservations about the quality of most of the trials, they did find that almost all of the studies reported positive results for the extract (most used 120 mg of extract for at least 4–6 weeks). They suggested that the presence of no negative trials within a large number of small and methodologically poor trials probably indicated a publication bias towards positive trials. They concluded in 1992 that overall the evidence for Ginkgo biloba was similar to that for a regulated drug then being used (co-dergocrine).

A Cochrane review conducted a decade after this first review (Birks *et al.*, 2002) provided more concrete support for the beneficial effects of Ginkgo biloba for cognitive impairment and dementia. The authors conducted a meta-analysis of all studies of Gingko biloba for cognitive impairment, including dementia, that met their quality criteria. The Ginkgo biloba was found to be safe, in that there were no more adverse events in the Ginkgo than in the placebo groups. The physician-determined Clinical Global Improvement scale showed statistically significant positive benefits for Gingko at doses above and below 200 mg/day at 12, 24 and 52 weeks. There were also significantly positive results for measures of mood and emotional function, and an index to measure capacity to cope with the activities of daily life. The authors concluded that Ginkgo is safe and that, despite the poor quality and small size of many of the early trials, it showed promising evidence of improvements in cognition and functioning. The one less than positive note was an observation that the three most modern trials showed inconsistent results.

Canter and Ernst (2002) identified nine short-term trials (maximum 30-day duration) that investigated the effects of Ginkgo extracts on normal healthy people to see if there was any justification for claims that it was a 'smart' drug that could improve cognition in people with no impairment. They found no indication that the Ginkgo extracts had any significant positive effects on any objective measures of cognitive function. They concluded that there was then no substantial evidence that Ginkgo extracts were able to enhance cognitive function in healthy people. Note that the authors were critical of the methodology of several of the trials and particularly noted the need for studies of longer duration.

Hilton and Stuart (2004) conducted a Cochrane review of Ginkgo biloba extracts for the management of tinnitus. They identified 12 trials, but excluded 10 of these on methodological grounds. They concluded that there was no evidence that Ginkgo was effective for the treatment of tinnitus as a primary complaint. Tinnitus also occurs as a symptom of 'cerebral insufficiency', but there were no trials of acceptable quality that had tested the efficacy of Ginkgo on the symptoms of tinnitus under these circumstances.

Horsch and Walther (2004) reviewed trials of the effectiveness of Ginkgo extract EGb 761 in the treatment of peripheral arterial occlusive disease, which leads to the symptom of intermittent claudication or ischaemic leg muscle pain brought on by walking. Seven of nine studies showed a statistically significant increase in the 'pain-free walking distance', which the authors also suggest was of real clinical relevance to the patients.

General descriptive reviews published in 2002 (Barnes, 2002a; Ernst, 2002) did appear to offer real grounds for believing that in controlled trials, standardised extracts of Ginkgo might offer the possibility of significant clinical benefits:

- Barnes suggested that they were more effective than the placebo in relieving symptoms associated with age-related cognitive deficiency, although Ernst expressed serious reservations about the evidence.
- Both authors suggested that Ginkgo might have some effect in improving cognition in dementia and Ernst thought that this could be clinically significant.
- There was no substantial evidence that Ginkgo leaf extracts reduce tinnitus.
- There was no good-quality evidence that Ginkgo leaf extracts had any memory-enhancing effect in people with normal cognitive function.
- Ernst also concluded that Ginkgo probably has a moderate but clinically significant beneficial effect in extending the pain-free walking distance in patients with intermittent claudication (Barnes only reviewed the Ginkgo in relation to cognitive aspects). Ernst concluded that it might have similar efficacy to the most common drug treatment used for this condition at the time, but that it was clearly less effective than regular walking exercise.

This means that when the first edition of this book was written in 2004, there were grounds for believing that Ginkgo supplements might offer useful benefits for people with dementia, age-related cognitive impairment and patients suffering from intermittent claudication. More recent trials and systematic reviews have tended not to support this earlier optimism and indeed, as outlined below, they seem to suggest that even good-quality defined ginkgo supplements offer little benefit for any of these conditions.

- A recent Cochrane review (Nicolai et al., 2009) found only, at best, a marginal effect of Ginkgo extracts on intermittent claudication, and they suggested that even this marginal effect was probably exaggerated by publication bias. They concluded that Ginkgo had no clinically significant benefits for patients with intermittent claudication.

- Birks and Grimley-Evans (2009) did a systematic review and meta-analysis of the effects of Ginkgo biloba on age-related cognitive impairment and dementia. They identified no fewer than 36 trials, but found that most were small and of less than three months' duration. They found nine more recent trials that were of six months' duration (total of over 2000 subjects) and generally conducted to a reasonable standard. The larger, later trials found inconsistent effects on measures of cognition, ability to perform everyday activities, mood and carer burden. When they confined their analysis to patients diagnosed with Alzheimer's disease, there was also no consistent benefit associated with the use of Ginkgo biloba.
- The review of Hilton and Stuart (2004), discussed earlier, was updated in 2009 without change to the conclusions that there was no evidential support for Ginkgo extracts having any beneficial effect in patients suffering from tinnitus.

Most clinical trials suggest that Ginkgo is well tolerated, without significantly more adverse events than in those taking the placebo. Mild gastrointestinal symptoms are occasionally reported in subjects taking Ginkgo biloba preparations. Occasional and fairly severe allergic skin reactions have occasionally been reported. In relation to allergic reactions, Barnes (2002a) notes that ginkgolic acids found in crude extracts are highly allergenic and thus that standard extracts should contain less than 5 ppm of these. Barnes also notes occasional reports of bleeding in people taking Gingko and that, given its effects on blood platelets, it might interact with anticoagulant therapies. She recommends that it should not be taken by people who are also taking anticoagulants or antiplatelet agents, and that Ginkgo treatment should be stopped 24–48 hours before any surgery. There is a lack of data on its safety in pregnancy and lactation, so Barnes recommends that it should not be used. There would seem to be no positive indication for its use in children and so it should not be given to children.

Most clinical trials of Ginkgo have used between 120 and 240 mg/day of the standardised extract. Commercial preparations usually contain 60–120 mg per tablet, equivalent to the flavonoid content of 3–6 g of whole Ginkgo leaves.

Ginseng

Several plants of the Panax genus are commonly referred to as ginseng. Ginseng (P. ginseng) was used by the Chinese as an aphrodisiac because its forked roots resemble the lower part of the human body. Native Americans brewed a type of tea from one species, P. quinquefolius, and they ate the roots of the dwarf ginseng, P. trifolius. Some plants referred to as Siberian, Manchurian and Brazilian ginseng do not belong to the Panax genus and so may not contain the agents in ginseng to which its effects are attributed. The term ginseng usually refers to Panax ginseng, also called Chinese or Korean ginseng, and this is the most commonly used and tested variety. It has been suggested that as many as six million Americans may use ginseng preparations.

The name of the genus Panax is derived from the Greek word for panacea, meaning 'all healing', and it is suggested that ginseng preparations have a number of diverse effects that promote general well-being. The active principles of ginseng are believed to be substances called ginsenosides, which are saponins consisting of a steroidal triterpene and a sugar residue; that is, triterpene glucuronides. Around a dozen of these ginsenosides have been identified in ginseng extracts.

Some of the claimed benefits for ginseng include:

- As a tonic to restore strength and promote general well-being.
- To improve physical performance.
- To improve memory and mental well-being.
- To help prevent cancer.
- To aid in the treatment of diabetes.

Vogler *et al.* (1999) conducted a systematic review of randomised controlled clinical trials of ginseng for a variety of possible uses. They identified 16 trials of sufficient quality to meet their inclusion criteria and they found that these trials provided no compelling evidence for the efficacy of ginseng for any of the indications tested:

- For enhancing physical performance.
- For improving mental performance or memory.
- For enhancing the immune system or for the treatment of infection with the Herpes simplex virus.
- In the management of diabetes.

Bucci (2000) lists (with references) a wide range of pharmacological activities that have been reported for the ginsenosides present in ginseng (extracts), usually on the basis of animal or *in vitro* studies, including the following:

- Some ginsenosides have CNS-stimulating effects while others have depressant effects.
- They cause increased release of corticotrophin from the pituitary and thus increased cortisol output (the so-called 'stress hormone') from the adrenal glands.
- They have modulating effects on the immune system.
- They have antioxidant effects via an increase in the glutathione content of the liver.
- They stimulate nitric oxide production at various sites.

Cardinal and Engels (2001) tested the effects of two doses of ginseng on 'psychological well-being' in a randomised controlled trial using 80 students. They measured the subjects' responses in psychological mood and well-being evaluation tests prior to and after two months of taking the ginseng or placebo. They found no significant effect of the ginseng at either dose. Lee *et al.* (2009), in a systematic review of the literature relating to the effects of ginseng on cognitive function in Alzheimer's disease, found only two studies that met their inclusion criteria. Both of these studies looked at the use of ginseng as an adjunct to conventional drug therapy, and while they did report positive findings, the reviewers suggested that they had serious methodological limitations. They concluded that evidence for the use of ginseng as a treatment for Alzheimer's disease was scarce and inconclusive.

Of all the herbs claimed to enhance physical athletic performance, ginseng is probably the most tested. There is a significant body of animal data suggesting that ginsenosides can induce improvements in exercise performance in controlled laboratory experiments with small mammals. However, most of these studies have used very large doses and/or injected the ginsenosides. Ginsenosides are known to undergo chemical conversion in the gut and so the injection studies, in particular, may have little application to oral use by people. Reviews by Bahrke and Morgan (1994 and 2000) and Bahrke *et al.* (2009) found no consistent evidence for an ergogenic effect of ginseng, which is consistent with the view of most reviewers. In the latest of these three reviews the authors noted that most of the methodological shortcomings found in earlier investigations were still present in more recent studies.

Bucci (2000) reviewed the literature relating to the effect of a number of herbal preparations on human performance. He provides an extensive tabulated list of studies that have tested the effects of Panax ginseng on human physical and mental performance. Like other reviewers, he notes the inconsistency of these trials, but goes on to suggest that those studies with positive outcomes have almost invariably used high doses (the equivalent of at least 2 g/day of dried root) and were of long duration (at least eight weeks). He further suggests from his overview of published trials that any benefits of ginseng may be largely confined to older, untrained subjects. He concludes that young, trained individuals probably get little if any benefit from ginseng on their physical performance, and that any effects there may be in older untrained subjects require large doses to be used over an extended period.

There is some evidence from case-control studies and from one cohort study that regular consumption of ginseng is associated with a reduced incidence of cancer (not site specific). Yun and Choi (1998) evaluated the ginseng intake of 4600 middle-aged and elderly Koreans and related this to their risk of developing cancer over the following five years. Those people who consumed ginseng had a significantly lower risk of developing cancer than those who did not. Over the five years of the study there were 48 cases of cancer per 1000 people in the 'no ginseng' group compared with 24 cases per 1000 in the ginseng group. While this data looks interesting, it should be borne in mind that epidemiological association does not necessarily indicate cause and effect. The Koreans who consumed the ginseng (70% of the sample) were a self-selecting group and, although they had a lower risk of cancer than those who did not, it would be very premature to attribute this effect to the ginseng *per se*. Yun (2001) has also reviewed evidence of the cancer-preventing effects of Panax ginseng. A more recent cohort study with almost 75 000 Chinese women (Kamangar *et al.*, 2007) found no evidence of a protective effect of ginseng on gastric cancer. There has been some speculation about a plausible mechanism by which ginseng might protect against the development of gastric cancer: it is said to inhibit the growth and suppress the chronic inflammatory effects of the bacterium

Helicobacter pylori, which is clearly implicated in the development of peptic ulcers and stomach cancer (see, for example, Lee *et al.*, 2008).

In a review of the risks and benefits of several herbal therapies, Ernst (2002) identified several serious but probably uncommon side-effects reported by people taking ginseng, including:

- Insomnia and nervousness.
- Diarrhoea.
- Skin eruptions.
- Headaches.
- Symptoms associated with oestrogenic activity, such as breast tenderness and vaginal bleeding in post-menopausal women (probably making it unsuitable for women with breast cancer).

There are some reports that ginseng may reduce the effectiveness of anticoagulant (warfarin) therapy (e.g. Yuan *et al.*, 2004). These potential side-effects need to be borne in mind if large supplemental doses are used for extended periods, but there is a long history of ginseng use in foods and drinks and so, provided usage is moderate, there seems no reason to discourage such use by most people. Those who enjoy its culinary use can be assured that there is no reason to stop using it and just the possibility that it might be beneficial. There is no established dose for supplemental use, but manufacturers recommend the equivalent of 0.5–3 g/day of the dried root. One quality UK supplier produces tablets that contain the equivalent of 600 mg of Korean ginseng root, guaranteed to contain at least 18 mg of ginsenosides.

Guarana

Guarana (Paullinia cupana) is a Brazilian climbing shrub whose seeds contain substantial amounts of caffeine, as well as two other alkaloids also found in tea and coffee, theobromine and theophylline; it also contains tannins. The seeds are used to make a paste that is employed medicinally and guarana is also the base for the most popular soft drink in Brazil. Natives of the Amazonian rain forest chewed the seeds or added them to foods or drinks in order to increase alertness and reduce fatigue. It is not widely used as a supplement in the UK, but one major chocolate manufacturer launched a chocolate bar in 2002 that contained guarana, promoting it as a 'tasty stimulating snack'.

Guarana seeds contain about twice as much caffeine as coffee beans and so, given the well-known stimulant effects of caffeine as well as theobromine and theophylline, it clearly would act as a general CNS stimulant. The caffeine in guarana is sometimes referred to as guaranine to make it sound unique. The caffeine content of guarana extracts may vary between 30 and 50% depending on brand; so one 200 mg tablet contains around 80 mg of caffeine and one cup of brewed coffee contains about 100 mg. A can of cola contains about half the caffeine in a cup of brewed coffee, but it varies according to brand and variety. Some other soft drinks marketed on their ability to boost energy levels and 'give you wings' contain several times the concentration of caffeine found in cola drinks.

Guarana is claimed to increase alertness, 'boost' energy levels and reduce fatigue. Given that caffeine and the other alkaloids in guarana and in tea and coffee are accepted to be CNS stimulants, such effects are to be expected from consuming any of these.

Caffeine and therefore guarana are known to have some capacity to boost athletic performance in large doses. For this reason, up until 2004 the International Olympic Committee classified caffeine as a restricted substance and set a threshold on the amount of caffeine (12 mg/L) that was permissible in competitors' urine samples. To exceed this threshold requires a large caffeine intake: about 8 cups of brewed coffee, ten 200 mg guarana tablets, 18 cans of cola or 800 mg of caffeine (note these figures are for illustrative purposes only and will obviously vary depending on body size and other factors).

Small trials have suggested that guarana extracts give short-term improvements in cognitive performance in healthy young volunteers (e.g. Haskell *et al.*, 2007) by more than can be accounted for than by merely the effects of the caffeine. Claims that tolerable doses of caffeine promote weight loss have not been substantiated.

The adverse effects of taking large doses of guarana are similar to those experienced when large amounts of strong coffee are consumed: nervousness, insomnia, palpitations, stomach irritation and a rise in blood pressure. Whether a supplemental source of caffeine is useful or desirable must be left for individual consumers to decide. Supplements typically contain up to 200 mg of guarana extract.

Kelp

Kelp is the name given to any brown or olive-green seaweed of the Laminariales and Fucales orders. Some large Pacific seaweeds are referred to as giant kelp. The Japanese dry and shred kelp and use it as a boiled vegetable or in soups and they call it kombu. A number of claims have been made regarding the value of kelp, but the main reason supplements are consumed in the UK is as a source of iodine (see Chapter 4). One problem with seaweed generally is that it may be contaminated with toxic metals, including arsenic, if harvested from polluted water.

Kelp supplements are consumed in the form of tablets, capsules or powders, which may contain the equivalent of 0.25–0.5 g of kelp. The iodine content of different kelp preparations varies and is often not stated on the packaging, but the recommended dose typically contains 150–300 µg of iodine, which compares with the adult RNI in the UK of 140 µg/day (US RDA 150 µg/day). The maximum dose of supplemental iodine recommended by FSA (2003) was 500 µg/day.

It was noted in Chapter 4 that overt iodine deficiency (goitre) is rarely seen in the affluent countries of Europe and the USA. Iodine deficiency is, however, one of the most common micronutrient deficiencies in the developing world, where it leads to retarded mental and physical development in children (cretinism) and high rates of still births and congenital abnormalities. Iodine deficiency is the most common cause of preventable mental retardation in children worldwide. It was also noted in Chapter 2 that average adult intakes of iodine in the UK are at or above the RNI, although 12% of young women in the UK have recorded iodine intakes deemed to be inadequate (Hoare *et al.*, 2004). As further noted in Chapter 4, a review by Zimmerman and Delange (2004) suggested that most women in Europe are iodine deficient during pregnancy, and the authors recommend that all pregnant women should receive iodine-containing supplements (150 µg/day) during pregnancy. However, they specifically counsel against the use of kelp or other seaweed supplements because of the unacceptable variability in their iodine content.

Persons with known thyroid disease should not take kelp supplements as it may interfere with the management of their condition. One concern raised by FSA (2003) about excessive iodine supplements was that they may precipitate thyroid disorders, usually hyperthyroidism. One small but well-controlled trial (Clark *et al.*, 2003) of kelp supplements in people with normal thyroid function did suggest that large kelp supplements raised both the basal levels of thyrotrophin (the pituitary hormone that stimulates thyroid activity) and the response to administration of thyrotrophin-releasing hormone (the hypothalamic factor that stimulates thyrotrophin output). This effect persisted two weeks after kelp supplementation had ceased in those receiving high doses of kelp. It is not possible to assess the long-term implications of this for kelp supplements as a potential cause of thyroid dysfunction. It would be prudent for consumers only to use kelp supplements with specified iodine content and to keep within the maximum dose recommended by FSA (2003).

In parts of the UK, especially in Wales, laver bread made from the purple laver seaweed (Porphyria umbicalis) is a local delicacy. It is also a rich source of iodine, as well as many other nutrients and carotenoids.

Milk thistle

Milk thistle (Silybum marianum) is a member of the daisy or aster family. No food use of milk thistle is given in Kiple and Ornelas (2000), although it has been used as a medicinal herb for thousands of years. On the list of herbal products on the borderline products section of the HMRA website, it is suggested that the fresh plant can be used in salads or as a substitute for green vegetables like cabbage or spinach, although it will no longer be sold as a food supplement within the EU from May 2011. The main use of milk thistle today is in the treatment of liver diseases or to protect the liver from damage by chemical (including alcohol) or viral damage. It is the ripe seeds or fruits of the plant that are usually used to make dietary supplements and herbal medicines.

The active constituents of milk thistle are referred to collectively as silymarin, which are a group of polymeric flavonoids known as flavonolignans. Three of the constituents of silymarin are silybin (which is assumed to be the most active ingredient), silydianin and silychristin. Extracts of milk thistle should be standardised to contain 70–80% silymarin. Silymarin is not readily soluble in water, so making tea from dried milk thistle is not an effective way of taking it.

In many experimental studies using isolated liver cells and a variety of animal species, milk thistle has been shown to protect the liver from several chemical insults, for example from hepatotoxic drugs like acetaminophen, from carbon tetrachloride and phenylhydrazine and from alcohol. In experimental studies with animals, silymarin has been shown to be effective in preventing the frequently fatal liver damage caused by poisoning with Amanita mushrooms (death caps). It inhibits the binding of mushroom toxins to liver cells. For example, Vogel *et al.* (1984) showed that silybarin administered up to 24 hours after a toxic dose of death cap fungus in dogs had the following effects:

- It suppressed the serum changes and changes in prothrombin that were indicative of liver damage in the control dogs.
- It reduced the amount of haemorrhagic liver necrosis.
- It reduced the death rate from 2/6 to 0/6.

There are several case reports (many not in English) suggesting that silymarin has been successful in reducing the expected consequences of accidental ingestion of these toxic mushrooms when administered up to 48 hours after poisoning. Silymarin is used and regarded as an effective emergency treatment for accidental Amanita poisoning in several European countries. There have been no controlled clinical trials of the use of milk thistle products for this purpose, and such studies would indeed be almost impossible to set up and probably impossible to justify ethically; Amanita poisoning is a relatively uncommon and acutely life-threatening occurrence. Hruby *et al.* (1983) identified case reports of Amanita poisoning where intravenous administration of a milk thistle-derived product had been used, often after the failure of other therapies, and they concluded that this intravenous use was an effective treatment for preventing serious liver damage when administered up to 48 hours after the mushroom ingestion.

More recently, Enjalbert *et al.* (2002) did a general retrospective analysis of over 2000 cases of poisoning by Amanita toxin and related toxins from other mushrooms. They concluded that although benzylpenicillin was the most frequently used chemotherapy, there was no evidence that it was effective. Their analysis did suggest that silybin, administered either alone or in combination with N-acetylcysteine, was the most effective treatment. While this discussion about its role as a hepatoprotective agent in the treatment of mushroom poisoning is of no direct relevance to the use of over-the-counter milk thistle preparations, it does confer some credibility on claims that it may have hepato-protective effects generally.

One of the more recent of the many *in vitro* and animal experimental studies of the hepato-protective effects of silymarin was conducted in baboons. Lieber *et al.* (2003) fed 12 baboons alcohol with or without silymarin for a period of three years. Several biochemical markers and morphological indicators of liver damage were reduced in the silymarin group. These results suggest that silymarin slows the development of alcohol-induced liver fibrosis in baboons. Lieber *et al.* (2003) propose that their results support the findings of several positive clinical trials in humans. They further suggest that some of the negative results from clinical trials may have been caused by poor compliance with the therapy, resulting in low or irregular silymarin intake. It is important to note that while silymarin appeared to slow the development of alcoholic cirrhosis in this primate study, it did not prevent it. Silymarin should not be regarded as a way of compensating for chronic alcohol abuse.

Valenzuela and Garrido (1994) suggest that silymarin may exert its hepatoprotective effects at three levels, as summarised below:

- By reducing oxidative liver damage by scavenging free radicals and raising the concentration of glutathione.
- By an effect on the hepatocyte cell membrane that reduces uptake of harmful chemicals and reduces cell breakdown.
- By increasing protein synthesis via an effect on DNA transcription.

It may also have an anti-inflammatory effect, which would reduce swelling of liver cells in response to injury.

The many experimental studies with isolated hepatocytes and with animal models of liver injury, together with the case reports on human Amanita poisoning, do suggest that milk thistle (silymarin) may be beneficial in some liver diseases, especially in prevention and in the very early stages of the disease. The results from many controlled clinical trials are generally mixed and inconclusive.

The Agency for Healthcare Research and Quality in the USA commissioned a major review of the efficacy of milk thistle in liver conditions (Lawrence *et al.*, 2000). This group identified 14 prospective, randomised, placebo-controlled trials of milk thistle for a variety of liver diseases up to the end of 1999. They also identified many other non-placebo-controlled trials. Their overall conclusion was that the efficacy of milk thistle was not established for any liver condition by the data then available. The most common outcomes measured were laboratory tests of liver function and, while there were several studies that did suggest benefit, the results were not consistent. Four of six studies of milk thistle in chronic liver disease showed a significant improvement in at least one measure of liver function or histology in the milk thistle group compared to the placebo group. There were some inconclusive suggestions of benefit in measures of liver function in chronic hepatitis. Trials in patients with cirrhosis were mixed, as were those where milk thistle was given in conjunction with hepato-toxic drugs. A meta-analysis of the 14 controlled trials was published in 2002 (Jacobs *et al.*, 2002). The only statistically significant effect from this meta-analysis was a greater reduction in alanine aminotransferase in patients with chronic liver disease when receiving milk thistle, which, they say, was of negligible clinical importance. As with many other reviewers of clinical trials of dietary supplements, these authors concluded that the poor quality and inadequate reporting of the data made proper analysis and interpretation difficult. The general conclusion was that milk thistle was safe and well tolerated.

A more recent large (177 patients), one-year study of Egyptian patients with chronic hepatitis C (Tanamaly *et al.*, 2004) found that silymarin had no more effect than multivitamin supplements on any objective outcome measure. Rambaldi *et al.* (2007) conducted a meta-analysis of published trials of milk thistle in patients with established alcoholic liver disease or liver disease caused by hepatitis B or C. They found 13 clinical trials (915 patients in total) and, when all of these studies were combined, discovered that milk thistle had no significant effect on total mortality, the complications of liver disease or liver histology, although it did lead to a significant reduction in liver-related mortality in those studies that reported this specifically. However, the decline in liver-related mortality became statistically non-significant when only the best studies were used for the analysis. These authors did not find high-quality evidence to support the use of milk thistle extracts in the treatment of established liver disease, although they did suggest the need for high-quality trials.

In general, clinical trials of milk thistle provide unconvincing support for the many *in vitro* and animal studies that have indicated a likely hepato-protective effect of silymarin, although it does seem to prevent the acute life-threatening liver damage induced by poisoning by Amanita phalloides and similar fungal toxins. There still seems to be a case for large multicentred trials of controlled doses of milk thistle in well-matched patients with specific liver conditions.

As a supplement, milk thistle is usually used to prevent liver damage rather than to treat clinical cases of liver disease. Even so, the current evidence is insufficient to recommend milk thistle as a useful dietary supplement; indeed, taking it in the expectation that it may protect the liver from alcohol or drug damage may be counter-productive by giving users a false sense of security and make them less likely to avoid the liver-damaging behaviour.

A 100 mg tablet of standardised milk thistle extract should provide about 80 mg of silymarin and this is equivalent to 3 g of seeds. Recommended doses of dietary supplements are 100 mg of extract per day, but doses used in clinical trials have been up to 10 times this daily amount. People who are allergic to members of the daisy or Asters should not take milk thistle. Barnes (2002) reports that about 1% of 3500 people taking 560 mg of silymarin daily for eight weeks reported usually mild and transient adverse effects, mainly gastrointestinal.

Saw palmetto

Saw palmetto, Serenoa repens, also known as the American dwarf palm tree, grows wild in the Southern states of the USA, especially in Florida and Georgia. It is an evergreen shrub, which grows up to 3 metres tall and has fan-shaped leaves. The plant was used as a food by the Native American populations in Florida and even today is still used as a food by the Seminole people; a sweetened traditional drink, 'shiope sofkee', is made from its juice.

Although saw palmetto has been used for a variety of medicinal purposes by Native Americans, it is now almost exclusively used to treat benign prostatic hyperplasia. It is easily the most commonly used herbal preparation for this condition worldwide, and in some European countries it is regarded as the first-line treatment for this condition and is considerably cheaper than conventional drugs. The fruit of the plant is used in modern dietary supplements and herbal medicines. It is consumed as a dried ground fruit or as an extract of the lipid fraction, where the pharmacological activity is thought to be found. Teas made from saw palmetto are consumed, but as the active ingredients are believed to be lipid soluble these will contain little of these ingredients. The lipid extract contains plant sterols (phytosterols), numerous free fatty acids and monoglycerides.

Benign prostatic hyperplasia (BHP) and saw palmetto

Benign prostatic hyperplasia (BHP) is an enlargement of the prostate gland that occurs frequently in older men. Perhaps a third of men in their 70s have symptomatic BHP. The enlarged prostate gland can interfere with the voiding of urine, which can produce a range of symptoms, such as:

- Difficulty in starting urination even when the bladder is full.
- Incomplete bladder emptying or the sensation of incomplete emptying.
- Slow flow of urine.
- Dribbling of urine after urination.
- Increased frequency of urination, including during the night.
- Urgency of urination.
- Discomfort when passing urine.

Occasionally this condition can result in acute chronic retention, where the patient is unable to pass urine even when the bladder is painfully full; this requires urgent catheterisation.

Neither the exact causes of BHP nor the mode of action of saw palmetto in its relief have been unequivocally established. It has been suggested that saw palmetto extracts might work by blocking adrenergic receptors (specifically the alpha1-adrenoreceptor) in the prostate, causing muscle relaxation and so assisting the passage of urine. Although saw palmetto extracts have been shown to have antagonistic effects on these receptors *in vitro*, Goepel *et al*. (2001) suggest that therapeutic doses of saw palmetto do not cause this effect *in vivo* in men. An alternative suggestion and one that is currently favoured is that saw palmetto extracts inhibit the enzyme (5-alpha reductase) that converts testosterone to its more active form, dihyrotestosterone; this effect has been demonstrated in isolated human prostate cells (Habib *et al*., 2004). Dihydrotestosterone stimulates growth of the prostate and there is speculation that hormonal imbalances in older men may be the cause of this prostatic hyperplasia. Saw palmetto may exert an anti-androgenic effect by blocking the binding of dihydrotestosterone to the androgen receptors in the prostate. Other less-documented pharmacological actions of saw palmetto are listed in the *United States Pharmacoepia* (USP, 2005).

There have been many clinical trials of saw palmetto for the treatment of BHP and several systematic reviews (Wilt *et al.*, 1998, 2000 and 2002). Wilt *et al.* (2000) identified 18 randomised trials of saw palmetto with a total of almost 3000 participants. Some trials compared saw palmetto with placebos in double-blind trials and some compared it to finasteride (a drug widely used to treat BPH, which is a known 5-alpha-reductase inhibitor). The main outcome measure was the patient's own assessment of their urinary symptoms using a standard validated scale. They concluded that the then available evidence suggested that saw palmetto performed significantly better than the placebo in reducing urological symptoms and improving urine flow. Its effects were comparable to those of the commonly used drug finasteride, but the saw palmetto was cheaper and better tolerated, with fewer adverse symptoms and fewer patient withdrawals. An update of this review (Wilt *et al.*, 2002) added three further trials, but essentially confirmed the original findings that saw palmetto provides mild to moderate symptomatic relief from the symptoms of BPH, with few adverse effects. None of the trials that were reviewed lasted longer than 48 weeks, so the long-term safety could not be established.

This review was updated again (Tacklind *et al.*, 2009) by a new panel of authors, including Wilt. This update found 12 new trials, of which 9 met their inclusion criteria; these 9 new studies had 2053 participants, which increased the total sample size by 65% compared to the 2002 review by Wilt *et al.* In contrast to the generally supportive conclusions of the earlier versions of this review, Tacklind *et al.* found that with the addition of the large number of extra participants, the saw palmetto was no more effective than a placebo in treating the urinary symptoms of BPH.

The standard dosage of saw palmetto is 320 mg/day of the lipid extract, taken in two aliquots each day, or 1–2 g of the dried fruit.

In the first edition of this book, the evidence available at that time did suggest some clinically useful benefit of this herb for treating BPH, but the evidence seems to have weakened substantially with the addition of newer trials. Tacklind *et al.* (2009) did point out that there had still been relatively few high-quality long-term trials (at least a year) of adequate doses of standardised preparations of saw palmetto for the treatment of BPH. They also suggested that such trials were clearly warranted by the high usage of this product for this purpose, both as a prescribed medication and as a dietary supplement, an estimated 2.5 million Americans using it in 2002. Self-medication should not be attempted without proper diagnosis of the condition and consultation with a physician. Some of the symptoms of BPH are common to prostatic cancer and other conditions. This general rule should apply for the use of supplements in most other symptomatic conditions as well.

Spirulina and Chlorella

Spirulina

Spirulina is a blue-green freshwater alga. Spirulina geitleri was known by the Aztecs as *tecuitlatl* and they harvested it from the surface of lakes, dried it and cut it into loaves that could be stored for extended periods. *Tecuitlatl* has a cheese-like texture and the paste was spread onto tortillas and eaten. Spirulina was also harvested by inhabitants of Chad in Africa, who called it *dihe*. In more recent years, it has attracted attention as a potential single-cell source of protein that can be produced by industrial-scale fermentation. Today, industrial plants are producing Spirulina in several Asian countries and in Mexico. It is used for both animal and human foodstuffs.

As a food Spirulina is high in protein (up to 70% of the dry weight) and low in fat. It is a good vegetarian source of available iron and some other minerals. Analysis of its composition also suggests that it has relatively large amounts of several B vitamins, including vitamin B_{12}, and is rich in carotenoids. Like other single-cell protein sources it is relatively high in nucleic acids (DNA and RNA) and consumption of large amounts of these may produce undesirable increases in uric acid levels. Uric acid crystals in joints are responsible for the symptoms of gout, and high blood levels of uric acid may be a risk factor for coronary heart disease.

In the UK, Spirulina is available as tablets, capsules or powders and the usual dose is 5–10 g per day. Spirulina has been marketed and used as a source of vitamin B_{12} (see Chapter 3) that is suitable for vegans (most dietary B_{12} comes from animal foods, with some coming from microbial contaminants).

It has been suspected for about 20 years that the vitamin B_{12} in Spirulina is not biologically active in humans. Dagnelie *et al.* (1991) showed that when vitamin B_{12}-deficient children were given Spirulina (or another vegetarian B_{12} source called nori), the haematological indicators of their deficiency continued to deteriorate even though their blood levels of B_{12} appeared to rise. The algal B_{12} was absorbed but did not improve the symptoms. The explanation for this is that the microbiological assays used to measure vitamin B_{12} also determine several inactive analogues of the vitamin. It has even been suggested that these analogues may exacerbate B_{12} deficiency by interfering with normal B_{12} metabolism. Watanabe *et al.* (1999) found that most of the vitamin B_{12} in Spirulina tablets as detected by microbiological assay is in the form of a compound they called pseudovitamin B_{12}, which is not biologically active in mammals. Spirulina is not a reliable source of vitamin B_{12} for vegetarians and should not be marketed or consumed as such.

Spirulina has been claimed to have a variety of beneficial effects on health, such as:

- Lipid lowering and hypoglycaemic effects in type 2 diabetes.
- Being a general tonic and improving stamina in athletes.
- Having value as a slimming aid.

There is very limited scientific evidence to back up these claims and certainly no reasonably sized, randomised, double-blind, placebo-controlled trials. Back in the 1970s, the American FDA found no evidence to support the claims then being made that Spirulina was a useful slimming aid.

Chlorella

Chlorella pyredinosa is another freshwater alga that has similar nutritional properties to Spirulina. It is available in the UK in the form of tablets, liquid extracts and powders, and typical daily doses would be 0.5–3 g. Unlike Spirulina, the vitamin B_{12} present in Chlorella is true vitamin B_{12} that is bioavailable for mammals (Kittaka-Katsura *et al.*, 2000).

As with Spirulina, many unsubstantiated health claims have been made for Chlorella, including:

- It is a general tonic.
- It promotes wound healing.
- It is an immune stimulant that, for example, aids in the treatment of colds and flu.
- It gives some relief from the symptoms of fibromyalgia.

Only one substantial randomised, double-blind, placebo-controlled trial of Chlorella was found in the scientific literature. Halperin *et al.* (2003) used 120 middle-aged and elderly adults receiving influenza vaccinations. These people were randomised to receive either a placebo, 200 mg of chlorella or 400 mg of chlorella for three weeks prior to the vaccination and for a further week after vaccination. There was no suggestion that the Chlorella supplements enhanced the immuno-logical response to the vaccine.

St John's wort (Hypericum perforatum)

St John's wort (Hypericum perforatum) is a native flowering plant of Europe and Asia, which produces attractive yellow flowers. According to Kiple and Ornelas (2000), its lemon-scented leaves have been used for thousands of years as human food and have also been used to make a form of tea, although it will cease to be sold as a food supplement from May 2011. Extracts of the flowers and leaves of this plant are now widely taken in the belief that they are mood enhancing and have beneficial effects in the treatment of clinical depression. In Germany, Hypericum extracts are widely prescribed by physicians for the treatment of clini-cal depression and it is the best selling antidepressant there.

What is depression?

Clinical depression is a common, painful and disabling condition that is more severe than the normal downward fluctuations in mood that we all regularly expe-rience. The American Psychiatric Association lists the following symptoms for depression:

- Depressed mood.
- Loss of interest in and lack of pleasure derived from activities that the patient usually finds pleasurable.
- Disturbed sleep patterns.
- Abnormal activity patterns, either agitation or being uncharacteristically inactive.
- Loss of drive and energy, loss of sex drive and reduced appetite.

To make a formal diagnosis of clinical depression, the first two of these symptoms must be present as well as most of the others. These symptoms should have been present for at least two weeks and should not be attributable to other disease, to drug use or be associated with bereavement. As many as one in five adults may be affected by depression during the course of their lives and rates are much higher in women than men.

Conventional drug treatment of depression

Medicinal drugs used to treat depression work by raising the amounts of serotonin (5HT or 5 hydroxy-tryptamine) and/or noradrenaline in synapses of the central nervous system. Monoamine oxidase (MAO) inhibitors such as iproniazid work by blocking the enzymes that are responsible for the breakdown of several nerve transmitters, including noradrenaline and serotonin. These drugs have now been largely superseded by other drugs with fewer side-effects. People taking MAO inhibitors were required to avoid consuming foods, like mature cheese and red wine, that contain a substance called tyramine, which could precipitate large and dangerous rises in blood pressure in those taking MAO inhibitors. Tricyclic antidepressants such as imipramine inhibit the reuptake of both serotonin and noradrenaline into the presynaptic terminals, which is the major route for curtailing the actions of these transmitters after release.

Together with the MAO inhibitors, the tricyclic antidepressants are termed first-generation antidepressants. The selective serotonin reuptake inhibitors (SSRIs) such as fluoxetine and paroxetine are examples of the so-called second-generation antidepressants and, as their name suggests, they selectively inhibit the reuptake of serotonin into pre-synaptic terminals, thus specifically increasing its actions. SSRIs are now by far the most widely used drugs in the treatment of depression; they have fewer side-effects than the first-generation tricyclics.

A readable account of antidepressants and their likely modes of action can be found in Parrott *et al.* (2004). The guidelines of the British Association for Psychotherapy for the diagnosis and treatment of depression can be found in Anderson *et al.* (2000).

Possible actions of Hypericum extracts

Hypericum extracts contain well over 20 bio-active substances, including the chemically complex polyphenols hypericin and pseudohypericin and the substance hyperforin, which is described as a prenylated phloroglucinol (the chemical structures of hypericin and hyperforin may be found in Barnes, 2002). Early studies in the 1980s suggested that hypericin was an MAO inhibitor and this led to widespread assumptions that hypericin was the active agent responsible for the antidepressant effects of Hypericum extracts and that MAO inhibition was its mode of action. Later studies failed to confirm this effect of hypericin, and have further suggested that hyperforin is probably the component responsible for most of the antidepressant effects of the extract.

It is no longer believed that Hypericum extracts have significant MAO-inhibitory effects. This early assumption that hypericin was the key ingredient has resulted in the standardisation of commercial preparations of Hypericum according to their hypericin content; that is, probably not to the active component(s). Most St John's wort preparations that are standardised on their hypericin content claim to supply between 300 and 1200 µg of hypericin per tablet. When a sample of tablets, purchased in London in 2003, was analysed they were found to contain between a third and two-thirds of the stated hypericin content, even when the total hypericin and pseudohypericin content was used (Lawrence, 2003). This means that not only were hypericum extracts standardised to the wrong component, even the claimed content of this ingredient often did not accurately reflect the true content. Linde *et al.* (2008) also noted that some preparations sold in Germany contain very low amounts of bioactive compounds, and De los Reyes and Koda (2002) found very large variability in the hyperforin content of eight brands of St John's wort marketed in the USA, with two brands having almost none. Now that hyperforin is considered to be the most bioactive component of St John's wort, it should be standardised to its hyperforin content, although in practice hypericin content is still often used.

Biochemical and pharmacological studies suggest that hyperforin acts as a nonselective reuptake inhibitor in the brain. It not only inhibits the reuptake of serotonin and noradrenalin, but also that of other brain transmitters, and does it in a different way to other antidepressant drugs (Nathan, 2001). Other reuptake inhibitors work by competing with the monoamine transmitter for the carrier molecules responsible for reuptake. Hyperforin, however, non-competitively inhibits the uptake of several monoamines by affecting the sodium-transporting system and raising the intracellular concentration of sodium in the pre-synaptic terminals. The reuptake of monoamine transmitters is sodium dependent; that is, it requires a low intracellular sodium concentration.

Testing the antidepressant effects of Hypericum extracts

There have been dozens of clinical trials of hypericum extracts that have tested its effects against a placebo and/or against first-generation antidepressant drugs like imipramine. In recent years there have also been several trials comparing its effectiveness to second-generation SSRIs. When testing the effectiveness of antidepressant treatments and other treatments for psychiatric or psychological problems, there are two major difficulties:

- There is almost always a large but variable placebo effect in such studies. At least a quarter of patients usually respond positively to the dummy treatment. This makes it more difficult to demonstrate a statistically significant effect of treatment and a statistically significant difference between the two moderately effective treatments.
- There are no objective measures of treatment efficacy, like a change in a blood parameter. The severity of depression is measured using a numerical scale that is based on patients' responses to a number of questions about the severity of a

list of symptoms, for example the Hamilton depression scale. This is measured prior to and at various times after the start of treatment. Other measures that may be used include the physician's and the patient's global assessment of the change in severity of their condition using a sliding scale from, say, 'very much improved' to 'very much worse'. The subjective nature of the outcome measures makes it particularly important that the double blinding of the different treatments is rigorous.

Does it work and is it safe?

Despite the dozens of clinical trials of St John's wort conducted since 1980, including several large multicentre studies, it is still not possible to make a definitive judgement on the usefulness and safety of Hypericum extracts for the treatment of mild to moderate depression. The confusion over the information available to members of the general public about St John's wort is exemplified from the following headlines taken from the BBC website over a six-year period:

- 10/12/1999 Herb 'helps ease depression'
- 1/3/2000 St John's wort warning (relating to its possible interaction with prescription drugs)
- 31/8/2000 Herb 'as effective as antidepressants'
- 9/4/2002 Herb ineffective as antidepressant
- 11/2/2005 Herb 'as good as depression drug'

There is fairly general agreement that St John's wort is not an appropriate treatment for severe depression (Barnes, 2002), and in general self-medication for severe depression is not appropriate because of the high suicide risk of sufferers. There also seems to be a consensus that the acute side-effects experienced by those taking Hypericum extracts are less than those experienced by patients taking the older tricyclic antidepressants like imipramine. However, in March 2000, the UK Department of Health issued a warning about the possible dangers of combining Hypericum extracts with several prescription drugs. This was based on evidence submitted to it from the independent Committee on the Safety of Medicines (DH, 2000). Patients were advised to tell their doctor or pharmacist if they were taking St John's wort and a prescription medicine. St John's wort induces detoxification enzymes in the liver, which can increase the rate at which a number of drugs are metabolised and thus render them less effective (see Zhou et al., 2004 for a review of the effects of St John's wort on drug metabolism). It may also interact with other drugs in different ways. For example, if taken with SSRI antidepressants it may induce 'serotonin syndrome', a potentially life-threatening drug reaction due to excess serotonin, with symptoms that include nausea and vomiting, loss of coordination, hyperthermia, tachycardia, rapid changes in blood pressure. Hypericum extracts should not be used together with:

- Anticoagulant drugs like warfarin
- The heart drug digoxin

- Oral contraceptives
- Antirejection drugs like cyclosporine
- Drugs used in the treatment of HIV infection
- Anticonvulsants used to treat epilepsy
- A number of drugs used to manage migraine
- Some anti-asthmatic drugs
- SSRI antidepressants

There are isolated reports that Hypericum extracts may increase photosensitivity (see Barnes, 2002) and some preparations now carry a warning to avoid direct sunlight exposure when taking St John's wort. This could be a particular problem for people suffering from seasonal affective disorder (SAD) who are also being treated with light therapy.

Prior to 2000, the bulk of the many published clinical trials supported the proposition that St John's wort did have beneficial effects in treating mild to moderate depression. Many of these studies were conducted in Germany, where St John's wort was and is one of the biggest selling antidepressant 'drugs'. These studies generally concluded that St John's wort was more effective than a placebo and of comparable efficacy to older antidepressant drugs like imipramine, and that it had less side-effects and lower drop-out rates than with these tricyclic antidepressants. Several systematic reviews and meta-analyses of these earlier clinical trials support these general conclusions (e.g. Linde *et al.*, 1996; Nangia *et al.*, 2000; Whiskey *et al.*, 2001). Many reviewers and commentators criticised these early clinical trials for a variety of reasons, such as those listed below:

- Many of these early trials were of short duration (often only about four weeks) and so the longer-term effectiveness could not be determined.
- Some of these trials used less than optimal dosing of antidepressant drugs.
- Variability of dosing and lack of standardisation for hyperforin in the different trials.
- Inadequate matching of baseline severity and several studies using patients who did not meet current formal diagnostic criteria for clinical depression.
- Some studies were said to have used inadequate outcome measures.
- That most comparative studies had compared St John's wort to older, first-generation antidepressants rather than to modern SSRIs.

In 1999, three major well-funded clinical trials of St John's wort were started in the USA, one of them funded by the National Institutes of Health (NIH; Bunk, 1999). The NIH-funded study was conducted by the same research group at Duke University Medical Center that published one of the positive meta-analyses of earlier St John's wort trials (Nangia *et al.*, 2001), but the conclusions were much less positive. The Hypericum Depression Trials Study Group (2002) had three groups, each with over 100 patients; one was treated with hypericum, one given a placebo and the third group given sertraline, an SSRI antidepressant. The first phase of the trial lasted for eight weeks, but patients who responded to initial treatment were offered a further 18 weeks of treatment in order that longer-term effects of treatment could be monitored. Neither the St John's wort nor the SSRI antidepressant produced statistically significant differences to the placebo when outcome was assessed using the Hamilton Depression Scale. The SSRI did produce a bigger improvement in the Clinical Global Impression- Improvements scale than either St John's wort or the placebo. The authors suggest that it is not uncommon in trials of antidepressant drugs for the active treatment not to produce a significant effect on Hamilton score ratings, which rather undermines the criticism of some early trials of St John's wort that have not used this outcome measure. To a non-psychiatrist, these data are hardly a ringing endorsement of either treatment, but they do emphasise the importance of a placebo control.

Werneke *et al.* (2004) attempted to sum up the position on the efficacy of St John's wort after the publication of the three recent large and largely negative trials. They reproduced a meta-analysis based on literature searches conducted in June 2000 and then reanalysed this data, adding to it the results of the more recent additional studies. The incorporation of the more recent data substantially reduced the apparent effect of St John's wort. They concluded that it may be less effective for treating depression than the earlier studies had suggested, and that if future trials followed the trend set by the other more recent trials, it may finally be shown to be ineffective. These negative conclusions are consistent with much of what has appeared in the British and American literature regarding St John's wort since 2002.

The most recent systematic review (Linde *et al.*, 2008) has attempted to address some of the criticisms of earlier reviews, including its own first version (Linde *et al.*, 1996). This group only included randomised controlled trials using adult patients who met the formal diagnostic criteria for major clinical depression. The authors included studies that had compared St John's wort to either a placebo or an adequate dose of an effective synthetic antidepressant, and the majority of these used a second-generation SSRI antidepressant drug. Only trials that were of at least four weeks duration and that included clinical outcomes for assessing depressive symptoms were used. They identified a total of 29 trials (5489 patients) that met all of their inclusion criteria. In those 18 trials that compared the effect of St John's wort to a placebo, these authors found that it was much more effective than the placebo. However, there was a marked variability between the trials and when they confined their analysis to just the more precise trials, when the effectiveness of St John's wort was substantially less, although still statistically significant.

Linde *et al.* (2008) had previously noted a tendency for trials from German-speaking countries (Austria, Germany and Switzerland) to be more positive about St John's wort than trials from other countries. When they separated trials on this basis, they found that the 11 trials from German-speaking countries were much more positive than the other 7 trials, which did not find a statistically significant effect for St John's wort (German-speaking risk ratio 1.78 with 95% confidence limits 1.42–2.25, and other studies risk ratio 1.07 and confidence limits 0.83–1.31, where a value of 1.0 implies that treatment and placebo effect were the same). The trials from the German-speaking countries showed much more variability in their outcomes and five were conducted before 2000, whereas all of the others were in 2000 or later.

Overall, in the comparisons of St John's wort to standard synthetic antidepressants they found that the herbal product was as effective as the standard drug, and two-thirds of these trials involved comparison to modern SSRIs. Once again, the trials from German-speaking countries were more favourable to the herb than those from other countries. While the authors (from Germany) could not satisfactorily explain the difference between the results obtained from different countries, they did suggest that it was possible that the German-speaking trials had selected slightly different types of patients, although they could not rule out the possibility that 'some smaller studies from German-speaking countries were flawed and reported overoptimistic results'. Note that in the earlier discussion of the review by Werneke et al. (2004) where adding in three new trials substantially diminished the apparent effectiveness of St John's wort, the three additional studies were from non-German-speaking areas.

St John's wort is marketed in Britain and the USA as a dietary supplement, but is a prescription drug in Germany and has now been banned for over-the-counter sale in Ireland and is only available there on prescription. The available data suggest that, even if it does have some benefit in treating depression, it should not be taken with other prescription medications and probably should not be used as a routine, long-term supplement for people not suffering from depression. It should be used as a medicine of herbal origin rather than a dietary supplement. It was included in this chapter largely because of the scale of its usage, with perhaps as many as two million Britons having tried it at some time. Note that high-quality clinical trials will have used well-defined extracts of St John's wort, whereas evidence discussed earlier from Germany, the USA and Britain suggest that readily available versions used for self-medication contain variable amounts of bioactive ingredients, and some contain almost none.

Tea extracts

Tea is a drink made from the dried leaves of Camellia sinensis. It is the most popular hot beverage in the world and is said to be the second most popular drink in the world after water. All tea starts as green, but if the rolled and cut leaves are allowed to stand and ferment for one to three days before drying, it becomes black. In green tea the enzyme that causes the blackening is inactivated by heat treatment, which prevents blackening. Oolong tea is fermented for a shorter period and its colour and taste are between green and black tea.

Tea leaves contain high quantities of polyphenols, which make up 20–30% of their dry weight. When tea leaves are rolled and crushed during processing, the enzyme polyphenol oxidase converts catechins (categorised earlier as flavonols) to polymeric forms, which give the fermented oolong and black teas their characteristic colours. Black tea is the form usually consumed in the UK, although green tea is available and extracts of green tea in tablet form are marketed. Tea contains some essential nutrients, but these probably provide only a tiny fraction of the adult requirement for these nutrients (with the exception of trace minerals like fluoride and manganese). Tea also contains the alkaloid caffeine and smaller amounts of theobromine, which are responsible for the stimulating effect of the beverage.

The components of tea and especially the polyphenols abundant in green tea have been shown to have potentially beneficial effects in animal models and *in vitro* systems (Duthie and Crozier, 2003), such as:

- Antioxidant effect including the ability to prevent oxidation of LDL.
- Antimutagenic effect and reduced tumour cell proliferation *in vitro* and prevention of chemically induced cancer in animal models.
- Reduced platelet aggregation by effects on the cyclo-oxygenase pathway (see Chapter 6).
- It may also reduce blood cholesterol, because flavonols reduce the absorption of cholesterol in the intestine.

There is some epidemiological evidence consistent with an association between high tea consumption and reduced rates of heart disease and cancer. However, this evidence is very inconsistent and sometimes even suggests a negative effect of tea. Animal studies consistently demonstrate the ability of green tea polyphenols to reduce chemically induced cancers in several animal models, but human epidemiological studies have produced mixed results. The epidemiological methods are probably too insensitive and too subject to confounding variables to be able to determine whether tea has disease-preventing properties or not.

Birt *et al.* (1999) have summed up the evidence of a cancer-preventing effect of tea extracts. These authors conclude that there are numerous experimental studies with animals suggesting that tea extracts can reduce the incidence of chemically induced cancers, and that oral or topical application of tea extracts can reduce the rate of skin cancer induced by exposure of animals to ultraviolet light. However, they also conclude that epidemiology provides no clear evidence for a relationship between tea consumption and human cancer: some suggest an increased risk associated with tea, some suggest no effect and some suggest a protective effect. The two factors listed below complicate this analysis:

- There is evidence that regular consumption of hot liquids, including tea, may increase the risk of oesophageal cancer.
- Green tea has higher concentrations of polyphenols than black tea, which is most commonly consumed in western countries. Green tea drinking is more prevalent in areas where micronutrient deficiencies are more common, and many of the epidemiological studies suggesting a beneficial effect of tea drinking were performed in these areas. Is there a difference between black and green tea? Is a protective effect of tea more likely in people who are micronutrient deficient?

Birt *et al.* (1999) quote a Dutch prospective study that found that black tea consumption was positively associated with breast cancer, not associated with risk of colorectal cancer and negatively associated (protective) with lung and stomach cancer. However, tea drinkers tended to smoke less than non-drinkers and also tended to eat more fruits and vegetables; when the results were corrected for this, the apparent protective effects of tea disappeared.

More recently, a major review by Boehm *et al.* (2009) has assessed evidence for an association between green tea consumption and risk of cancer and cancer mortality in humans. They found 51 studies involving over 1.5 million people that had addressed this issue and all but one of these were observational case-control or cohort studies. Most of these studies were conducted in Asia, where green tea drinking is very common and, as with the review by Birt *et al.* (1999), they found that the evidence was conflicting and did not allow them to make any firm recommendations regarding the use of green tea to prevent cancer.

Similar mixed findings have been reported for the association between tea consumption and heart disease.

Thus at present there is a lot of experimental data, using animals and *in vitro* systems, which point towards the potential for tea, particularly green tea, to have protective effects against cancer and heart disease. While such experiments may be of great value in generating hypotheses about the protective potential of agents in tea, they are not sufficient to make firm conclusions about the long-term benefits of these chemicals in people or to make public health recommendations. There is little substantial or consistent corroborating evidence from human studies that this theoretical potential actually translates into real benefits. It seems reasonable to say that if you are a regular tea drinker, there is some conflicting evidence that you may get some benefit from it provided you don't drink it too hot. It seems unreasonable on the basis of the evidence available to encourage people to drink more tea for health reasons or to take extracts of tea as a supplement. Those who enjoy tea can continue to enjoy it with the knowledge that it just may also have some long-term beneficial effects. Boehm *et al.* (2009) confirmed that moderate, habitual consumption of green tea appeared to be safe. Theoretically it might be expected that there would be substantial differences between green and black tea, with most of the animal and *in vitro* studies suggesting that green tea is more likely to have a beneficial effect.

The dose of tea extract is not clearly established, but 200–400 mg of extract is commonly used. These extracts should be standardised to contain a high level of polyphenols (up to 95%), with 40% of this as the catechin, epigallocatechin gallate. This is the equivalent of drinking 4–6 cups of green tea per day.

9 Functional Foods

Introduction and scope of the chapter

It is difficult to define exactly what constitutes a functional food, but they almost inevitably carry some sort of health claim in their marketing and they have components or ingredients in them that are designed to provide a specific medical or physiological benefit. They are sometimes also termed nutraceuticals, to imply that they have both nutritional and pharmaceutical functions. The Institute of Medicine in Washington defined them as 'those foods that encompass potentially healthful products including any modified food or ingredient that may provide a health benefit beyond the traditional nutrients it contains'. In other words, they are foods that are said to have health-promoting or disease-preventing properties that are over and above their usual nutritional value. They are sold as foods and so in the UK they cannot make claims that they are capable of preventing, treating or curing human disease. Even more general claims about their effects on physiological or biochemical parameters are now being subjected to scrutiny and approval by the European Foods Standards Agency, as discussed in Chapter 1.

The issues surrounding vitamin, mineral and/or antioxidant supplements, whether they come from pills or food fortification, have been dealt with in Chapters 2–5 and so they will not be readdressed here. Likewise, the effects of changing the balance between the intakes of the different fatty acid types was discussed in Chapter 6; whether this is achieved by taking oil supplements or functional foods with modified fatty acid profiles does not essentially change the arguments. This means that even though the items in the categories listed below could justifiable be included in a list of functional foods, they will not be discussed in this chapter because the substantial issues have been dealt with in earlier chapters:

- Foods like breakfast cereals, bread or margarine that have been fortified with vitamins and/or minerals with the aim of helping to ensure dietary adequacy.
- Foods fortified with specific nutrients or antioxidants with the aim of gaining a specific health benefit, such as calcium-enriched foods or drinks to promote bone health or food fortified with folic acid to prevent neural tube defects in the newborn.

Dietary Supplements and Functional Foods, 2nd Edition. Geoffrey P. Webb.
© 2011 Blackwell Publishing Ltd.

- Foods enriched with omega-3 fatty acids (e.g. eggs in which the omega-3 content has been raised by manipulating the diets of the hens).
- Conventional foods that are promoted on the basis of their nutrient or anti-oxidant content (see next section on superfoods) or the promotion of new varieties with enhanced levels of such compounds, e.g. the promotion of milk as a source of calcium or tomato products as a source of lycopene and other carotenoids.
- Foods marketed as low in calories, such as:
  o Foods where the sugar present in the standard version of the food has been replaced with an essentially calorie-free artificial sweetener such as saccharin or aspartame.
  o Foods containing synthetic and indigestible fats like olestra, which are said to have the taste and mouth-feel properties of foods made with natural fats. However, as olestra is not digested or absorbed, the foods that contain it are lower calorie and from a nutritional viewpoint low in fat. At the time of writing, olestra is not available within the EU, but is permitted to be used in the USA for savoury snack foods like crisps.

Perhaps the one substantial issue that separates food fortification and supplement taking is that in the case of fortification, everyone who consumes that food gets the added nutrient or component without always actively choosing to take it. This is particularly the case when it becomes the usual practice to fortify a category of food or where fortification is a legal requirement. The likely maximum intake of people who consume high amounts of these foods needs to be estimated to make sure that it does not exceed safe upper levels. As we saw in Vhapter 3 with the discussion of the impact of folic acid supplements or food fortification on the incidence of neural tube defects, (mandatory) food fortification may be the only way of achieving a substantial increase in the intake of a nutrient within a reasonable period. The issue of fortification of food with nutrients to help a specific subgroup also raises ethical issues about whether it is reasonable to fortify common foods that everyone eats for the benefit of a relatively small number of people, such as fortification of foods with folic acid for the benefit of those few pregnant women at risk of having a baby with a neural tube defect (see Chapter 3).

Estimates of the size of the market for functional foods will obviously vary with decisions about exactly which food and drinks are included in the definition. In a review of the global market for functional foods, Just-food (2008) estimated that by 2013 the total global market would reach a value of $90.5 billion. What is undisputed is the extremely rapid growth in the market for functional foods in the last decade. IGD (2007) estimated that in the UK the market for functional foods increased from £134 million in 1998 to £1.72 billion in 2007, which represents a tenfold increase even after allowing for inflation. In the USA sales of functional foods have been estimated at $20–30 billion per year, which represents about 5% of the overall US food market. The US market for functional foods is growing at 10–20% per year compared to overall growth in the food industry of 1–4% (PWC, 2009).

Having consciously excluded the categories listed earlier from this chapter, this leaves those given below, which have been selected for specific discussion:

- Margarine and other products with high levels of certain plant sterols (phytosterols and phytostanols), which inhibit the absorption (and the reabsorption) of cholesterol in the gut and thus can lower blood cholesterol levels.
- Foods and supplements containing high levels of phyto-oestrogens. These are a group of phytochemicals that partially mimic the action of the female hormone oestrogen and have been claimed to be beneficial for both ameliorating consequences of the menopause and for preventing hormone-dependent cancers.
- Probiotics, fermented dairy products containing live cultures of bacteria that are claimed to 'improve the microbial balance of the body' and thus reduce the risk of certain infections. Some of these cultures are now available in pill form, but will be dealt with as an extension of functional foods rather than a dietary supplement.
- Prebiotics are non-digestible food ingredients that are said to promote the growth of certain bacteria within the body and thus to beneficially change the microbial balance of the body in a similar way to probiotics.

A note about 'superfoods'

Many 'ordinary; foods are now marketed on the basis of some proposed health benefit, for example green tea, tomato products, fortified cereals, many fruits and berries. Some of these have been given the unofficial classification of being a 'superfood'. According to Bender (2007), the concept of superfoods originated in the USA around 2003 and was introduced into Britain at the end of 2005 in an article in a national newspaper (*Daily Mail*). He defines superfoods as ordinary foods that are marketed as being particularly rich in conventional nutrients, antioxidants, polyunsaturated fatty acids, dietary fibre or specific phytochemicals/secondary plant metabolites. While there is no definitive list, a quick search using the search engine Google will generate several different but overlapping lists produced by different individuals and organisations. Using this approach, Bender (2007) generated a list of 40 foods. Since that article was written, a number of other foods have been termed superfoods, including several exotic fruits and vegetables that would not previously have been seen on the shelves of ordinary British supermarkets, such as Goji berries, Acai berries and pomegranate juice, as well as the more familiar turmeric and walnuts. In many cases, extracts of these so-called superfoods are now being marketed in pill form as dietary supplements, including pomegranates, Goji berries, Acai berries, green tea, turmeric, garlic, ginger, bilberries, cranberries, broccoli and fish oil.

While these superfoods are not discussed here, some of them have been individually discussed in earlier chapters and there has been extensive discussion of vitamins, minerals, polyunsaturated fatty acids, antioxidants and plant secondary metabolites. Listed below are examples of superfoods with an indication of the justification for classifying them in this way (in some cases there may be multiple 'beneficial' components). This list is not claimed to be definitive, merely illustrative:

- Broccoli and several other cruciferous vegetables like cabbage and sprouts. These vegetables are a source of the sulphur-containing secondary metabolites known as glucosinolates. It is suggested that substances generated from these glucosinolates may inhibit the activation of potential carcinogens and thus have a protective effect against cancer.
- Garlic and other members of the Allium or onion family. These all contain S-alkyl cysteine sulphoxides, which are another class of sulphur-containing secondary plant metabolites. In particular, the allicin in garlic has been claimed to have antibacterial activity, anticancer effects, and antithrombotic and blood cholesterol-lowering effects.
- Several berry fruits, including blueberries, cranberries, strawberries and several other more recently introduced types like Goji berries and acai berries. These are marketed on their high content of anthocyanins, which have antioxidant activity.
- Foods that are rich in pigments from the carotenoid group of tetraterpenoids. These include carrots (β-carotene), tomatoes (lycopene) and red peppers (lutein). A few carotenoids such as β-carotene have vitamin A activity, but all of them have antioxidant activity, with lycopene (no vitamin A activity) regarded as the most powerful antioxidant.
- Salmon and some other oily fish, because of their high content of omega-3 polyunsaturated fatty acids, especially those with long hydrocarbon chains.
- A variety of other fruits, such as apples, kiwi, mango and red grapes, usually as a combination of antioxidant effects due to the presence of antioxidant nutrients and flavonoids of various types.
- Olive oil, because of its high level of monounsaturated fatty acids and also because of the presence of lipid soluble antioxidants.
- Soy, largely because of the presence of phyto-oestrogens, as discussed later in this chapter. Flaxseeds and other cereal seeds also contain lignans, which have oestrogenic activity.
- Green tea, because of the presence of polyphenols that may have antioxidant and antimutagenic effects. Cocoa is also rich in phenolic compounds.
- Red wine is said to have cardio-protective effects because of its content of polyphenols, including resveratrol, which act as antioxidants. Small amounts of alcohol in general seem to afford some protection against cardiovascular disease, although the well-documented and severe deleterious health and social effects of excess alcohol need to be considered before promoting the consumption of any alcoholic drink on health grounds.
- Walnuts and several other types of tree nuts. There is epidemiological evidence to link high nut consumption with a reduced risk of cardiovascular disease and most are rich in polyunsaturated fatty acids. Brazil nuts are considered a rich source of selenium, but this probably depends on where they are grown.

Phytosterols and phytostanols

Plants do not produce cholesterol, it is only found in foods of animal origin. Plants do, however, produce similar steroid compounds, known as phytosterols. β-sitosterol and campesterol are the most abundant phytosterols in the human diet and make up over 80% of the total phytosterol intake, which is typically 100–300 mg/day; that is, similar to the average daily intake of cholesterol (note that vegetarians consume more phytosterols than omnivores). Other phytosterols include stigmasterol and the sterol ergosterol, which is made by yeast and other fungi and can also act as a precursor for vitamin D if irradiated with ultraviolet light.

Most dietary phytosterols, like cholesterol, have a double bond within the steroid nucleus; they are structurally very similar to cholesterol and have just an extra one or two carbon atoms in their side chain, for example β-sitosterol is 24 ethyl cholesterol and differs from cholesterol only in having an extra ethyl group attached to carbon 24 in the cholesterol side chain. A small proportion of the normal dietary load of phytosterols are compounds without a double bond in the steroid nucleus; these 'saturated phytosterols' are now generally known as phytostanols, for example, if the double bond in the steroid nucleus of β-sitosterol is hydrogenated then the resulting compound is called β-sitostanol (see Figure 9.1). Note that in this discussion the term phytosterol is used to include both the saturated (stanols) and unsaturated plant sterols.

Phytosterols are in general poorly absorbed from the gut and phytostanols are especially poorly absorbed; less than 1% of ingested β-sitostanol is absorbed. It has been known for around 50 years that although these phytosterols are themselves poorly absorbed from the gut, they are nonetheless able to inhibit the absorption of dietary cholesterol and the reabsorption of biliary cholesterol, probably by displacing cholesterol from micelles in the gut; micelles are the minute suspension particles from which lipids and fat-soluble vitamins are absorbed in the gut. They thus have the potential to lower blood cholesterol by increasing the amount of dietary and biliary cholesterol that is lost in the faeces. There has been much speculation about whether phytosterols lower LDL cholesterol levels by additional mechanisms to these well-established ones. It has been suggested that they have effects on cholesterol metabolism within enterocytes and hepatocytes, and that they lead to increased expression of the LDL receptor, thus enhancing clearance of cholesterol from plasma (see Plat and Mensink, 2005; Calpe-Berdiel et al., 2009).

The basic science described above is well established and the potential of high dietary loads of phytosterols to have some effect of lowering blood cholesterol is generally accepted. β-sitosterol was used as a cholesterol-lowering 'drug' as early as the 1970s. However, interest in the potential use of these compounds for lowering blood cholesterol has attracted greatly increased attention and research since the launch in Finland in 1995 of a margarine with a high content of β-sitostanol esters, which is claimed to lower the blood cholesterol of consumers. It is claimed specifically to lower LDL cholesterol without affecting HDL cholesterol or blood triglycerides (see Chapter 6 for details of blood lipoprotein fractions). This product has been launched across the world (UK launch in 1999). There are now

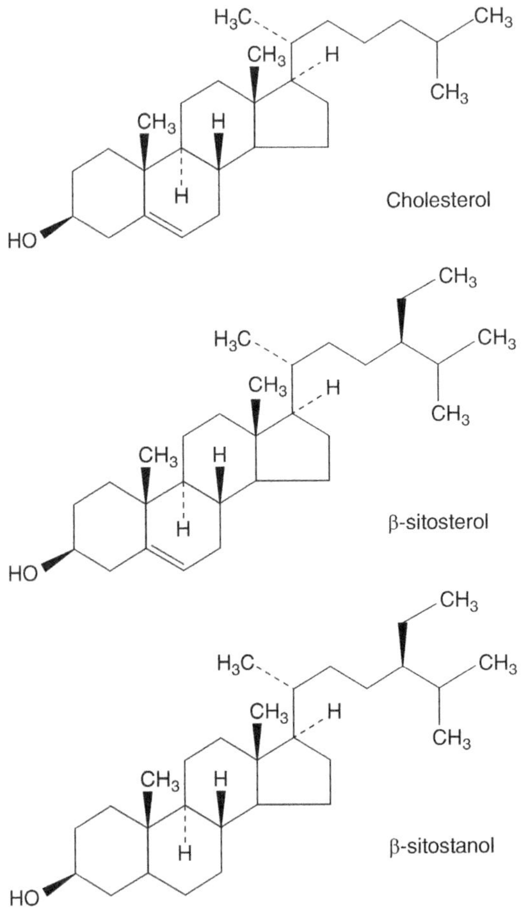

Figure 9.1 The chemical structures of cholesterol, β-sitosterol and β-sitostanol.

competing brands of margarine that are also marketed on the basis of their phytosterol content and cholesterol-lowering ability, and other phytosterol-enriched products such as yoghurts, yoghurt drinks, cream cheeses and salad dressings have been developed.

Large amounts of unsaturated phytosterols are produced as a byproduct of the wood-pulping and paper-making industries and these are then hydrogenated to produce saturated stanols, principally β-sitostanol. These stanols are very insoluble and so they are esterified with fatty acids to improve their lipid solubility so that they can be incorporated into foods like margarine, which typically contain around 12 g of stanol ester per 100 g of margarine.

In the year that the first stanol-containing margarine was launched in Finland, a much-quoted paper appeared in the prestigious *New England Journal of Medicine* (Miettinen *et al.*, 1995), which provided convincing evidence that consuming β-sitostanol-containing margarine could significantly lower both total plasma cholesterol concentration and LDL cholesterol concentration. This was the report of a year-long, randomised, double-blind trial with 150 mildly hyperc-holesteraemic men; 50 controls and two groups of 50 consuming one of two doses of stanol ester (1.8 or 2.6 g/day). There was a 10% reduction in the total blood cholesterol concentration in the treated groups (i.e. reduced by 24 mg/100 ml or 0.62 mmol/L) and a 14% reduction in the LDL cholesterol concentration; the effect of the stanol was dose dependent and there were no such changes in the control group.

Numerous other controlled trials have since confirmed the cholesterol-lowering effects of stanols or unsaturated phytosterols using a variety of age groups, both sexes and in trials of much shorter duration than the one-year study of Miettinen *et al.* (Law, 2000 lists 14 such trials). They have also been shown to augment the effects of statins, the modern group of potent cholesterol-lowering drugs. Unsaturated phytosterols are as effective as stanols, but the absorption of β-sitostanol (<1%) is even less than that of β-sitosterol (5%), which reduces the chance of adverse systemic consequences. There is a rare inherited condition, phy-tosterolaemia, in which there is increased absorption of phytosterols and, once absorbed, they accelerate atherosclerosis, just like cholesterol.

Law (2000), in a review of the use of phytosterol-enriched margarine, concluded that the consumption of around 2 g/day of plant sterol in margarine would result in substantial reductions in average plasma LDL cholesterol concentrations. The effect on LDL cholesterol would increase progressively with age (up to 0.54 mmol/L in those aged 50–59 years). Law estimated that this reduction in average LDL cho-lesterol was greater than could be expected from achievable reductions in saturated fat intake and might cut heart disease risk by 25%. He highlighted the high cost of these margarines (at that time around four times that of ordinary polyunsaturated margarine) as a major limiting factor in their general use. He 'welcomed' their introduction as 'an important innovation in the primary prevention of ischaemic heart disease' and expressed the hope that 'in the longer term these plant sterols and stanols will become cheap and plentiful so will be able to be added to foods eaten by the majority of the population'.

More recent meta-analyses tend to confirm the conclusions in Law (2000). Katan *et al.* (2003), in a meta-analysis of 41 trials, suggested that a daily dose of 2 g/day of either phytosterols or phytostanols reduced LDL cholesterol by about 10%. They found that eating a diet low in saturated fat and cholesterol together with phytosterols could reduce LDL cholesterol by about 20%. The effect of combin-ing phytosterols with statins enhanced the cholesterol-lowering effect more than doubling the statin dose. Phytosterols did not adversely affect the blood levels of vitamin A or D. Demonty *et al.* (2009) were able to establish a dose–response rela-tionship for the cholesterol-lowering effect of phytosterols when delivered in vari-ous types of food. At higher doses of phytosterols, solid foods appeared to be more effective than liquid ones and there were indications that the phytosterols were more effective when given in multiple doses rather than single ones.

There is thus compelling evidence that in controlled trials, 2–3 g/day of phyto-sterol administered in margarine or other functional foods lead to significant reduc-tions in total plasma cholesterol concentration and LDL cholesterol concentration within a few weeks in both men and women. There are still, however, some unresolved issues or questions (see list below), which suggest the need for caution and further research before phytosterols can be given unqualified endorsement for universal usage. Some of these issues were discussed by Law (2000) and some of the others were raised by correspondents to the *British Medical Journal* after publication of Law's review (which can be accessed free of charge via the British Medical Journal website, www.bmj.com).

- The availability of phytosterol from natural sources as byproducts of vegetable oil refining and wood pulping for papermaking is limited and, according to Law (2000), could only supply 10% of people in western countries. Hence the relatively high cost of products that are fortified with them.
- Although sterols occur naturally in the diet, the amounts being advocated (around 2 g/day) in functional foods is around 100 times the average intake from 'normal' foods; it might well be considerably higher in those consuming large amounts or multiple types of phytosterol-fortified products. It is difficult to be sure that such levels of consumption over the whole of the human life span would not have any adverse effects, either for people in general or for some specific subgroup(s) of the population.
- It may well be that the degree of cholesterol-lowering achieved by general use of phytosterol-supplemented products by free-living populations will be less than that achieved in controlled trials. This is the general experience of other dietary interventions aimed at lowering blood cholesterol concentrations (Oliver, 1981).
- There is little direct evidence that the reductions in plasma cholesterol due to phytosterol supplementation will translate into holistic health benefits; that is, reduced ischaemic heart disease and improved longevity and quality of life. The reduction in coronary heart disease prevalence predicted by Law (2000) is dependent on several unproven assumptions. Prior to the introduction of the statin group of cholesterol-lowering drugs, it was the common experience that it was difficult to demonstrate any significant reduction in total mortality or even heart disease mortality as a result of cholesterol-lowering interventions; some interventions seemed to increase total mortality (Smith *et al.*, 1993). More recent trials with statins (a group of drugs that inhibit the rate-limiting enzyme in cholesterol synthesis) have shown that they not only lead to large and sustained reductions in both total and LDL cholesterol in plasma, but also to significant reductions in both heart disease and total mortality (e.g. SSSS Group, 1994; Shepherd *et al.*, 1995). If a large decline in blood cholesterol caused by statins leads to reductions in mortality, then cholesterol lowering by other means should produce the same benefits.
- Phytosterols not only reduce the absorption of cholesterol and its concentration in blood, they also reduce the blood levels of some other lipid-soluble substances, in particular the carotenoids and vitamin E (although not apparently vitamin A or D).
- There are a few people with rare genetic defects who are susceptible to high phytosterol intakes (e.g. those with phytosterolaemia, described earlier in this

section). It is possible that the larger number of people who are heterozygous for such conditions may also have some increased susceptibility to large phyto-sterol intakes.

Most of the above, largely theoretical reasons for being (over?) cautious in advocating universal use of these products would diminish or disappear if they are used by adults who do have elevated plasma cholesterol concentrations or have had previous episodes of heart disease.

Phyto-oestrogens

The phyto-oestrogens are plant substances that, although they are not steroids, do have structural similarities to human oestrogen and bind to the human oestrogen receptor. They are classified as partial agonists because they bind to the oestrogen receptor, but only exert a small oestrogen-like effect (even the most potent of them, genistein, has less than one ten-thousandth the potency of oestradiol). This means that they can paradoxically be used either to boost the effects of endogenous oestrogen or to reduce them, depending on the hormone status of the recipient. When endogenous oestrogen production is very low, as in post-menopausal women, their small oestrogen-like effect will boost overall oestrogenic activity. Thus in post-menopausal women they could potentially fulfil similar functions to hormone (oestrogen) replacement therapy (HRT) and reduce both the immediate and chronic consequences of the menopause. When body oestrogen levels are high, they will compete for oestrogen receptor sites with the more potent endogenous hormones and thus perhaps moderate the oestrogen response. It has been suggested that this might reduce the risk of developing breast cancer.

Soy products contain a class of phyto-oestrogens known as isoflavins, which includes the most active phyto-oestrogens, diadzein and genistein. Although these compounds are found in other legumes, the levels in soybeans (2–4 mg isoflavin per gram soy protein) are at orders of magnitude greater than in these other foods. There are other classes of phyto-oestrogens, namely the lignans found in whole grains, fruits, vegetables and flaxseed and the coumestins found in clover and alfalfa sprouts. These other phyto-oestrogens generally have much less oestrogenic activity than the soy isoflavins.

The amount of isoflavin present in soy products depends on the processing methods: alcohol extraction or defatting lowers the final isoflavin content. Soy foods that contain isoflavins are:

- Textured soy protein, which is sometimes used in meat substitutes or used as partial replacement for meat in some meat products; that is, used as 'meat stretchers' – around 5 mg total isoflavin per gram soy protein
- Soy flour – 5 mg/g
- Tofu – 2 mg/g
- Soy milk 2 mg/g

- Soy sauce – none
- Extracts of soy and some other plant extracts that are sold as dietary supplements with high levels of phyto-oestrogens, e.g. red clover (black cohosh contains phyto-oestrogens but from May 2011 will no longer be sold as a food supplement)

There are four suggested benefits that may be gained from consuming soy products or other extracts rich in phyto-oestrogens:

- They could reduce acute menopausal symptoms that result from the fall in oestrogen secretion by the ageing ovary: such as hot flushes, night sweats, insomnia, depression, vaginal dryness and possibly reduced memory.
- They might reduce the acceleration in bone mineral loss that accompanies the decline in oestrogen production at the time of the menopause. This menopausal decline in sex hormone output is the reason why elderly women are four to five times more susceptible to osteoporosis fractures than men; if loss of sex hormones does occur in men it also increases fracture risk. Phyto-oestrogens could thus help to maintain bone density in older women and reduce the risk of osteoporosis-related fractures of the wrist, vertebrae and hip in older women.
- It is well established in controlled trials that increased soy protein intake has the potential to lower LDL cholesterol levels and thus also perhaps to reduce the risk of heart disease, particularly in post-menopausal women.
- Phyto-oestrogens may reduce the long-term risk of cancer when consumed throughout life; breast cancer has been the focus of attention and study, but there are also claims that they might reduce the risk of prostate and colon cancer.

It is well established that HRT greatly reduces the acute menopausal symptoms, especially hot flushes. For example, in a meta-analysis of 24 published trials lasting at least three months, MacLennan et al. (2004) found that HRT reduced hot flush frequency by 75% compared to a placebo and also significantly reduced the severity of symptoms. They concluded that HRT was highly effective in alleviating hot flushes and night sweats in menopausal women. HRT also prevents the acceleration in the rate of bone mineral loss that occurs around the menopause and so maintains bone density and protects against osteoporosis-related bone fractures (e.g. Nelson et al., 2002). Millions of women across the industrialised world have been prescribed various types of HRT for these reasons over the last few decades. Prior to the menopause, women have lower rates of heart disease than men and have lower plasma concentrations of LDL cholesterol. After the menopause, average concentrations of LDL cholesterol in women rise towards and perhaps even beyond those in men and rates of coronary heart disease also move towards the higher levels seen in men.

For many years, it was widely believed that HRT might also protect post-menopausal women from the usual rise in heart disease risk. However, a large and widely publicised study has stated that in fact the opposite is the case and that HRT actually increases rates of heart disease in post-menopausal women (Nelson et al.,

2002). Note that this study has been criticised because most of the subjects were elderly and thus, because they had existing heart disease, were unlikely to benefit from the cardio-protective effects of HRT. These critics have suggested that HRT may still have cardio-protective effects if instigated in younger women at the time menopausal symptoms first appear.

For many years there have also been persistent reports of some increased risk of breast cancer associated with long-term use of HRT. This seems to have been confirmed in a recent extensive review of the risks and benefits of HRT (Nelson *et al.*, 2002) and a more specific study involving one million women that looked specifically at the relationship between breast cancer and use of HRT (Beral, 2003).

Although discussion of the merits and risks of HRT is outside the remit of this book, one of the reasons for the current upsurge in interest in phyto-oestrogens is the hope that they might be able to afford some of the undoubted benefits of HRT with fewer of the associated risks. Phyto-oestrogens are seen as a more 'natural alternative' to HRT; the term natural in this case refers to the mode of administration, by eating soy foods or other plant extracts rather than taking human oestradiol in pill form or via hormone patches. Although these phyto-oestrogens have only a tiny fraction of the potency of natural oestradiol, they would nonetheless be taken in much higher doses than HRT (typical dose 50 µg/day of oestradiol whereas soy, black cohosh and other supplements might typically contain 40 mg of total phyto-oestrogen).

Relief from menopausal symptoms, especially hot flushes, has been a major stimulus for women to seek medical help and to try HRT. It is generally accepted that HRT is the most effective treatment for hot flushes and decreases them by around 75%. There has been much speculation, supported in the main by low-quality evidence, that soy supplements or eating a soy-enriched diet also leads to a significant reduction in hot flushes. However, even if it does have some effect it is clearly considerably less effective than conventional HRT. One of the problems with such studies is that placebos produce substantial reductions in reported hot flushes and this varies from study to study (this large placebo effect was highlighted by MacLennan *et al.*, 2004). Although the reported reduction in some of the early studies looks impressive, it is often not markedly greater than the placebo effect despite being statistically significant in some of these studies (Vincent and Fitzpatrick, 2000). This underlines the need for high-quality, double-blind, placebo-controlled trials, which were again highlighted by MacLennan *et al.* (2004) as essential for testing any treatments for menopausal symptoms.

Lethaby *et al.* (2007) assessed the evidence for a beneficial effect of foods or supplements containing high levels of phyto-oestrogens in reducing hot flushes and night sweats in menopausal women. They identified 30 trials of at least 12 weeks' duration that met their inclusion criteria. Very few of these trials reported data that were suitable for including in a meta-analysis, but five trials of a red clover extract of phyto-oestrogens were combined and showed no effect greater than the placebo for these symptoms. Overall, they concluded that there was no evidence that phyto-oestrogen-based treatments were no more effective than a placebo in alleviating these symptoms.

The numbers of fractures caused by osteoporosis has reached epidemic proportions in many western countries. The National Osteoporosis Society (NOS, 2010) estimates that about three million people in the UK are affected by osteoporosis, with 50 000 wrist fractures, 70 000 hip fractures and 120 000 vertebral fractures attributable to osteoporosis each year. One quarter of all orthopaedic beds in the UK are occupied by patients with osteoporosis and it results in many deaths and much long-term disability. Fracture rates have increased both as a result of population ageing and because of 'real', age-specific increases in prevalence. The projected increases in the numbers of elderly people, particularly very elderly women, in industrialised countries means that this problem will continue to grow unless the age-specific fracture prevalence can be reduced. It is well known and generally accepted that HRT maintains bone density and, if take-up were high enough, HRT would afford a real hope of reducing age-specific rates of fractures due to osteoporosis. HRT has therefore been widely promoted and prescribed as a useful public health intervention for reducing osteoporosis.

Persistent concerns about the long-term safety of HRT (e.g. Beral *et al.*, 2003), as well as the short-term side-effects experienced by many women, have limited long-term usage. Recent adverse publicity about HRT safety has led to many women abandoning HRT and has made most family doctors reluctant to continue long-term prescription. In 2003, the Medicine and Healthcare Products Regulatory Authority issued advice to doctors that HRT should no longer be used for the long-term prevention of osteoporosis in women over 50 years.

Could phyto-oestrogens offer a safer long-term alternative to HRT for maintaining bone health in elderly women? In a review of phyto-oestrogens and bone health (Valtuena *et al.*, 2003), it was suggested that studies of the effects of phyto-oestrogens on bone health were still at an early stage and that supporting data was largely from *in vitro* experiments, animal studies and epidemiological associations. Those studies directly investigating the effects of phyto-oestrogens on human bones *in vivo* have been of short duration, small size and have used various doses and preparations of phyto-oestrogens. This review thus focused mainly on the appropriate design and investigative approaches that should be used for future studies of the effects of phyto-oestrogens on bone health.

Branca (2003) also reviewed the evidence that phyto-oestrogens might improve bone health and summed up the various lines of evidence thus:

- In *in vitro* studies with isolated bone cells, genistein seems to reduce bone resorption by osteoclasts and to stimulate bone-forming osteoblasts. Silwinski *et al.* (2005) showed that genistein from soy reduces the formation of osteoclasts (cells involved in bone breakdown) when added to *in vitro* cultures of bone marrow cells, as does a drug with oestrogenic activity.
- In animal studies, soybean feeding generally leads to increases in bone density, bone mass or other measures of bone health in female rats whose ovaries have been surgically removed (an animal model of the human post-menopausal state). This effect was confirmed by Mathey *et al.* (2007).

- In cross-sectional epidemiological studies with South East Asian populations who have high average spontaneous intakes of soy phyto-oestrogens, women with the highest intakes have higher bone mineral density. This effect is not seen where the spontaneous intake of soy is low, which implies that a high dose may be needed to produce a measurable effect.
- A review of seven studies that lasted for six months or more concluded that there was some support for a positive influence of phyto-oestrogens on bone mineral density in the lumbar spine. These studies used various doses and sources of phyto-oestrogens. In a more recent meta-analysis, Liu *et al.* (2009) found 10 eligible studies that had looked at the effect of soy isoflavones on bone mineral density. They found that a mean dose of 87 mg/day of soy isoflavones used for at least a year did not have significant beneficial effects on bone density, although there was some suggestion that in studies using the highest doses there may have been some effect on bone mineral density in the lumbar spine. They concluded that it was unlikely that soy isoflavone supplements would have any significant favourable effect on bone mineral density at the hip or lumbar spine in women.

An extensive review of phyto-oestrogens published by the Food Standards Agency in the UK (COT, 2002) also concluded that short-term human studies do suggest a small protective effect of phyto-oestrogens on bone density in the lumbar spine. There is no firm evidence for benefit at other sites.

The weight of evidence from large numbers of controlled clinical trials of soy-based diets strongly suggests that they do significantly lower total and LDL cholesterol levels (Vincent and Fitzpatrick, 2000). A meta-analysis of 38 controlled trials found that an average of intake of around 50 g of soy protein per day resulted in a 13% reduction in LDL cholesterol (Anderson *et al.*, 1995). The weight of evidence was substantial enough to persuade the FDA in the USA to permit the use on food labels of the health claim that soy protein can reduce the risk of coronary heart disease. However, purified phyto-oestrogens do not produce this effect and this has led both the FDA and COT (2003) in the UK to conclude that the beneficial effects of soy protein on blood lipoprotein profiles are not related to their phyto-oestrogen content. One suggestion is that soy protein itself (or the soluble fibre in soy products) may chelate bile acids in the gut and thus increase the faecal excretion of cholesterol (Vincent and Fitzpatrick, 2000). Cassidy *et al.* (2006) also concluded that whole soybeans and soybean protein isolates have some beneficial effect on lipid markers of cardiovascular disease, but that consumption of isolated isoflavones does not affect blood lipid levels or blood pressure.

Soy products are staple foods in China and Japan and the high intake of soy products in these Asian populations is associated with much lower rates of breast cancer than in most western countries, where soy consumption is much lower. Average soy intakes in these Asian populations range from 10–50 g/day, compared to adult intakes of 1–3 g/day in the USA and UK. Such observations led to the hypothesis that high consumption of soy foods and phyto-oestrogens in particular might afford some protection against breast cancer. In Chinese and Japanese migrants to the west, breast cancer rates remain low but rise in subsequent generations, which has led to suggestions that exposure to these phyto-oestrogens in early life or even *in utero* affords the later protection against breast cancer. Of course, it also possible that new migrants take some time to adopt the dietary patterns of their new country and that only in subsequent generations is this acculturation largely completed. More recent epidemiological studies relating either soy consumption or phyto-oestrogen intake to risk of breast cancer have produced inconclusive and contradictory results. Studies with chemically induced breast tumours in animals do seem to indicate a protective effect of phyto-oestrogens. Asian women have 40% lower plasma oestradiol concentrations and significantly longer menstrual cycles than Caucasian women. Some controlled studies suggest that large phyto-oestrogen supplements produce favourable changes in steroid hormone profiles in women. The information in this paragraph is reviewed by COT (2003), Limer and Speirs (2004) and Rice and Whitehead (2006). The evidence that dietary phyto-oestrogens help to prevent human breast cancer is at present inconclusive. Warri *et al.* (2008) discuss possible mechanisms by which early exposure to soy foods might reduce breast cancer risk.

COT (2003) also reviewed the possible harmful consequences of high phyto-oestrogen intake. There are at least two areas of possible concern:

- Possible adverse consequences of high phyto-oestrogen by infants who are fed on soy milk formula.
- The possibility that phyto-oestrogens might accelerate the growth of existing mammary tumours.

Concerns about the safety of phyto-oestrogen-rich diets first emerged in the 1940s when it was observed that some Australian sheep became infertile when allowed to graze on a type of clover. This infertility has been attributed to the high phyto-oestrogen content of their diet and is sometimes called 'red clover disease'. Similar effects have not been observed when other farmed species have been fed high soy and phyto-oestrogen rich diets, although they have been reported in quail. Babies fed on soy-based formula are probably the population group that have the highest exposure to phyto-oestrogens, certainly in western countries. COT (2003) estimated their exposure to be around 4 mg/kg body weight/day, which on a weight-for-weight basis is at least four times higher than the adult exposure in high soy-consuming countries of the Far East.

Despite the fact that soy-based infant formula has been available for around 80 years, there is no evidence of any adverse effects on human sexual development or fertility, although there have been very few published studies that have addressed this issue. Very high doses of phyto-oestrogens, often administered by injection, have been reported to lead to some changes in rates of sexual maturation in rodents, but it is very difficult to judge their significance for humans. The COT (2003) working group recommended that soy-based infant formula should only be fed to infants when indicated clinically. It noted that similar guidance had been issued in other countries. Allergy to cow milk would be a clinical reason for using soy formula, although many children who are allergic to cow milk are also allergic to soy milk. Osborn and Sinn (2006) found that when babies were started with soy formula rather than cow milk-based formula it did not seem to reduce subsequent allergies in infants and children; that is, there is nothing to suggest that soy formula is inherently less allergenic than cow milk-based formula.

This recommendation not to use soy-based formula unless clinically necessary may seem unduly conservative in view of the absence of any real evidence of harm for a product used very widely (up to perhaps 25% of bottle-fed babies in the USA) and in use for such a considerable length of time. Perhaps one reason for this extreme caution lies in memories of the effects of exposure of babies to diethylstilbestrol (DES). DES is a non-steroidal oestrogenic compound with structural similarities to the phyto-oestrogens that was widely used in the USA to prevent miscarriage and to treat other complications of pregnancy. In the 1970s it became clear that babies exposed to this compound *in utero* had higher levels of abnormalities of the genital tract and high levels of uterine, vaginal and perhaps other genital cancers. DES had been in use for over 30 years and more than four million American babies were exposed to it before these side-effects became clear; some people are still developing cancers as a result of DES exposure before 1971. The implications of exposure of babies to phyto-oestrogens *in utero* via high soy or supplement consumption by their mothers is unclear and largely unexamined. Merritt and Jenks (2004) and the Canadian Paediatric Society (2009) have since both concluded that soy-based formula does not adversely affect human growth, development or reproduction for most babies. However, the Canadian Paediatric Society did say that soy-based formula may not adequately promote growth in premature infants and thus that its use in this group was not recommended.

Some soy formula used in the past and made with soy flour was goitrogenic (inhibited thyroid function), but this problem does not occur with current soy formula, which uses soy protein isolate and is enriched with iodine.

There is evidence from short-term studies of women with breast disease that phyto-oestrogens may have a proliferative effect. In animal studies there are also indications that the rate of growth of implanted breast tumours may be accelerated by phyto-oestrogens. So there is another paradox, that phyto-oestrogens that have been widely studied and promoted as being able to reduce the risk of developing breast cancer are also being investigated for possible adverse effects on the progression of breast cancer. Barnes (2003) and COT (2003) have reviewed the safety of phyto-oestrogens.

Probiotics, prebiotics and synbiotics

Definitions and scale of usage

Probiotics are live cultures of micro-organisms, usually bacteria that survive passage through the upper parts of the gut, particularly the acid environment of the stomach, and adhere to and colonise the bowel, where they favourably alter the microbial balance. When they colonise the bowel they displace other potentially pathogenic bacteria and create an environment that is unfavourable for pathogen multiplication. Most of the organisms used as probiotics are lactic acid bacteria, which are a large group of bacteria that produce lactic acid as the end products of their fermentation of carbohydrate. The lactic acid bacteria include the lactobacilli, the bifidobacteria and some streptococci and other gram-positive cocci; a few yeasts have also been used as probiotics. More than a decade ago, over 20 different species were already listed by Fuller and Gibson (1999) as having been used as probiotics and others have been added since they compiled this list. Although mainly consumed as fermented milk drinks or yoghurts, other foods and drinks are now being used as vehicles for probiotic bacteria and they are also available in powders or pills that contain live, freeze-dried bacteria.

According to RTS (2005), the western European market for probiotics increased from €825 million in 2000 to €1.45 billion in 2005, an annual growth rate of around 12%, which compares with 1–2% growth in the total food market. The vast majority of probiotics were sold as yoghurts, other desserts or fermented milk drinks. It further estimated that the market would continue to grow at an annual rate of 8% to reach well over €2 billion per year by 2010.

Prebiotics are indigestible oligosaccharides (small carbohydrate polymers) that enter the large bowel and selectively enhance the growth of certain bacteria within the bowel, so again favourably altering the microbial balance in the bowel. They are made up of a variety of non-digestible carbohydrates that include oligosaccharides like inulin, fructo-oligosaccharides (FOS), galacto-oligosaccharides (GOS) and lac-tulose (a synthetic dimer of glucose and galactose). The western European market for prebiotics was €365 million in 2000, but had grown to €880 million in 2005, an annual growth rate of almost 20% (RTS, 2005). This market was predicted to continue growing at almost 10% per annum to reach almost €1.4 billion by 2010.

Synbiotics are live cultures of bacteria combined with a prebiotic, which enhances the colonisation of the bowel by the probiotic bacteria.

The lactic acid bacteria

Lactic acid bacteria are widely used in the production of traditional fermented foods like yoghurt, cheese, kefir, koumiss, sauerkraut, sourdough bread, salami and some sausages. The resulting acidity of the food and other products of the fermentation help to preserve the food by inhibiting the growth of spoilage organisms and reduce the risk of food poisoning by inhibiting the growth of potential pathogens. The fermentation process also adds distinctive flavours to the food and, in the case of milk, alters its texture by curdling the milk protein. Yoghurt is usually made by fermenting milk with a mixed culture of Lactobacillus bulgaricus and Streptococcus thermophilus; in the USA, the FDA requires that these two species must have been used if the food is to be called yoghurt, although it does allow the addition of other lactic acid bacteria.

Even if 'live natural yoghurt' is eaten, it has limited value as a probiotic unless organisms other than the traditional ones have been added, because these particular bacterial strains have low survival in the acid environment of the stomach, so other, more resistant lactobacilli and bifidobacteria are used in probiotic preparations.

Breast milk and the 'bifidus factor'

Up to 99% of the bacteria in the stools of breast-fed babies are bifidobacteria, whereas in formula-fed babies there is a much more diverse gut microflora. Breast milk contains oligosaccharides and perhaps other substances that stimulate the growth of bifidobacteria and this has been dubbed the 'bifidus factor' – nature's prebiotic? Breast-fed babies have a lot fewer gut and respiratory infections than bottle-fed babies; in developing countries, hygiene problems with bottle feeds are a major reason for this difference. However, the difference is still seen in developed countries, where the anti-infective properties of breast milk are thought to be the main reason for it (Filteau and Tomkins, 1994). This 'bifidus factor' is one of several agents in breast milk that may directly or indirectly have anti-infective properties. Anything that might contribute to reduced rates of diarrhoea in babies is of great significance, because diarrhoeal disease is a major cause of infant mortality. Mortality rates in bottle-fed babies in developing countries are much higher than those of breast-fed babies.

What makes a good probiotic?

Goldin (1998) suggested that the number of organisms that had then been identified as probiotics represented only a tiny fraction of those potentially available. He lists the following as the ideal characteristics of a good probiotic and thus as criteria for the selection of new probiotic organisms:

- Species compatibility. Ideally, probiotic organisms intended for humans should be isolated from human intestines, because those isolated from different species are generally less effective. In practice, the origin of some probiotics is unknown.
- The ability to survive passage through the gut and reach the intestines in a viable state.
- Good ability to adhere to the intestinal epithelium.
- A short generation time so that they can colonise the bowel rapidly. Some bacteria with poor adherence to the intestinal epithelium are still able to colonise the bowel temporarily because of their short generation time.
- Production of antimicrobial agents that will kill or inhibit the growth of pathogens.
- Good survival in foods or powdered supplements so that the product has a reasonable shelf life.
- No pathogenicity itself. Current probiotics are generally recognised as safe and are non-pathogenic and non-toxin-producing organisms, although on very rare

occasions they might be a source of infection in people whose immune systems have been compromised.

- Antigenotoxic properties; that is, the ability to reduce mutation and carcinogenesis, for example by reducing the production of mutagenic substances by other organisms in the intestine.

Suggested benefits of probiotics

This section discusses some of the many claims for the health benefits of probiotics.

They increase the nutrient content or nutrient availability in fermented food or even produce nutrients within the gut. Fermentation by lactic acid bacteria can increase the B vitamin content of dairy foods, including the folic acid content; it can also partially digest proteins and fats. It is difficult to establish the contribution to the host of intestinal production of vitamins by the gut microflora. The improved nutrient availability, together with reduced infection rates, may account for the increased weight gain reported in several studies when probiotics have been added to the food of young animals and bottle-fed babies (Goldin, 1998).

They reduce the symptoms of lactose intolerance. Milk is the only natural source of lactose and in around 70% of the world population, the ability to digest lactose declines markedly after about four years of age and lactase production is not reinduced by lactose consumption. High consumption of lactose in people with this 'primary lactase non-persistence' can precipitate unpleasant symptoms such as diarrhoea, bloating and flatulence, caused by the osmotic effects of lactose in the large bowel and its fermentation by colonic bacteria. It is well established that fermented milk products like yoghurt decrease the symptoms of lactose intolerance and improve lactose digestion in people with lactose intolerance.

The presence of traditional lactic acid bacteria in live yoghurt depletes the lactose content during the fermentation process (by up to 50%) and after consumption (Montalto et al., 2006). However, adding L.acidophilus to unfermented milk does not significantly reduce the symptoms of lactose intolerance or affect objective measures of lactose intolerance (breath hydrogen content). According to Montalto et al. (2006) this is probably because there is insufficient availability of bacterial lactase in the intestine to be effective. Adding probiotics to unfermented milks has produced mixed results. In a systematic review, Levry et al. (2005) specifically addressed the question of whether adding probiotic bacteria to unfermented dairy products reduced lactose intolerance in adults at that meal. They concluded that in general, probiotics did not reduce the symptoms or an objective measure of lactose intolerance, although there was some evidence that some specific strains or preparations were effective.

They reduce the rates or severity of intestinal infections. Claims have been made that probiotics can help to prevent or treat a number of different categories of diarrhoeal disease, including infectious diarrhoea in children and adults, traveller's diarrhoea and diarrhoea associated with antibiotic treatment. This suggested benefit of probiotics is discussed in more detail later in the chapter.

They may lower blood cholesterol concentrations and thus reduce atherosclerotic changes in arteries and, ultimately, the risk of coronary heart disease. The Masai of East Africa eat a diet rich in saturated fat and cholesterol but have low rates of coronary heart disease. Observational and experimental studies of the Masai in the 1970s led to the suggestion that live fermented milk might contain a factor that lowered blood cholesterol (see McGill, 1979 for a summary of this early work on the Masai).

More recent human experimental studies that have used more reasonable quantities of fermented milk have produced inconsistent results. In a review of several earlier studies, Taylor and Williams (1998) concluded that if probiotics do have any cholesterol-lowering effect, then it is weak and it would require large samples to get sufficient statistical power to detect such small changes against the background of wide intra-individual variation in serum cholesterol and significant technical errors in measurement. More recently, Greany et al. (2008) found that capsules containing Bifidobacterium longum, Lactobacillus acidophilus and a prebiotic had no effect on blood lipid levels in healthy young men and women when administered for two months. Agerholm-Larsen et al. (2000) did a small meta-analysis of studies that had investigated a milk fermented with a specific probiotic culture (one strain of Enterococcus faecium and two strains of Streptococcus thermophilus), marketed by the Danish company that sponsored the study as GAIO®. They found that short-term use of this product (4–8 weeks) could reduce plasma LDL cholesterol by around 5%. Of course, these apparent contradictions between different trials may be due to different effects of different strains of bacteria or different formulations, and this problem applies generally to trials of probiotics.

They have been claimed to reduce the incidence of vaginal infections, particularly vaginal candidiasis (thrush) caused by the yeast Candida albicans, which is the most common vaginal infection. Lactic acid bacteria, particularly Lactobacillus acidophilus, predominate in the normal microflora of the vagina, as they do in the intestine. L. acidophilus generates an acid pH of 4, which inhibits the growth of other organisms that can cause vaginal infections. A number of factors predispose to changes in the gut microflora that favour colonisation by candida or one of the other organisms that cause vaginal infections, including pregnancy, oral contraceptive use, diabetes and antibiotic use.

The theoretical case for consuming probiotic preparations (especially L. acidophilus) to treat or prevent vaginal infections is essentially very similar to their use to against intestinal infections; that is, that they restore or maintain a healthy balance to the vaginal microflora that reduces the risk of colonisation by pathogenic organisms. About 15 years ago, Elmer et al. (1996) concluded that at that time there was only limited evidence to support their effectiveness, although several studies have since shown that oral consumption of probiotics can alter the vaginal microflora (Reid et al., 2004). Preparations containing probiotic bacteria can also be applied directly to the vaginal area. Vaginitis frequently occurs after antibiotic therapy. In a large trial of both oral and direct application of lactobacilli in non-pregnant women after antibiotic therapy, Pirotta et al. (2004) found that neither oral nor vaginal lactobacilli reduced the incidence of vaginitis after antibiotic

treatment. Senok *et al.* (2009) did a systematic review of trials of probiotic preparations for the treatment of bacterial vaginosis and found no evidence that they were
effective when given alone or that they increased the efficacy of standard antibiotics. This contrasts with a more general systematic review of treatments for bacterial
vaginosis, which found that lactobacilli were effective in treatment and that they
enhanced the efficacy of the antibiotic metronidazole (Oduyebo *et al.*, 2009).

It is suggested that long-term consumption of probiotics might afford some protection against bowel cancer. This proposition is discussed further later in the
chapter.

Another suggestion is that when taken by pregnant women and infants, they may
reduce the risk of childhood eczema. This proposition is also discussed further later
in the chapter.

Effect of probiotics on incidence and severity of diarrhoea

Diarrhoea is not only a common, incapacitating and unpleasant condition of adults
and children, diarrhoeal diseases are also a major cause of infant mortality in the
world. While diarrhoea-associated mortality is most common in developing countries, it also causes the deaths of many babies in developed countries. Mortality
rates from diarrhoea are much higher in developing countries in those babies who
are bottle fed compared to those who are breast fed.

The normal gut microflora provides protection against infection by pathogenic
organisms and it is suggested that probiotics alter the balance of the gut microflora
so as to maximise this effect. This idea is given general support by the major differences between the gut microflora in breast-fed and bottle-fed babies, already briefly
discussed. Up to 99% of the bacterial population in the gut of a breast-fed baby are
bifidobacteria and most of the rest are other lactic acid bacteria. Bottle-fed babies
have a much more diverse flora, with higher levels of Bacteroides, Clostridia and
E. coli, some of which are potentially pathogenic and may have other adverse
effects, such as the production of potential carcinogens and intestinal putrefaction.
The faeces of bottle-fed babies are similar in colour and odour to those of adults,
whereas those of breast-fed babies are paler, looser and have a cheese-like odour.
This unique microflora associated with breastfeeding is considered to be generally
beneficial and is thought to contribute to the lower infection rates of breast-fed
babies, which is apparent even in countries where hygiene standards are good. It is
suggested that a number of different mechanisms could contribute to the reduced
risk of pathogen infection that results from the presence of high levels of lactic acid
and other 'good bacteria' in the gut. Several of these are listed below:

- They may compete with other bacteria for key nutrients, even though one would
  expect the gut to be a nutrient-rich environment.
- They produce an acidic environment that inhibits the growth and survival of
  pathogens. The pH of the stools of breast-fed babies is acidic with a pH of
  5–5.5, whereas that of bottle-fed babies is close to neutral (pH 7).

- They secrete antimicrobial substances that kill or inhibit the growth of other bacteria. Many lactic acid bacteria produce peptides or bacteriocins that inhibit the growth of other bacteria, but these tend to be active against other lactic acid bacteria.
- They compete with pathogens for adhesion sites on the intestinal epithelium and thus speed up their elimination and reduce the chances of them colonising the gut.
- They may break down toxins that are responsible for the adverse symptoms that a pathogen produces.
- It is suggested that lactic acid bacteria bind strongly to epithelial membranes and may provoke an immune response. This could enhance the host's ability to combat both enteric and systemic infections.

From simple observational comparisons of the infection rates of breast- and bottle-fed babies, one can only speculate on the contribution made by the unique gut microflora of breast-fed babies to the overall reduction in infection risk. Differences in hygiene risks and other anti-infective agents in breast milk also contribute to this reduced risk. Use of probiotics in bottle-fed babies is one way of trying to make their gut microflora more like that of 'naturally' fed babies. Probiotic manufacturers also advocate the use of probiotic supplements, even in breast-fed babies.

Szajewska and Mrukowicz (2001) published a systematic review of 10 randomised, controlled trials of the treatment of acute infectious diarrhoea in infants and young children with various probiotics. Overall, these studies indicated that probiotics significantly reduced the duration of the diarrhoea compared to those receiving the placebo, and that this effect was most marked for diarrhoea associated with human rotavirus, a very common cause of infant diarrhoea. They also looked at three studies investigating the preventive effect of probiotics for childhood diarrhoea, but the data did not enable them to draw any firm conclusions about the preventive benefits; just one of the three studies showed a significant beneficial effect. In a more recent long-term study, Saavedra et al. (2004) fed formula containing live probiotic organisms (B. lactis and S. thermophilus) to around 80 babies for up to a year and found that it was well tolerated; there was reduced reporting of colic or irritability and reduced antibiotic use in those receiving the probiotics as compared to those receiving the placebo (unsupplemented formula). Binns et al. (2007) also reported that in 1–3-year-old children attending childcare centres in Australia, a milk product containing both probiotics and prebiotics reduced by 20% compared to a placebo the number of days on which children were reported as passing four or more stools.

Diarrhoea is a frequent side-effect of antibiotic therapy. The antibiotic not only kills the targeted bacteria but also kills many of those that make up the normal gut microflora. This distorts the gut microflora and increases the chances of pathogenic bacteria colonising the gut and producing diarrhoea. The organism Clostridium difficile is now known to be a major cause of antibiotic-associated diarrhoea. This diarrhoea can be treated with other antibiotics, but there are grounds for believing that probiotics might offer an alternative or an adjunct to this further antibiotic use. D'Souza *et al.* (2002) conducted a meta-analysis of nine randomised controlled trials of the use of probiotics and concluded that they did help to prevent this type of diarrhoea. Lactobacilli and the yeast Saccharomyces boulardii have been identified as having particular potential in this regard. A more recent meta-analysis by McFarland (2010) supported the proposition that S. boulardii could significantly reduce the incidence of C. difficile diarrhoea and that other probiotics might be effective against other causes of antibiotic-associated diarrhoea. Tung *et al.* (2009) investigated the effect of S. boulardii preparations in the recurrence of C. difficile infections in populations with this infection at baseline. They found two studies that tended to support the use of S. boulardii to prevent the recurrence of C. difficile infections in patients receiving antibiotic therapy.

Many people experience a bout of 'traveller's diarrhoea' when they travel abroad on holiday or business. This susceptibility seems to occur even in people who travel from traditional summer holiday destinations to colder climes. A high proportion of these cases of diarrhoea are caused by strains of Escherichia coli to which the visitor has less immunity than the local population. A large number of other organisms can, of course, cause any particular outbreak or case of diarrhoea in travellers. Several studies have looked at the potential of probiotics taken before and/or during a foreign visit to reduce the risk of suffering a bout of diarrhoea. There have been some studies that have reported significant, even substantial, reductions in diarrhoea risk associated with the use of probiotics, but there have also been others that have not shown any beneficial effect (for examples see Goldin, 1998 or Macfarlane and Cummings, 1999). Conflicting results are perhaps inevitable given the variety of probiotics and the range of potential organisms capable of causing traveller's diarrhoea, such that a variety of preventives have been tested on their ability to prevent a variety of different infections. There has been nothing published in the scientific literature since the first edition of this book that has materially altered these conclusions.

When looking at individual causes and types of diarrhoea, much of the evidence is inconclusive. However, taken overall there does seem to be support on both theoretical and experimental grounds for expecting that some probiotics could be helpful in the treatment and/or prevention of some types of diarrhoea. There are almost no reports of significant adverse effects of using probiotics in a normal population. Allen *et al.* (2003) reviewed 23 trials that had tested the effect of probiotics in cases of acute diarrhoea caused by an infectious agent in adults and children. They found that probiotics overall reduced the risk of diarrhoea still being present at three days and reduced the mean duration of diarrhoea by over 30 hours.

Possible effects of probiotics on the risk of developing bowel cancer

In the UK and the USA, the bowel is the second most common cancer site for both men and women. Internationally, rates of bowel cancer vary by as much as fifteen-fold and evidence from studies with migrants, as well as recent large and rapid increases in bowel cancer rates in some genetically stable populations (e.g. Japan), suggest that most of this international variation is due to environmental factors, including diet. Populations or groups who eat diets that are low in meat and fat but high in starch, fibre, fruits and vegetables have low rates, whereas those who eat typical western diets that are high in meat and fat but low in starch, fibre, fruit and vegetables have high bowel cancer rates. It is suggested that diet could alter susceptibility to bowel cancer by a number of mechanisms:

- Substances present in food and food degradation products could have mutagenic effects.
- Substances produced from the breakdown of bile acids could be mutagenic.
- Some products of bacterial fermentation in the colon could have a protective effect, e.g. butyrate is known to have an antiproliferative effect that may inhibit tumour development.
- An acid pH in the colon generated by bacterial fermentation may prevent the production of mutagenic substances from bile acids or prevent the growth of mutagen-generating bacterial species.
- Increases in stool bulk and more rapid clearance of waste might reduce the exposure of colonic epithelium to mutagens that are demonstrably present in faeces.

At least two observations have encouraged nutritionists to speculate that regular probiotic consumption might afford some protection against developing bowel cancer:

- The growing evidential support for the protective effect of probiotics against acute pathogen colonisation of the bowel and thus against intestinal infections.
- That several of the mechanisms proposed above by which diet might alter bowel cancer risk would be affected by differences in the gut microflora and differences in the end products of bacterial fermentation in the gut.

It has proved difficult to get consistent evidence for the ability of probiotics to produce significant short-term benefits on infection rates and blood cholesterol. It is therefore likely to be some years before a substantial body of consistent direct evidence is able to provide a convincing case for or against a protective effect of probiotics on bowel cancer risk. Reddy (1998) reviews evidence to suggest that probiotics can reduce rates of chemically induced bowel cancers in animal models of human cancer, but there is no direct evidence that fermented food consumption prevents cancer in people. More recently, Fotiadis *et al.* (2008) have come to similar conclusions. They confirm that there is no direct evidence that probiotics or prebiotics prevent bowel cancer in humans. However, some but by no means all epidemiological studies suggest an association between consumption of large quantities of fermented milk and lower incidence of bowel cancer. Fotiadis *et al.* (2008) discuss evidence that probiotics and prebiotics are capable of bringing about the mechanistic changes that might ultimately lead to a modification of bowel cancer risk.

Probiotics and the prevention of childhood eczema

There has been considerable media and scientific attention devoted to the apparent large and rapid increases in the incidence of atopic (allergic) diseases in recent years; that is, asthma, allergic rhinitis (hayfever) and eczema. In some developed countries it is estimated that half of all children may develop one or more of these conditions. There has been much speculation about why these increases have occurred and many factors have been blamed, including:

- reduced breast-feeding of infants
- maternal smoking
- atmospheric pollution
- high number of immunisations
- overly hygienic home environments

It has also been hypothesised that 'optimising' the gut microflora might reduce the risk of allergic disease by preventing increases in gut permeability associated with infection, and so improving the barrier to antigen penetration, and/or by stimulating anti-allergenic immunological processes.

Two papers from a group working in Finland suggested that there were grounds for considerable optimism that probiotics taken by pregnant and lactating women and/or added to bottle feeds might substantially reduce the toll of at least one atopic disease, eczema. Kalliomaki *et al.* (2001) published the results of a large, double-blind, placebo-controlled trial of a probiotic bacterium (Lactobacillus rhamnosus GG) on the development of eczema in infants. They identified over 150 pregnant women whose babies had a close family history of atopic disease. These were randomly assigned to receive either a placebo or a capsule containing the probiotic. The identical capsules were taken by the mothers two to four weeks prior to due date, and for six months after delivery they were either given directly to the baby or taken by the breast-feeding mother. The frequency of atopic eczema at 2 years of age was halved in the babies receiving the probiotic compared to those receiving the placebo. Note that the manufacturers of the capsules coded them and did not release details of which were placebos or probiotics until after all the data had been collected. The chances of this being a chance finding was estimated at less than 1 in 100 (p = 0.008). This means that it is highly probable either that this is a real treatment effect or that there was some flaw or bias in the design or execution of the study. These authors found no difference in the apparent beneficial effect of the probiotic whether it was taken directly by the baby or by the breast-feeding mother. In a follow-up paper (Kalliomaki *et al.*, 2003), these authors reported that the apparent beneficial effect of the probiotic on eczema prevalence was still apparent when the children were 4 years old. They were not able to demonstrate any significant protective effect of the probiotic on allergic rhinitis or asthma, although this may be because asthma and allergic rhinitis usually present after 4 years of age.

Since that time, the balance of evidence has still favoured the belief that neonatal exposure to probiotics (especially L. rhamnosus) may lead to some reduction in the incidence of childhood eczema, and may also have some beneficial symptomatic effects in babies and young children with eczema. However, the evidence is by no means unequivocal and it would seem unlikely from the results discussed below that a 50% reduction in prevalence would be a general outcome.

Osborn and Sinn (2007a) performed a meta-analysis of five studies (c. 1500 infants) that did suggest that a modest but significant reduction in infant eczema was seen in high-risk infants who had been given a probiotic containing L. rhamnosus. However, these reviewers also found significant and substantial inconsistency between the studies. When the meta-analysis was restricted to those infants with atopic eczema, confirmed by a skin prick test or specific IgE, then the effect of the probiotic was no longer significant. These authors also found insufficient evidence to support the addition of probiotics to infant feeds with the aim of preventing allergic disease and food hypersensitivity. They noted a very large loss of patients in follow-up in the trials that they reviewed, which would reduce confidence in any positive findings.

Some studies published since this 2007 review have also reported no protective effect of probiotics (which included L. rhamnosus) against atopic eczema (e.g. Soh et al., 2009). A recent and large controlled trial (Wickens et al., 2008) reported that supplementation with L. rhamnosus (but not another probiotic) from 35 weeks of gestation until 2 years of age did significantly reduce the incidence of eczema when compared to a placebo. Neither probiotic reduced sensitivity to common allergens in a skin prick test. Betsi et al. (2008) found that in several trials, probiotics containing L. rhamnosus did significantly reduce the severity of atopic dermatitis in children with the condition although in most trials probiotics did not significantly reduce objective inflammatory markers for the disease.

Prebiotics

Prebiotics are intended to favourably alter the gut microflora in much the same way as probiotics. If they actually achieve this aim, then much of the evidence of favourable effects of probiotics could also be used to support the use of prebiotics. Most prebiotics are oligosaccharides (polymers of various monosaccharides containing 'a few' sugar units – that is, less than 20 – that are not digestible by human gut enzymes. Much attention has recently been focused on polymers of fructose, oligofructose and inulin, which can be extracted commercially from chicory root but are also present in other foods like bananas, onions, asparagus and artichokes. Although inulin and fructo-oligosaccharides (FOS) are not digested in the small intestine, they are fermented by bacteria in the colon. None of the component monosaccharides is absorbed as such. They can be regarded as part of the 'dietary fibre'.

In vitro, it can be shown that FOS selectively stimulate the growth of Bifidobacteria. Gibson et al. (1995) were also able to show the same effect in vivo. They were able to show that in human volunteers, replacing 15 g of sucrose in a controlled diet with 15 g of FOS for 15 days increased the proportion of bifidobacteria in the subjects' stools from 17% to 82% of the total bacterial count, and halved the proportion made up of Clostridia from 2% to 1%. Inulin, which has more fructose residues than FOS, had a qualitatively similar effect. Palframan *et al.* (2003) developed a quantitative index for assessing the possible value of potential prebiotics based on the changes they produce to key bacterial groups during fermentation. Osborn and Sinn (2007b) reviewed the small number of trials testing the effects of prebiotics added to infant formula feeds in preventing allergic disease and food hypersensitivity. They found inconsistent results from published trials, which did not overall suggest a significant benefit.

Synbiotics

The aim of mixing a prebiotic with a probiotic is to 'improve the survival and implantation of live microbial supplements in the gastrointestinal tract, by selectively stimulating the growth and/or activating the metabolism of one or more of a limited number of health-promoting bacteria' (Roberfroid, 1998). The prebiotic component thus either increases colonisation by the probiotic organisms(s) or stimulates the growth of endogenous Bifidobacteria. Roberfroid suggests that it may well be difficult to demonstrate any amplification of Bifidobacterial colonisation of the intestine if the effect of the probiotic alone is already large. There is some limited evidence that addition of prebiotics may prolong the colonisation by Bifidobacteria after consumption of the probiotic is stopped.

References

ABC (2010) *The Commission E Monographs of Approved Herbs*. The American Botanical Council. Sample monographs available free at: http://cms.herbalgram.org/commissione/index.html.

ACSM, ADA & DC (American College of Sports Medicine, American Dietetic Association, Dietitians of Canada) (2000) Joint position statement: Nutrition and athletic performance. *Medical Science for Sports and Exercise*, **32**, 2130–45.

Agerholm-Larsen, L., Bell, M.L., Grunwald, G.K. & Astrup, A. (2000) The effect of a probiotic milk product on plasma cholesterol: A meta-analysis of short-term intervention studies. *European Journal of Clinical Nutrition*, **54**, 856–60.

Ahlemeyer, B. & Krieglstein, J. (2003) Neuroprotective effects of Ginkgo biloba extract. *Cellular and Molecular Life Sciences*, **60**, 1779–92.

Allen, S.J., Okoko, B., Martinez, E.G., Gregorio, G.V. & Dans, L.F. (2003) Probiotics for treating infectious diarrhoea. *Cochrane Database of Systematic Reviews*, Issue 4. Art. No.: CD003048. DOI: 10.1002/14651858.CD003048.pub2.

Allied Dunbar National Fitness Survey (1992) *A Report on Activity Patterns and Fitness Levels*. Sports Council, London.

Althuis, M.D., Jordan, N.E., Ludington, E.A. & Wittes, J.T. (2002) Glucose and insulin responses to dietary chromium supplements: A meta-analysis. *American Journal of Clinical Nutrition*, **76**, 148–55.

Anderson, I.M., Nutt, D.J. & Deakin, J.F.W. (2000) Evidence-based guidelines for treating depressive disorders with antidepressants: A revision of the 1993 British Association for Psychopharmacology guidelines. *Journal of Psychopharmacology*, **14**(1), 3–20.

Anderson, J.W., Johnstone, B.M. & Cook-Newell, M.E. (1995) Meta-analysis of the effects of soy protein intake on serum lipids. *New England Journal of Medicine*, **333**, 276–82.

Anon (1980) Preventing iron deficiency. *Lancet*, **i**, 1117–8.

Aso, K., Kanno, S., Tadano, T., Satoh, S. & Ishikawa, M. (2004) Inhibitory effect of propolis on the growth of human leukaemia U937. *Biological and Pharmaceutical Bulletin*, **27**, 727–30.

Avenell, A., Gillespie, W.J., Gillespie, L.D. & O'Connell, D. (2009) Vitamin D and vitamin D analogues for preventing fractures associated with involutional and post-menopausal osteoporosis. *Cochrane Database of Systematic Reviews*, Issue 2. Art. No.: CD000227. DOI: 10.1002/14651858.CD000227.pub3.

Dietary Supplements and Functional Foods, 2nd Edition. Geoffrey P. Webb.
© 2011 Blackwell Publishing Ltd.

Bahrke, M.S. & Morgan, W.P. (1994) Evaluation of the ergogenic properties of ginseng. *Sports Medicine*, **18**, 229–48.

Bahrke, M.S. & Morgan, W.P. (2000) Evaluation of the ergogenic properties of ginseng: An update. *Sports Medicine*, **29**, 113–33.

Bahrke, M.S., Morgan, W.P. & Stegner, A. (2009) Is ginseng an ergogenic aid? *International Journal of Sport Nutrition and Exercise Metabolism*, **19**, 298–322.

Ball, G.F.M. (2004) *Vitamins: Their Role in the Human Body*. Blackwell, Oxford.

Barnes, J. (2002a) Herbal therapeutics (2) Depression. *The Pharmaceutical Journal*, **268**, 908–10. www.pharmj.com/pdf/cpd/pj_20020629_herbal2.pdf.

Barnes, J. (2002b) Herbal therapeutics (8) Gastrointestinal system and liver disorders. *The Pharmaceutical Journal*, **269**, 848–50. www.pharmj.com/pdf/cpd/pj_20021214_herbal8.pdf.

Barnes, J. (2003) Herbal therapeutic: Women's Health. *The Pharmaceutical Journal*, **270**, 16–19. www.pharmj.com/pdf/cpd/pj_20030104_herbal9.pdf.

Barrett, B.P., Brown, R.L., Locken, K., Mayberry, R., Bobula, J.A. *et al.* (2002) Treatment of the common cold with unrefined Echinacea. A randomised, double-blind, placebo-controlled trial. *Annals of Internal Medicine*, **137**, 939–46.

Bassleer, C., Rovati, L. & Franchimont, P. (1998) Stimulation of proteoglycan production by glucosamine sulphate in chondrocytes isolated from human osteoarthritic articular cartilage in vitro. *Osteoarthritis and Cartilage*, **6**, 427–34.

Bazzano, L.A., Reynolds, K., Holder, K.N. & He, J. (2007) Effect of folic acid supplementation on risk of cardiovascular diseases: A meta-analysis of randomized controlled trials. *Journal of the American Medical Association*, **296**, 2720–26.

Bender, D.A. (2007) Health Watch position paper: Functional foods. Health Watch, London. www.healthwatch-uk.org/Functional%20foods.pdf.

Beral, V. for Million Women Study Collaborators (2003) Breast cancer and hormone-replacement therapy in the Million Women Study. *Lancet*, **362**, 419–27.

Betsi, G.I., Papadavid, E. & Falagas, M.E. (2008) Probiotics for the treatment and prevention of atopic dermatitis: A review of the evidence from randomized controlled trials. *American Journal of Clinical Dermatology*, **9**, 93–103.

Beyer, F.R., Dickinson, H.O., Nicolson, D., Ford, G.A. & Mason, J. (2006) Combined calcium, magnesium and potassium supplementation for the management of primary hypertension in adults. *Cochrane Database of Systematic Reviews*, Issue 3. Art. No.: CD004805. DOI: 10.1002/14651858.CD004805.pub2.

Binns, C.W., Lee, A.H., Harding, H., Gracey, M. & Barclay, D.V. (2007) The CUPDAY study: Prebiotic-probiotic milk product in 1–3-year-old children attending childcare centres. *Acta Paediatrica*, **96**, 1646–50.

Birks, J. & Grimley Evans, J. (2009) Ginkgo biloba for cognitive impairment and dementia. *Cochrane Database of Systematic Reviews*, Issue 1. Art. No.: CD003120. DOI: 10.1002/14651858.CD003120.pub3.

Birks, J., Grimley, E.V. & Van Dongen, M. (2002) Ginkgo biloba for cognitive impairment and dementia. *Cochrane Database of Systematic Reviews*, Issue 4. Art. No.: CD003120.

Birt, D.F., Shull, J.D. & Yaktine, A.L. (1999) Chemoprevention of cancer. In: *Modern Nutrition in Health and Disease* (eds M.E. Shils, M. Shike & J. Olson), 9th edn. pp. 1283–95. Lippincott, Williams and Wilkins, Philadelphia.

Bjelakovic, G., Nikolova, D., Gluud, L.L., Simonetti, R.G. & Gluud, C. (2007) Mortality in randomized trials of antioxidant supplements for primary and secondary prevention. Systematic review and meta-analysis. *Journal of the American Medical Association*, **297**, 842–57.

Bjelakovic, G., Nikolova, D., Gluud, L.L., Simonetti, R.G. & Gluud, C. (2008) Antioxidant supplements for prevention of mortality in healthy participants and patients with various diseases. *Cochrane Database of Systematic Reviews*, Issue 2. Art. No.: CD007176. DOI: 10.1002/14651858.CD007176.

Black, C., Clar, C., Henderson, R., MacEachern, C., McNamee, P. *et al.* (2009) The clinical effectiveness of glucosamine and chondroitin supplements in slowing or arresting progression of osteoarthritis of the knee: A systematic review and economic evaluation. *Health Technology Assessment*, 13, 1–148.

Bliddal, H., Rosetsky, A., Schlichting, P., Weidner, M.S., Andersen, L.A. *et al.* (2000) A randomized, placebo-controlled, cross-over study of ginger extracts and ibuprofen in osteoarthritis. *Osteoarthritis and Cartilage*, 8, 9–12.

Blot, W.J., Li, J.Y., Taylor, T.D., Guo, W., Dawsey, S. *et al.* (1993) Nutrition intervention trials in Linxian, China: Supplementation with specific vitamin, mineral combinations, cancer incidence and disease-specific mortality in the general population. *Journal of the National Cancer Institute*, 85, 1483–92.

Boehm, K., Borrelli, F., Ernst, E., Habacher, G., Hung, S.K. *et al.* (2009) Green tea (Camellia sinensis) for the prevention of cancer. *Cochrane Database of Systematic Reviews*, Issue 3. Art. No.: CD005004. DOI: 10.1002/14651858.CD005004.pub2.

Bokura, H. & Kobayashi, S. (2003) Chitosan decreases total cholesterol in women: A randomized, double-blind, placebo-controlled trial. *European Journal of Clinical Nutrition*, 57, 721–5.

Borrelli, F., Capasso, R., Aviello, G., Pittler, M.H. & Izzo, A.A. (2005) Effectiveness and safety of ginger in the treatment of pregnancy-induced nausea and vomiting. *Obstetrics and Gynecology*, 105, 849–56.

Botto, L.D., Lisi, A., Robert-Gnansia, E., Erickson, J.D., Vollset, S.E. *et al.* (2005) International retrospective cohort study of neural tube defects in relation to folic acid recommendations: Are the recommendations working? *British Medical Journal*, 330, 571.

Branca, F. (2003) Dietary phyto-oestrogens and bone health. *Proceedings of the Nutrition Society*, 62, 877–87.

Branch, J.D. (2003) Effect of creatine supplementation on body composition and performance: A meta-analysis. *International Journal of Sport Nutrition and Exercise Metabolism*, 13, 198–226.

Breslow, J.L. (2006) n-3 fatty acids and cardiovascular disease. *American Journal of Clinical Nutrition*, 83(6 Suppl), 1477S–82S.

Broad, E.M., Maughan, R.J. & Galloway, S.D. (2005) Effects of four weeks L-carnitine L-tartrate ingestion on substrate utilization during prolonged exercise. *International Journal of Sport Nutrition and Exercise Metabolism*, 15, 665–79.

Brown, K.H., Peerson, J.M., Baker, S.K. & Hess, S.Y. (2009) Preventive zinc supplementation among infants, preschoolers, and older prepubertal children. *Food and Nutrition Bulletin*, 30(1suppl), S12–S40.

Bucci, L.R. (2000) Selected herbals and exercise performance. *American Journal of Clinical Nutrition*, 72, 624–36S. Full text available free at www.ajcn.org/cgi/content/full/72/2/624S.

Buchman, A.L. (2006) Manganese. In: *Modern Nutrition in Health and Disease* (eds M.E. Shils, M. Shike & J. Olson), 10th edn. pp. 326–31. Lippincott, Williams and Wilkins, Philadelphia.

Budeiri, D., Li Wan Po, A. & Dornan, J.C. (1996) Is evening primrose oil of value in the treatment of premenstrual syndrome? *Controlled Clinical Trials*, 17, 60–68.

Bunk, S. (1999) St John's wort set for U.S. clinical trials. *The Scientist*, **13**(3), 10–14.

Burdge, G. (2004) Alpha-linolenic acid metabolism in men and women: Nutritional and biological implications. *Current Opinion in Clinical Nutrition and Metabolic Care*, 7, 137–44.

Burgess, J.R., Steven, L., Zhang, W. & Peck, L. (2000) Long-chain polyunsaturated fatty acids in children with attention-deficit hyperactivity disorder. *American Journal of Clinical Nutrition*, **71**(1Suppl), 327S–30S.

Burk, R.F. & Levander, O.A. (2006) Selenium. In: *Modern Nutrition in Health and Disease* (eds M.E. Shils, M. Shike & J. Olson). 10th edn. pp. 312–25. Lippincott, Williams and Wilkins, Philadelphia.

Burr, M.L., Fehily, A.M., Gilbert, J.F., Rogers, S., Holliday, R.M. *et al.* (1991) Effects of changes in fat, fish and fibre intakes on death and myocardial infarction: Diet and reinfarction trial (DART). *Lancet*, **ii**, 757–61.

Buttriss, J. (1999) *n-3 Fatty Acids and Health*. British Nutrition Foundation briefing paper. British Nutrition Foundation, London.

Calpe-Berdiel, L., Escola-Gil, J.C. & Blanco-Vaca, F. (2009) New insights into the molecular actions of plant sterols and stanols in cholesterol metabolism. *Atherosclerosis*, **203**, 18–31.

Canadian Paediatric Society (2009) Concerns for the use of soy-based formulas in infant nutrition. *Paediatrics and Child Health*, **14**, 109–13.

Canter, P.H. & Ernst, E. (2002) Ginkgo biloba: A smart drug? A systematic review of controlled trials of the cognitive effects of ginkgo biloba extracts in healthy people. *Psychopharmacology Bulletin*, **36**, 108–23.

Cappuccio, F.P. & MacGregor, G.A. (1991) Does potassium supplementation lower blood pressure? A meta analysis of published trials. *Journal of Hypertension*, **9**, 465–73.

Cappuccio, F.P., Markandu, N.D., Beynon, G.W., Shore, A.C., Sampson, B. *et al.* (1985) Lack of effect of oral magnesium on high blood pressure: A double blind study. *British Medical Journal*, **291**, 235–8.

Cardinal, B.J. & Engels H.J. (2001) Ginseng does not enhance psychological well-being in healthy young adults: Results of a double-blind, placebo-controlled, randomized clinical trial. *Journal of the American Dietetic Association*, **101**, 655–60.

Carmel, R. (2006) Folic acid. In: *Modern Nutrition in Health and Disease* (eds M.E. Shils, M. Shike & J. Olson). 10th edn. pp. 470–81. Lippincott, Williams and Wilkins, Philadelphia.

Casey, A. & Greenhaff, P.L. (2000) Does dietary creatine supplementation play a role in skeletal muscle metabolism and performance? *American Journal of Clinical Nutrition*, **72**, 607S–17S.

Cassidy, A., Albertazzi, P., Lise Nielsen, I., Hall, W., Williamson, G. *et al.* (2006) Critical review of health effects of soyabean phyto-oestrogens in post-menopausal women. *Proceedings of the Nutrition Society*, **65**, 76–92.

Castilla, E.E., Orioli, I.M., Lopez-Camelo, J.S., Dutra Mda, G. & Nazer-Herrera, J.(2003) Preliminary data on changes in neural tube defect prevalence rates after folic acid supplementation in South America. *American Journal of Medical Genetics A*, **123**, 123–8.

Chaiyakunapruk, N., Kitikannakorn, N. Nathisuwan, S., Leepakobboon, K. & Leelasettagool, C. (2006) The efficacy of ginger for the prevention of postoperative nausea and vomiting: A meta-analysis. *American Journal of Obstetrics and Gynecology*, **194**, 95–9.

Chapuy, M.C., Arlot, M.E., Delmas, P.D. & Meunier, P.J. (1994) Effects of calcium and cholecalciferol treatment for three years on hip fractures in elderly women. *British Medical Journal*, **308**, 1081–2.

Clark, C.D., Bassett, B. & Burge, M.R. (2003) Effects of kelp supplementation on thyroid function in euthyroid subjects. *Endocrine Practice*, 9, 363–9.

Colter, A.L., Cutler, C. & Meckling, K.A. (2008) Fatty acid status and behavioural symptoms of attention deficit hyperactivity disorder in adolescents: A case-control study. *Nutrition Journal*, 7, 8.

COMA (Committee on Medical Aspects of Food Policy) (1989) *The Diets of British Schoolchildren*. Report on Health and Social Subjects No. 36. HMSO, London.

COMA (1991) *Dietary Reference Values for Food Energy and Nutrients for the United Kingdom*. Report on Health and Social Subjects No. 41. HMSO, London.

COMA (1994) *Nutritional Aspects of Cardiovascular Disease*. Report on Health and Social Subjects No. 46. HMSO, London.

COMA (1998a) *Nutritional Aspects of the Development of Cancer*. Report on Health and Social Subjects No. 48. HMSO, London.

COMA (1998b) *Nutrition and Bone Health with Particular Reference to Calcium and Vitamin D*. Report on health and social subjects No. 49. HMSO, London.

COMA (2000) *Folic Acid and the Prevention of Disease*. HMSO, London.

Corrada, M.M., Kawas, C.H., Hallfrisch, J., Muller, D., & Brookmeyer, R. (2005) Reduced risk of Alzheimer's disease with high folate intake: The Baltimore Longitudinal Study of Aging. *Alzheimer's and Dementia*, 1, 11–18.

COT (2002) *Draft report of the Committee on Toxicology on Phyto-estrogens*. Food Standards Agency, London. Available at www.food.gov.uk/multimedia/webpage/phytoreportworddocs.

Coulter, I., Hardy, M., Shekelle, P. Morton, S.C. & Hardy, M. (2003) *Effect of the Supplemental Use of Antioxidants Vitamin C, Vitamin E, and the Coenzyme Q10 for the Prevention and Treatment of Cancer*. Summary, Evidence Report/Technology Assessment: Number 75. AHRQ Publication Number 04 -E002, October 2003. Agency for Healthcare Research and Quality, Rockville, MD. www.ahrq.gov/clinic/epcsums/aoxcansum.htm.

Crowther, C.A., Crosby, D.D. & Henderson-Smart, D.J. (2010) Vitamin K prior to preterm birth for preventing neonatal periventricular haemorrhage. *Cochrane Database of Systematic Reviews*, Issue 1. Art. No.: CD000229. DOI: 10.1002/14651858.CD000229.pub2.

Crozier, A. (2003) Classification and biosynthesis of secondary plant products: An overview. In: *Plants: Diet and Health. Report of the British Nutrition Task Force* (ed. G. Goldberg). pp. 27–48. Blackwell, Oxford.

Cunha, D.F., Cunha, S.F., Unamuno, M.R. & Vannucchi, H. (2001) Serum levels assessment of vitamin A, E, C, B_2 and carotenoids in malnourished and non-malnourished elderly patients. *Clinical Nutrition*, 20, 167–70.

Curtis, C.L., Harwood, J.L., Dent, C.M. & Caterson, B. (2004) Biological basis for the benefit of nutraceutical supplementation in arthritis. *Drug Discovery Today*, 9, 165–72.

Curtis, C.L., Rees, S.G., Cramp, J., Flannery, C.R. & Hughes, C.E. (2002) Effects of n-3 fatty acids on cartilage metabolism. *Proceedings of the Nutrition Society*, 61, 381–9.

Cutler, R.R. & Wilson, P. (2004) Antibacterial activity of a new, stable, aqueous extract of allicin against methicillin-resistant Staphylococcus aureus. *British Journal of Biomedical Science*, 61, 71–4.

Czeizel, A.E. (2009) Periconceptual folic acid and multivitamin supplementation for the prevention of neural tube defects and other congenital abnormalities. *Birth Defects Research Part A: Clinical and Molecular Teratology*, 85, 260–68.

Czeizel, A.F. & Dudas, I. (1992) Prevention of first occurrence of neural tube defects by periconceptual vitamin supplementation. *New England Journal of Medicine*, 327, 1832–5.

Dagnelie, P.C., van Staveren, W.A. & van den Berg, H. (1991) Vitamin B$_{12}$ from algae appears not to be bioavailable. *American Journal of Clinical Nutrition*, 53, 695–7.

Dangour, A.D., Allen, E., Elbourne, D., Fasey, N., Fletcher, A. *et al.* (2009) Fish consumption and cognitive function among older people in the UK: Baseline data from the OPAL study. *Journal of Nutrition, Health and Aging*, 13, 198–202.

Daniele, C., Thompson Coon, J., Pittler, M.H. & Ernst, E. (2005) Vitex agnus castus: A systematic review of adverse events. *Drug Safety*, 28, 319–32.

Dawson-Hughes, B. (2006) Osteoporosis. In: *Modern Nutrition in Health and Disease* (Eds M.E. Shils, M. Shike & J. Olson). 10th edn. pp. 1339–52. Lippincott, Williams and Wilkins, Philadelphia.

DCCT (Diabetes Control and Complications Trial Research Group) (1993) The effect of intensive treatment of diabetes on the development and progression of long term complications in insulin-dependent diabetes mellitus. *New England Journal of Medicine*, 329, 977–86.

Dedov, V.N., Tran, V.H., Duke, C.C., Connor, M., Christie, M.J. *et al.* (2002) Gingerols: A novel class of vanilloid receptor (VR1) agonists. *British Journal of Pharmacology*, 137, 793–8.

De los Reyes, G.C. & Koda, R.T. (2002) Determining hyperforin and hypericin content in eight brands of St John's wort. *American Journal of Health-System Pharmacy*, 59, 545–7.

Demonty, I., Ras, R.T., van der Knaap, H.C., Duchateau, G.S., Meijer, L. *et al.* (2009) Continuous dose-response relationship of the LDL-cholesterol-lowering effect of phytosterol intake. *Journal of Nutrition*, 139, 271–84.

DH (1992) *Folic Acid and the Prevention of Neural Tube Defects. Report from an Expert Working Group*. Department of Health, London.

DH (2000) New advice on St John's wort. Department of Health, London. The contents of this press release can be accessed at http://news.bbc.co.uk/1/hi/health/662481.stm.

DHSS (Department of Health and Social Security) (1969) *The Fluoridation Studies in the United Kingdom and the Results Achieved after Eleven Years*. Reports on Public Health and Medical Subjects No. 122. HMSO, London.

Dickinson, H.O., Nicolson, D., Campbell, F., Cook, J.V., Beyer, F.R. *et al.* (2006) Magnesium supplementation for the management of primary hypertension in adults. *Cochrane Database of Systematic Reviews*, Issue 3. Art. No.: CD004640. DOI: 10.1002/14651858. CD004640.pub2.

Dorant, E., van den Brandt, P.A. & Goldbohm, R.A. (1996) A prospective cohort study on the relationship between onion and leek consumption, garlic supplement use and the risk of colorectal carcinoma in the Netherlands. *Carcinogenesis*, 17, 477–84.

D'Souza, A.L., Rajkumar, C., Cooke, J. & Bulpitt, C.J. (2002) Probiotics in prevention of antibiotic associated diarrhoea: Meta-analysis. *British Medical Journal*, 324, 1361–6. Available free online at: http://bmj.bmjjournals.com/cgi/content/full/324/7350/1361.

Dunn, J.T. (2006) Iodine. In: *Modern Nutrition in Health and Disease* (eds M.E. Shils, M. Shike & J. Olson). 10th edn. pp. 300–11. Lippincott, Williams and Wilkins, Philadelphia.

Duthie, G. & Crozier, A. (2003) Beverages. In: *Plants: Diet and Health. Report of the British Nutrition Task Force* (eds G. Goldberg). pp. 147–82. Blackwell, Oxford.

Dyerberg, J. & Bang, H.O. (1979) Haemostatic function and platelet polyunsaturated fatty acids in Eskimos. *Lancet*, ii, 433–5.

Eberhart, L.H., Mayer, R., Betz, O., Tsolakidis, S., Hilpert, W. *et al.* (2003) Ginger does not prevent postoperative nausea and vomiting after laparoscopic surgery. *Anaesthesiology and Analgesia*, 96, 995–8.

Eckhert, C.D. (2006) Other trace elements. In: *Modern Nutrition in Health and Disease* (eds M.E. Shils, M. Shike & J. Olson). 10th edn. pp. 338–50. Lippincott, Williams and Wilkins, Philadelphia.

Egger, M., Davey Smith, G., Schneider, M. & Minder, C. (1997) Bias in meta-analysis detected by a simple graphical test. *British Medical Journal*, **315**, 629–34.

Eklund, H., Finnstrom, O., Gunnarskog, J., Kallen, B. & Larsson, Y. (1993) Administration of vitamin K to newborn infants and childhood cancer. *British Medical Journal*, **307**, 89–91.

Elmer, G.W., Surawicz, C.M. & McFarland, L.V. (1996) Biotherapeutic agents. A neglected modality for the treatment and prevention of selected intestinal and vaginal infections. *Journal of the American Medical Association*, **275**, 29–30.

Enjalbert, F., Rapior, S., Nouguier-Soule, J., Guillon, S., Amouroux, N. *et al.* (2002) Treatment of amatoxin poisoning: A 20-year retrospective analysis. *Journal of Toxicology – Clinical Toxicology*, **40**, 715–57.

Ernst, E. (2002) The risk-benefit profile of commonly used herbal therapies: Gingko, St John's Wort, Ginseng, Echinacea, Saw palmetto, and Kava. *Annals of Internal Medicine*, **136**, 42–53.

Ernst, E. & Pittler, M.H. (2000) Efficacy of ginger for nausea and vomiting: A systematic review of randomized clinical trials. *British Journal of Anaesthesia*, **84**, 367–71.

Eskes, T.K.A.B. (1998) Neural tube defects, vitamins and homocysteine. *European Journal of Pediatrics*, **157**(supplement 2), S139–41.

EVM (2000) Current usage of vitamin and mineral supplements (VMS) in the UK. Discussion paper produced by the Expert Group on Vitamins and Minerals, 21 July. www.food.gov.uk/multimedia/pdfs/evm0005p.pdf.

Filteau, S. & Tomkins, A. (1994) Infant feeding and infectious disease. In *Infant Nutrition* (eds A.F. Walker & B.A. Rolls). pp. 143–62. Chapman and Hall, London.

Finch, S., Doyle, W., Lowe, C., Bates, C.J., Prentice, A. *et al.* (1998) *National Diet and Nutrition Survey: People aged 65 Years and Over.* HMSO: London.

Forbes, A.L. & McNamara, S.H. (2006) Food labelling, health claims and dietary supplement legislation. In: *Modern Nutrition in Health and Disease* (eds M.E. Shils, M. Shike & J. Olson). 10th edn. pp. 1875–82. Lippincott, Williams and Wilkins, Philadelphia.

Forman, J.P., Curhan, G.C. & Taylor, E.N. (2008) Plasma 25-hydroxyvitamin D levels and risk of incident hypertension among young women. *Hypertension*, **52**, 828–32.

Fotiadis, C.I., Stoidis, C.N., Spyropoulos, B.G. & Zografos, E.D. (2008) Role of probiotics, prebiotics and synbiotics in chemoprevention for colorectal cancer. *World Journal of Gastroenterology*, **14**, 6453–7.

FSA (Food Standards Agency) (2003) *Safe Upper Levels for Vitamins and Minerals. Report of the Expert Group on Vitamins and Minerals.* HMSO, London. Available free online at www.food.gov.uk/multimedia/pdfs/vitmin2003.pdf.

Fuller, R. & Gibson, G. (1999) Probiotics and prebiotics: Definition and role. In *The Encyclopaedia of Human Nutrition Volume 3* (eds M.J. Sadler, J.J. Strain& B. Caballero). Academic Press, London.

Gades, M.D. & Stern, J.S. (2003) Chitosan supplementation and fecal fat excretion in men. *Obesity Research*, **11**, 683–8.

Gaullier, J.M., Halse, J., Hoye, K., Kristiansen, K., Fagertun, H. *et al.* (2004) Conjugated linoleic acid supplementation for 1y reduces body fat mass in healthy overweight humans. *American Journal of Clinical Nutrition*, **79**, 1118–25.

Gerritson, A.A., de Kram, M.C., Struljs, M.A., Scholten, R.J., de Vet, H.C. *et al.* (2002) Conservative treatment options for carpal tunnel syndrome: A systematic review of randomised controlled trials. *Journal of Neurology*, **249**, 272–80.

Gesch, C.B., Hammond, S.M., Hampson, S.E., Eves, A. & Crowder, M.J. (2002) Influence of supplementary vitamins, minerals and essential fatty acids on the antisocial behaviour of young adult prisoners. Randomised, placebo-controlled trial. *British Journal of Psychiatry*, **181**, 22–8.

Gey, K.F., Puska, P., Jordan, P. & Moser, U.K. (1991) Inverse correlation between plasma vitamin E and mortality from ischemic heart disease in cross cultural epidemiology. *American Journal of Clinical Nutrition*, 53(suppl1), 326S–34S.

Gibson, G.R., Beatty, E.B., Wang, X. & Cummings, J.H. (1995) Selective stimulation of bifidobacteria in the human colon by oligofructose and inulin. *Gastroenterology*, **108**, 975–82.

GISSI-Prevenzione Investigators (1999) Dietary supplementation with n-3 polyunsaturated fatty acids and vitamin E after myocardial infarction: Results of the GISSI-Prevenzione trial. *The Lancet*, **354**, 447–55.

Goel, V., Lovlin, R., Barton, R., Lyon, M.R., Bauer, R. *et al.* (2004) Efficacy of a standardized Echinacea preparation (Echinilin) for the treatment of the common cold: A randomized, double-blind, placebo-controlled trial. *Journal of Clinical Pharmacology and Therapeutics*, **29**, 75–83.

Goepel, M., Dinh, L., Mitchell, A., Schafers, R.F., Rubben, H. *et al.* (2001) Do saw palmetto extracts block human alpha 1–adrenoreceptor subtypes in vivo? *Prostate*, **46**, 226–32.

Goldin, B.R. (1998) Health benefits of probiotics. *British Journal of Nutrition*, **80**, S203–7.

Greany, K.A., Bonorden, M.J., Hamilton-Reeves, J.M., McMullen, M.H., Wangen, K.E. *et al.* (2008) Probiotic capsules do not lower plasma lipids in young women and men. *European Journal of Clinical Nutrition*, **62**, 232–7.

Gregory, J.R., Collins, D.L., Davies, P.D.W., Hughes, J.M. & Clarke, P.C. (1995) *National Diet and Nutrition Survey: Children aged 11/2 to 41/2 years. Volume 1.* HMSO, London.

Gregory, J., Foster, K., Tyler, H. & Wiseman, M. (1990) *The Dietary and Nutritional Survey of British Adults.* HMSO, London.

Gregory, J., Lowe, S., Bates, C.J., Prentice, A., Jackson, L.V. *et al.* (2000) *National Diet and Nutrition Survey: Young People aged 4 to 18 Years. Volume 1: Findings.* HMSO, London.

Grontved, A., Brask, T., Kambskard, J. & Hentzer, E. (1988) Ginger root against seasickness. A controlled trial on the open sea. *Acta Otolaryngolica*, **105**, 45–9.

Group (Alpha-Tocopherol, Beta Carotene Cancer Prevention Study Group) (1994) The effect of vitamin E and Beta Carotene on the incidence of lung cancer and other cancer in male smokers. *New England Journal of Medicine*, **330**, 1029–35.

Guerciolini, R., Radu-Radulescu, L., Boldrin, M., Dallas, J. & Moore, R. (2001) Comparative evaluation of fecal fat excretion induced by orlistat and chitosan. *Obesity Research*, **9**, 364–7.

Habib, F.K., Ross, M.K.H., Ho, C., Lyons, V. & Chapman, K. (2004) Serenoa repens (Permixon®) inhibits the 5alpha-reductase activity of human prostate cancer cell lines without interfering with PSA expression. *International Journal of Cancer*, **114**, 190–94.

Hall, K., Whiting, S.J. & Comfort, B. (2000) Low nutrient intake contributes to adverse clinical outcomes in hospitalized elderly patients. *Nutrition Reviews*, **58**, 214–17.

Halperin, S.A., Smith, B., Nolan, C., Shay, J. & Kralovac, J. (2003) Safety and immunoenhancing effect of a Chlorella-derived dietary supplement in healthy adults undergoing influenza vaccination: Randomised, double-blind, placebo-controlled trial. *Canadian Medical Association Journal*, **169**, 111–17.

Hamblin, T. (2006) The secret life of Dr Chandra. *British Medical Journal*, **332**, 369.

Hardy, M., Coulter, I., Morton, S.C., Favreau, J., Venuturupalli, S. *et al.* (2002) S-Adenosyl-L-Methionine for Treatment of Depression, Osteoarthritis, and Liver Disease. Evidence Report/Technology Assessment Number 64. AHRQ Publication No. 02-E034 Rockville, MD: Agency for Healthcare Research and Quality. www.ncbi.nlm.nih.gov/books/bv. fcgi?rid=hstat1a.chapter.2159.

Harper, A.E. (1999) Defining the essentiality of nutrients. In: *Modern Nutrition in Health and Disease* (eds M.E. Shils, M. Shike & J. Olson). 9th edn. pp. 3–10. Lippincott, Williams and Wilkins, Philadelphia.

Harper, A.E. & Rolls, B.A. (1992) Recommended dietary allowances of nutrients: Basis, policy and politics. In *Nutrition and the Consumer* (ed. A.F. Walker & B.A. Rolls). pp. 1–16. Elsevier, London.

Harper, C.R., Edwards, M.J., DeFilippis, A.P. & Jacobson, T.A. (2006) Flaxseed oil increases the concentrations of Cardioprotective (n-3) fatty acids in humans. *Journal of Nutrition*, **136**, 83–7.

Harris, R.C., Soderlund, K. & Hultman, E. (1992) Elevation of creatine in resting and exercised muscle of normal subjects by creatine supplementation. *Clinical Science*, **83**, 367–74.

Haskell, C.F., Kennedy, D.O., Wesnes, K.A., Milne, A.L., & Scholey, A.B. (2007) A double-blind, placebo-controlled, multi-dose evaluation of the acute behavioural effects of guarana in humans. *Journal of Psychopharmacology*, **21**, 65–70.

Hathcock, J. (2001) Dietary supplements: How they are used and regulated. *Journal of Nutrition*, **131**, 1114S–17S.

Hayes, C.E. (2000) Vitamin D: A natural inhibitor of multiple sclerosis. *Proceedings of the Nutrition Society*, **59**, 531–5.

He, K., Song, Y., Daviglus, M.L., Liu, K., Van Horn, L. *et al.* (2004) Accumulated evidence on fish consumption and coronary heart disease mortality: A meta-analysis of cohort studies. *Circulation*, **109**, 2705–11.

He, Z., Chen, R., Zhou, Y., Geng, L., Zhang, Z. *et al.* (2009) Treatment for premenstrual syndrome with Vitex agnus castus: A prospective, randomized, multi-center placebo controlled study in China. *Maturitas*, **63**, 99–103.

Hegsted, D.M. (1986) Calcium and osteoporosis. *Journal of Nutrition*, **116**, 2316–19.

Hemila, H., Chalker, E., Treacy, B. & Douglas, B. (2007) Vitamin C for preventing and treating the common cold. *Cochrane Database of Systematic Reviews*, Issue 3. Art. No.: CD000980. DOI:10.1002/14651858.CD000980.pub.3.

Henderson, L., Irving, K., Gregory, J., Bates, C.J., Prentice, A. *et al.* (2003) *The National Diet and Nutrition Survey: Adults aged 19 to 64 Years. Volume 3. Vitamin and Mineral Intakes and Urinary Analytes.* HMSO, London. Available at www.food.gov.uk/multimedia/pdfs/ndnsv3.pdf.

Hennekens, C.H., Buring, J.E., Manson, J.E., Stampfer, M., Rosner, B. *et al.* (1996) Lack of effect of long-term supplementation with beta-carotene on the incidence of malignant neoplasms and cardiovascular disease. *New England Journal of Medicine*, **334**, 1145–9.

Higdon, J. (2002) L-carnitine. A review published by the Micronutrient Information Center of The Linus Pauling Institute at Oregon State University. http://lpi.oregonstate.edu/infocenter/othernuts/carnitine/.

Higdon, J. (2003a) Coenzyme Q_{10}. A review published by the Micronutrient Information Center of The Linus Pauling Institute at Oregon State University. http://lpi.oregonstate.edu/infocenter/othernuts/coq10/index.html.

Higdon, J. (2003b) Alpha-lipoic acid. A review published by the Micronutrient Information Center of The Linus Pauling Institute at Oregon State University. http://lpi.oregonstate.edu/infocenter/othernuts/la/index.html.

Higgins, J.P.T. & Flicker, L. (2000) Lecithin for dementia and cognitive impairment. *Cochrane Database of Systematic Reviews*, Issue 4. Art. No.: CD001015. DOI: 10.1002/14651858.CD001015.

Hilton, M.P. & Stuart, E.L. (2004) Ginkgo biloba for tinnitus. *Cochrane Database of Systematic Reviews*, Issue 2. Art. No.: CD003852. DOI: 10.1002/14651858.CD003852. pub2.

HMSO (2003) Food Supplements (England) Regulations 2003. HMSO, London. www. legislation.hmso.gov.uk/si/si2003/20031387.htm.

Ho, M.J., Bellusci, A. & Wright, J.M. (2009) Blood pressure lowering efficacy of coenzyme Q10 for primary hypertension. *Cochrane Database of Systematic Reviews*, Issue 4. Art. No.: CD007435. DOI: 10.1002/14651858.CD007435.pub2.

Hoare, C., Li Wan Po, A. & Williams, H. (2000) Systematic review of treatments for atopic eczema. *Health Technology Assessments*, 4(37) 1–191.

Hoare J., Henderson L., Bates C.J., Prentice A., Birch, M. *et al.* (2004) *National Diet and Nutrition Survey: Adults aged 19 to 64 Years. Volume 5: Summary Report.* HMSO, London.

Holick, M.F. (2006) Vitamin D. In: *Modern Nutrition in Health and Disease* (eds M.E. Shils, M. Shike & J. Olson). 10th edn. pp. 386–95. Lippincott, Williams and Wilkins, Philadelphia.

Holick, M.F. & Chen, T.C. (2008) Vitamin D deficiency: A worldwide problem with health consequences. *American Journal of Clinical Nutrition*, 87(suppl), 1080S–6S.

Honein, M.A., Paulozzi, L.J., Mathews, T.J., Erickson, J.D., Wong, L.C. (2001) Impact of folic acid fortification of the US food supply on the occurrence of neural tube defects. *Journal of the American Medical Association*, 285, 2981–6.

Horrobin, D. (2003) Nutrition discussion forum. Why do we not make more medical use of nutritional knowledge? How an inadvertent alliance between reductionist scientists, holistic dietitians and drug-orientated regulators and governments has blocked progress. *British Journal of Nutrition*, 90, 233–8.

Horsch, S. & Walther, C. (2004) Ginkgo biloba special extract EGb 761 in the treatment of peripheral arterial occlusive disease (PAOD) – a review based on randomized, controlled studies. *International Journal of Clinical Pharmacology and Therapeutics*, 42, 63–72.

Horvath, K., Noker, P.E., Somfai-Relle, S., Glavits, R., Financsek, I. *et al.* (2002) Toxicity of methylsulfonylmethane in rats. *Food and Chemical Toxicology*, 40, 1459–62.

Hruby, K., Csomos, G., Fuhrmann, M. & Thaler, H. (1983) Chemotherapy of Amanita phalloides poisoning with intravenous silibinin. *Human Toxicology*, 2, 183–95.

Hughes, R. & Carr, A. (2002) A randomized, double-blind, placebo-controlled trial of glucosamine sulphate as an analgesic in osteoarthritis of the knee. *Rheumatology*, 41, 279–84.

Hultman, E., Harris, R.C. & Spriet, L.L. (1999) Diet in work and exercise performance. In: *Modern Nutrition in Health and Disease* (eds M.E. Shils, M. Shike & J. Olson). 9th edn. pp. 761–82. Lippincott, Williams and Wilkins, Philadelphia.

Hypericum Depression Trial Study Group (2002) Effect of Hypericum perforatum (St John's wort) in major depressive disorder: A randomised controlled trial. *Journal of the American Medical Association*, 287, 1807–14.

IGD (2007) Functional foods. Free IGD factsheet. IGD, Watford. www.igd.com/index.asp?id=1&fid=1&sid=4&tid=46&cid=118.

Ionescu-Ittu, R., Marelli, A.J., Mackie, A.S. & Pilote, L. (2009) Prevalence of severe congenital heart disease after folic acid fortification of grain products: A time trend analysis in Quebec, Canada. *British Medical Journal*, 338, b1673.

Isaac M, Quinn, R. & Tabet, N. (2008) Vitamin E for Alzheimer's disease and mild cognitive impairment. *Cochrane Database of Systematic Reviews*, Issue 3. Art. No.: CD002854. DOI: 10.1002/14651858.CD002854.pub2.

Jackson, J. (2003) Potential mechanisms of action of bioactive substances found in plants. In: *Plants: Diet and Health. Report of the British Nutrition Task Force* (eds G. Goldberg). pp. 65–75. Blackwell, Oxford.

Jacobs, B.P., Dennehy, C., Ramirez, G., Sapp, J. & Lawrence, V.A. (2002) Milk thistle for the treatment of liver disease: A systematic review and meta-analysis. *American Journal of Medicine*, **113**, 506–15.

Jadad, A.R., Moore, R.A., Carroll, D., Jenkinson, C., Reynolds, D.J. *et al.* (1996) Assessing the quality of randomized clinical trials: Is blinding necessary? *Controlled Clinical Trials*, **17**, 1–12.

Jarry, H., Leonhardt, S., Gorkow, C. & Wuttke, W. (1994) In vitro prolactin but not LH or FSH is inhibited by compounds in extracts of Agnus castus: Direct evidence for a dopaminergic principle by the dopamine receptor assay. *Experimental and Clinical Endocrinology and Diabetes*, **102**, 448–54.

Jewell, D. & Young, G. (2003) Interventions for nausea and vomiting in early pregnancy. *Cochrane Database of Systematic Reviews*, Issue 4. Art. No.: CD000145. DOI: 10.1002/14651858.CD000145.

Johnson, I. (2003) Influence of the gut microflora. In: *Plants: Diet and Health. Report of the British Nutrition Task Force* (ed. G. Goldberg). pp. 76–85. Blackwell, Oxford.

Jones, P.J.H. & Kubow, S. (2006) Lipids, sterols and their metabolites. In: *Modern Nutrition in Health and Disease* (eds M.E. Shils, M. Shike & J. Olson). 10th edn. pp. 92–120. Lippincott, Williams and Wilkins, Philadelphia.

Josling, P. (2001) Preventing the common cold with a garlic supplement: A double-blind, placebo-controlled survey. *Advances in Therapy*, **18**, 189–93.

Jull, A.B., Ni Mhurchu, C., Bennett, D.A., Dunshea-Mooij, C.A.E. & Rodgers, A. (2008) Chitosan for overweight or obesity. *Cochrane Database of Systematic Reviews*, Issue 3. Art. No.: CD003892. DOI: 10.1002/14651858.CD003892.pub3.

Just-Food (2008) Global Market review of functional foods – forecasts to 2013. Just-Food, Bromsgrove. www.just-food.com/store/product.aspx?id=62137.

Kalliomaki, M., Salminen, S., Arvilommi, H., Kero, P., Koskinen, P. *et al.* (2001) Probiotics in the primary prevention of atopic disease: A randomised placebo-controlled trial. *Lancet*, **357**, 1076–9.

Kalliomaki, M., Salminen, S., Poussa, T., Arvilommi, H., Kero, P. *et al.* (2003) Probiotics and the prevention of atopic disease: 4-year follow-up of a randomised placebo-controlled trial. *Lancet*, **361**, 1869–71.

Kamangar, F., Yu-Tang, G., Xiao-Ou, S., Kahkeshani, K., Ji, B.-T. *et al.* (2007) Ginseng intake and gastric cancer risk in the Shanghai women's health study cohort. *Cancer Epidemiology, Biomarkers and Prevention*, **16**, 629.

Katan, M.B., Grundy, S.M., Jones, P., Law, M., Miettinen, T. *et al.* (2003) Efficacy and safety of plant stanols and sterols in the management of blood cholesterol levels. *Mayo Clinic Proceedings*, **78**, 965–78.

Keele, A.M., Bray, M.J., Emery, P.W., Duncan, H.D. & Silk, D.B. (1997) Two phase randomised controlled clinical trial of postoperative oral dietary supplements in surgical patients. *Gut*, **40**, 393–9.

Khoo, Y.S. & Aziz, Z. (2009) Garlic supplementation and serum cholesterol: A meta analysis. *Journal of Clinical Pharmacology and Therapeutics*, **34**, 133–45.

King, J.C. & Cousins, R.J. (2006) Zinc. In: *Modern Nutrition in Health and Disease* (eds M.E. Shils, M. Shike & J. Olson). 10th edn. pp. 271–85. Lippincott, Williams and Wilkins, Philadelphia.

King, J.C. & Keen, C.L. (1999) Zinc. In: *Modern Nutrition in Health and Disease* (eds M.E. Shils, M. Shike & J. Olson). 9th edition. Lippincott Williams and Wilkins, Philadelphia.

Kiple, K.F. & Ornelas K.C. (2000) *The Cambridge World History of Food*. Cambridge University Press, Cambridge.

Kittaka-Katsura, H., Fujita, T., Watanabe, F. & Nakano, Y. (2002) Purification and characterization of a corrinoid compound from Chlorella tablets as an algal health food. *Journal of Agricultural and Food Chemistry*, 50, 4994–7.

Kiuchi, F., Iwakami, S., Shibuya, M., Hanaoka, F. & Sankawa, U. (1992) Inhibition of prostaglandin and leukotriene biosynthesis by gingerols and diarylheptanoids. *Chemical and Pharmaceutical Bulletin*, 40, 387–91.

Kleijnen, J. & Knipschild, P. (1992) Ginkgo biloba for cerebral insufficiency. *British Journal of Clinical Pharmacology*, 34, 352–8.

Krell, R. (1996) *Value-added Products from Beekeeping*. FAO Agricultural Services bulletin No 124. www.fao.org/docrep/w0076e/w0076e00.htm#con.

Kremer, J.M. (2000) n-3 fatty acid supplements in rheumatoid arthritis. *American Journal of Clinical Nutrition*, 71(suppl), 349S–51S.

Kremer, J.M., Bigauoette, J., Mickalek, A.V., Timchalk, M.A., Lininger, L. *et al.* (1985) Effects of manipulation of dietary fatty acids on clinical manifestation of rheumatoid arthritis. *Lancet*, i, 184–7.

Kris-Etheron, P.M., Harris, W.S. & Appel, L.J. (2003) Omega-3 fatty acids and cardiovascular disease. New recommendations from the American Heart Association. *Atherosclerosis, Thrombosis, and Vascular Biology*, 23, 151.

Kritchevsky, D. (2000) Antimutagenic and some other effects of conjugated linoleic acid. *British Journal of Nutrition*, 83, 459–65.

Kromhout, D. (1990) n-3 fatty acids and coronary heart disease: Epidemiology from Eskimos to Western populations. *British Nutrition Foundation Nutrition Bulletin*, 15, 93–102.

Langer, G., Schloemer, G., Knerr, A., Kuss, O. & Behrens, J. (2003) Nutritional interventions for preventing and treating pressure ulcers. *Cochrane Database of Systematic Reviews*, Issue 4 Art. No.: CD003216. DOI: 10.1002/14651858. CD 003216.

Law, M. (2000) Plant sterol and stanol margarines and health. *British Medical Journal*, 320, 861–4.

Lawrence, P. (2003) Analysis on herbal and botanical supplements. St John's wort. Laboratory of the Government Chemist, London.

Lawrence, V., Jacobs, B., Dennehy, C., Sapp, J., Ramirez, G. *et al.* (2002) *Milk Thistle: Effects on Liver Disease and Cirrhosis and Clinical Adverse Effects*. Evidence Report/Technology Assessment No 21. AHRQ publication No 01-E025. Available at http://www.ncbi.nlm.nih.gov/bookshelf/br.fcgi?book=erta21.

Lawson, R.E., Moss, A.R. & Givens, D.I. (2001) The role of dairy products in supplying conjugated linoleic acid to man's diet: A review. *Nutrition Research Reviews*, 14, 153–72.

Lee, I.M., Cook, N.R., Gaziano, J.M., Gordon, D., Ridker, P.M. *et al.* (2005) Vitamin E in the primary prevention of cardiovascular disease and cancer: The Women's Health Study: A randomized controlled trial. *Journal of the American Medical Association*, 294, 56–65.

Lee, M.S., Yang, E.J., Kim, J.I. & Ernst, E. (2009) Ginseng for cognitive function in Alzheimer's disease: A systematic review. *Journal of Alzheimer's Disease*, 18, 399–44.

Lee, S.Y., Shin, Y.W. & Hahm, K.B. (2008) Phytoceuticals: Mighty but ignored weapons against Helicobacter pylori infection. *Journal of Digestive Diseases*, 9, 129–39.

Leeb, B.F., Schweitzer, H., Montag, K. & Smolen, J.S. (2000) A meta-analysis of chondroitin sulphate in the treatment of osteoarthritis. *Journal of Rheumatology*, 27, 205–11.

Lethaby, A., Marjoribanks, J., Kronenberg, F., Roberts, H. & Eden, J. (2007) Phyto-estrogens for vasomotor menopausal symptoms. *Cochrane Database of Systematic Reviews*, Issue 4. Art. No.: CD001395. DOI: 10.1002/14651858.CD001395.pub3.

Leung, R., Ho, A., Chan, J., Choi, D. & Lai, C.K. (1997) Royal jelly consumption and hypersensitivity in the community. *Clinical and Experimental Allergy*, 27, 333–6.

Levry, K.M., Ketvertis, K., Deramo, M., Merenstein, J.H. & D'Amico, F. (2005) Do probiotics reduce adult lactose intolerance? A systematic review. *Journal of Family Practice*, 54, 613–20.

Lieber, C.S. (2006) Nutrition in liver disorders and the role of alcohol. In: *Modern Nutrition in Health and Disease* (eds M.E. Shils, M. Shike & J. Olson). 10th edn. pp. 1235–59. Lippincott, Williams and Wilkins, Philadelphia.

Lieber, C.S., Leo, M.A., Cao, Q., Ren, C. & DeCarli, L.M. (2003) Silymarin retards the progression of alcohol-induced hepatic fibrosis in baboons. *Journal of Clinical Gastroenterology*, 37, 336–9.

Lien, H.C., Sun, W.M., Chen, Y.H., Kim, H., Hasler, W. *et al.* (2003) Effects of ginger on motion sickness and gastric slow wave dysrhythmias induced by circular vection. *American Journal of Physiology. Gastrointestinal and Liver Physiology*, 284, G481–9.

Lim, W.S., Gammack, J.K., Van Niekerk, J.K. & Dangour, A. (2006) Omega 3 fatty acid for the prevention of dementia. *Cochrane Database of Systematic Reviews*, Issue 1. Art. No.: CD005379. DOI: 10.1002/14651858.CD005379.pub2.

Limer, J.L. & Speirs, V. (2004) Phyto-oestrogens and breast cancer chemoprevention. *Breast Cancer Research*, 6, 119–27.

Linde, K., Barrett, B., Wolkart, K., Bauer, R. & Melchart, D. (2006) Echinacea for preventing and treating the common cold. *Cochrane Database of Systematic Reviews*, Issue 1. Art. No.: CD000530. DOI: 10.1002/14651858.CD000530.pub2.

Linde, K., Berner, M.M. & Kriston, L. (2008) St. John's wort for major depression. *Cochrane Database systematic Reviews*, issue 4. Art. No.: CD000448. DOI 10.1002/14651858. CD000448.pub3.

Linde, K., Ramirez, G., Mulrow, C.D. & Melchart, D. (1996) St John's wort for depression – an overview and meta-analysis of randomised clinical trials. *British Medical Journal*, 313, 253–8. Available free online at http://bmj.bmjjournals.com/cgi/content/full/313/7052/253.

Lissiman, E., Bhasale, A.L. & Cohen, M. (2009) Garlic for the common cold. *Cochrane Database of Systematic Reviews*, Issue 3. Art. No.: CD006206. DOI: 10.1002/14651858. CD006206.pub2.

Liu, J., Ho, S.C., Su, Y.X., Chen, W.Q., Zhang, C.X. *et al.* (2009) Effect of long-term intervention of soy isoflavones on bone mineral density in women: A meta-analysis of randomized controlled trials. *Bone*, 44, 948–53.

Loehrer, F.M.T., Schwab, R., Angst, C.P., Haefeli, W.E. & Fowler, B. (1997) Influence of oral S-adenosylmethionine on plasma 5-methyltetrahydrofolate, S-adenosylhomocysteine, homocysteine and methionine in healthy humans. *Journal of Pharmacology and Experimental Therapeutics*, 282, 845–50.

McAlindon, T.E., La Valley, M.P., Gulin, J.P. & Felson, D.T. (2000) Glucosamine and chondroitin for treatment of osteoarthritis: A systematic quality assessment and meta-analysis. *Journal of the American Medical Association*, 283, 1469–75.

McFarland, L.V. (2010) Sytematic review and meta-analysis of Saccharomyces boulardii in adult patients. *World Journal of Gastroenterology*, 16, 2202–22.

Macfarlane, G.T. & Cummings, J.H. (1999) Probiotics and prebiotics: Can regulating the activities of intestinal bacteria benefit health? *British Medical Journal*, 318, 999–1003.

McGill, H.C. (1979) The relationship of dietary cholesterol to serum cholesterol concentration and to atherosclerosis in man. *American Journal of Clinical Nutrition*, 32, 2664–702.

MacLean, C.H., Mojica, W.A., Morton, S.C., Pencharz, J., Hasenfeld Garland, R. *et al.* (2004) Effects of Omega-3 Fatty Acids on Lipids and Glycemic Control in Type II Diabetes and the Metabolic Syndrome and on Inflammatory Bowel Disease, Rheumatoid Arthritis, Renal Disease, Systemic Lupus Erythematosus, and Osteoporosis. Evidence Report/Technology Assessment. No. 89 (Prepared by Southern California/RAND Evidence-based Practice Center, under Contract No. 290–02–0003). AHRQ Publication No. 04-E012–2. Rockville, MD: Agency for Healthcare Research and Quality. Available at: www.ncbi.nlm.nih.gov/bookshelf/br.fcgi?book=hserta&part=A131668.

MacLennan, A.H., Broadbent, J.L., Lester, S. & Moore, V. (2004) Oral oestrogen and combined oestrogen/progestogen therapy versus placebo for hot flushes. *Cochrane Database of Systematic Reviews*, Issue 4. Art. No.: CD002978. DOI: 10.1002/14651858.CD002978.pub2.

Malouf, R. & Areosa Sastre, A. (2003) Vitamin B12 for cognition. *Cochrane Database of Systematic Reviews*, Issue 3. Art. No.: CD004394. DOI: 10.1002/14651858.CD004394.

Malouf, R. & Grimley Evans, J. (2008) Folic acid with or without vitamin B12 for the prevention and treatment of healthy elderly and demented people. *Cochrane Database of Systematic Reviews*, Issue 4. Art. No.: CD004514.DOI: 10.1002/14651858.CD004514.pub2.

Manson, J.J. & Rahman, A. (2004) This house believes that we should advise our patients with osteoarthritis of the knee to take glucosamine. *Rheumatology*, 43, 100–101.

Marcoff, L. & Thompson, P.D. (2007) The role of coenzyme Q10 in statin-associated myopathy: A systematic review. *Journal of the American College of Cardiology*, 49, 2231–7.

Marti-Carvajal, A.J., Sola, I., Lathyris, D. & Salanti, G. (2009) Homocysteine lowering interventions for preventing cardiovascular events. *Cochrane Database of Systematic Reviews*, Issue 4. Art. No.: CD 006612.DOI: 10.1002/14651858.CD006612.pub2.

Mason, J.B., Dickstein, A., Jacques, P.F., Haggarty, P., Selhub, J. *et al.* (2007) A temporal association between folic acid fortification and an increase in colorectal cancer rates may be illuminating important biological principles: A hypothesis. *Cancer Prevention, Epidemiology and Biomarkers*, 16, 1325–9.

Mason, P. (2007) *Dietary Supplements*. 3rd edn. Pharmaceutical Press, London.

Mathers, J.C. (2009) Folate intake and bowel cancer risk. *Genes and Nutrition*, 4, 173–8.

Mathews, F. (1996) Antioxidant nutrients in pregnancy: A systematic review of the literature. *Nutrition Research Reviews*, 9, 17595.

Mathey, J., Mardon, J., Fokialakis, N., Puel, C., Kati-Coulibaly, S. *et al.* (2007) Modulation of soy isoflavones bioavailability and subsequent effects on bone health in ovariectomised rats: The case for equol. *Osteoporosis International*, 18, 671–9.

Maughan, R.J. (1994) Nutritional aspects of endurance exercise in humans. *Proceedings of the Nutrition Society*, 53, 181–8.

Maughan, R.J. & Evans, S.P. (1982) Effects of pollen extract upon adolescent swimmers. *British Journal of Sports Medicine*, 16, 142–5.

Meier, B., Berger, D., Hoberg, E., Sticher, O. & Schaffner, W. (2000) Pharmacological activities of Vitex agnus-castus extracts in vitro. *Phytomedicine*, 7, 373–81.

Melchart, D., Linde, K., Fischer, P. & Kaesmayr, J. (2000) Echinacea for preventing and treating the common cold. *Cochrane Database of Systematic Reviews*, CD000530. (Updated version is Linde *et al.*, 2006.)

Merritt, R.J. & Jenks, B.H. (2004) Safety of soy-based infant formulas containing isoflavones: The clinical evidence. *Journal of Nutrition*, **134**, 1220S–24S.

MHRA (2007) *A Guide to What Is a Medicinal Product*. MHRA Guidance Note No. 8. Medicines and Healthcare Products Regulatory Authority, London. Available free at www.mhra.gov.uk/home/groups/is-lic/documents/publication/con007544.pdf.

Mhurchu, C.N., Poppitt, S.D., McGill, A.T., Leahy, F.E., Bennett, D.A. *et al.* (2004) The effect of the dietary supplement, Chitosan, on body weight: A randomised controlled trial in 250 overweight and obese adults. *International Journal of Obesity and Related Metabolic Disorders*, **28**, 1149–56.

Miettinen, T.A., Puska, P., Gylling, H., Vanhanen, H. & Vartiainen, E. (1995) Reduction of serum cholesterol with sitostanol-ester margarine in a mildly hypercholesteremic population. *New England Journal of Medicine*, **333**, 1308–12.

Milewicz. A., Gejdel, E., Sworen, H., Sienkiewicz, K., Jedrzejak, J. *et al.* (1993) Vitex agnus castus extract in the treatment of luteal phase defects due to latent hyperprolactinaemia. Results of a randomized placebo-controlled double-blind study. *Arzneimittelforschung*, **43**, 752–6. (Article in German but English abstract is available.)

Mintel (2001) *Vitamins and Mineral Supplements*. Mintel International Group, London.

Mintel (2009) *Vitamins and Supplements – UK – May 2009*. Mintel International Group, London.

Moher, D., Pham, B., Jones, A., Cook, D.J., Jadad, A.R. *et al.* (1998) Does quality of reports of randomised trials affect estimates of intervention efficacy reported in meta-analyses? *Lancet*, **352**, 609–13.

Montalto, M., Curigliano, V., Santoro, L., Vastola, M., Cammarota, G. *et al.* (2006) Management and treatment of lactose malabsorption. *World Journal of Gastroenterology*, **12**, 187–91.

Morse, P.F., Horrobin, D.F., Manku, M.S., Stewart, J.C., Allen, R. *et al.* (1989) Meta-analysis of placebo-controlled studies of the efficacy of Epogam in the treatment of atopic eczema. Relationship between plasma essential fatty acid changes and clinical response. *British Journal of Dermatology*, **121**, 75–90.

Mowe, M., Bohmer, T. & Kindt, E. (1994) Reduced nutritional status in elderly people is probable before disease and probably contributes to the development of disease. *American Journal of Clinical Nutrition*, **59**, 317–24.

MRC (MRC Vitamin Study Group) (1991) Prevention of neural tube defects: Results of the Medical Research Council Vitamin Study. *Lancet*, **338**, 131–7.

MSM (2010) *The MSM Miracle*. The 'official' website of the MSM – Medical Information Foundation. www.msm-info.com.

Mulrow, C., Lawrence, V., Ackerman, R., Ramirez, G., Morbidoni, L. *et al.* (2000) *Garlic: Effects on Cardiovascular Risks and Disease, Protective Effects Against Cancer, and Clinical Adverse Effects*. Evidence report/technology assessment number 20. AHRQ publication N. 01-E022. Rockville MD: Agency for Healthcare Research and Quality. www.ncbi.nlm.nih.gov/bookshelf/br.fcgi?book=hserta&part=A29362.

Nangia, M., Syed, N. & Doraiswamy, P.M. (2000) Efficacy and safety of St John's Wort for the treatment of major depression. *Public Health Nutrition*, **3**, 487–93.

NAS (2004) *Dietary Reference Intakes (DRIs)*. Food and Nutrition Board, Institute of Medicine, National Academy of Sciences, Washington, DC.

Nasser, M., Javaheri, H., Fedorowicz, Z. & Noorani, Z. (2009) Carnitine supplementation for inborn errors of metabolism. *Cochrane Database of Systematic Reviews*, Issue 2. Art. No.: CD006659. DOI: 10.1002/14651858.CD006659.pub2.

Nathan, P.J. (2001) Hypericum perforatum (St. John's wort): A non-selective reuptake inhibitor? A review of the recent advances in its pharmacology. *Journal of Psychopharmacology*, 15(1), 47–54.

Naylor, C.D. (1997) Meta-analysis and the meta-epidemiology of clinical research. *British Medical Journal*, 315, 617–19.

NCCAM (National Center for Complimentary and Alternative Medicine) (2008) The NIH glucosamine/chondroitin arthritis intervention trial (GAIT). *Journal of Pain and Palliative Care Pharmacotherapy*, 22, 39–43.

Nelson, H.D., Humphrey, L.L., Nygren, P., Teutsch, S.M. & Allan, J.D. (2002) Postmenopausal hormone replacement therapy. *Journal of the American Medical Association*, 288, 872–81.

Neuringer, M., Connor, W.E., Lin, D.S., Barstad, L. & Luck, S. (1986) Biochemical and functional effects of prenatal and postnatal omega 3 fatty acid deficiency on retina and brain in rhesus monkeys. *Proceedings of the National Academy of Sciences*, 83, 4021–5.

Nicolaï, S.P.A., Kruidenier, L.M., Bendermacher, B.L.W., Prins, M.H. & Teijink, J.A.W. (2009) Ginkgo biloba for intermittent claudication. *Cochrane Database of Systematic Reviews*, Issue 2. Art. No.: CD006888. DOI: 10.1002/14651858.CD006888.pub2.

NOS (2010) The website of the National Osteoporosis Society, www.nos.org.uk.

NRC (National Research Council) (1989) *Recommended Dietary Allowances*. 10th edn. National Academy of Sciences, Washington, DC.

Oduyebo, O.O., Anorlu, R.I. & Ogunsola, F.T. (2009) The effects of antimicrobial therapy on bacterial vaginosis in non-pregnant women. *Cochrane Database of Systematic Reviews*, Issue 3. Art. No.: CD006055. DOI: 10.1002/14651858.CD006055.pub2.

Oliver, M.F. (1981) Diet and coronary heart disease. *British Medical Bulletin*, 37, 49–58.

Omenn, G.S., Goodman, G.E., Thornquist, M.D., Balmes, J., Cullen, M.R. *et al.* (1996) Combination of beta-carotene and vitamin A on lung cancer and cardiovascular disease. *New England Journal of Medicine*, 334, 1150–5.

Oosthuizen, W., Virster, H.H., Vermaak, W.J., Smuts, C.M., Jerling, J.C. *et al.* (1998) Lecithin has no effect on serum lipoprotein, plasma fibrinogen and macro molecular protein complex levels in hyperlipidaemic men in a double-blind controlled study. *European Journal of Clinical Nutrition*, 52, 419–24.

Osborn, D.A. & Sinn, J.K.H. (2006) Soy formula for prevention of allergy and food intolerance in infants. *Cochrane Database of Systematic Reviews*, Issue 4. Art. No.: CD003741. DOI: 10.1002/14651858.CD003741.pub4.

Osborn, D.A. & Sinn, J.K.H. (2007a) Probiotics in infants for prevention of allergic disease and food hypersensitivity. *Cochrane Database of Systematic Reviews*, Issue 4. Art. No.: CD006475. DOI: 10.1002/14651858.CD006475.pub2.

Osborn, D.A. & Sinn, J.K.H. (2007b) Prebiotics in infants for prevention of allergic disease and food hypersensitivity. *Cochrane Database of Systematic Reviews*, Issue 4. Art. No.: CD006474. DOI: 10.1002/14651858.CD006474.pub2.

Palframan, R., Gibson, G.R. & Rastall, R.A. (2003) Development of a quantitative tool for comparison of the prebiotic effects of dietary oligosaccharides. *Letters in Applied Microbiology*, 37, 281–4.

Paolini, M., Cantelli-Forti, G., Perocco, P., Pedulli, G.F., Abdel-Rahman, S.Z. *et al.* (1999) Co-carcinogenic effect of β-carotene. *Nature*, 398, 760–61.

Papakostas, G.I. (2009) Evidence for S-adenosyl-L-methionine (SAM-e) for the treatment of major depressive disorder. *Journal of Clinical Psychiatry*, 70(Suppl 5), 18–22.

Parker, J., Hashmi, O., Dutton, D., Mavrodaris, A., Stranges, S. *et al.* (2010) Levels of vitamin D and cardiometabolic disorders: Systematic review and meta-analysis. *Maturitas*, 65, 225–36.

Parrott, A., Morinan, A., Moss, M. & Scholey, A. (2004) *Understanding Drugs and Behaviour.* John Wiley, Chichester.

Pavelka, K., Gatterova, J., Olejarova, M., Machacek, S., Giacovelli, G. *et al.* (2002) Glucosamine sulphate use and delay of progression of knee osteoarthritis: A 3-year, randomized, placebo-controlled, double-blind study. *Archives of Internal Medicine*, 162, 2113–23.

Phillips, F. (2003) *Diet and Bone Health. Fair-Flow 4 Synthesis Report.* INRA: Paris. Available at www.functionalfoodnet.eu/images/site/assets/a-Diet%20and%20bone%20 health-hp-syn5.pdf.

Pilz, S., Tomaschitz, A., Ritz, E. & Pieber, T.R. (2009) Vitamin D status and arterial hypertension: A systematic review. *Nature Reviews Cardiology*, 6, 621–30.

Pirotta, M., Gunn, J., Chondros, P., Grover, S., Hurley, S. *et al.* (2004) Effect of lactobacillus in preventing post-antibiotic vulvovaginal candidiasis: A randomised controlled trial. *British Medical Journal*, 329, 548.

Pittler, M.H., Abbot, N.C., Harkness, E.F. & Ernst, E. (1999) Randomized, double-blind trial of chitosan for body weight reduction. *European Journal of Clinical Nutrition*, 53, 379–81.

Plat, J. & Mensink, R.P. (2005) Plant stanol and sterol esters in the control of blood cholesterol levels: Mechanism and safety aspects. *American Journal of Cardiology*, 96(1A), 15D–22D.

Poston, L., Briley, A.L., Seed, P.T., Kelly, F.J. & Shennan, E.H. (2006) Vitamin C and vitamin E in pregnant women at risk for pre-eclampsia (VIP trial): Randomised placebo-controlled trial. *Lancet*, 367, 1145–54.

Prentice, A. (1997) Is nutrition important in osteoporosis? *Proceedings of the Nutrition Society*, 56, 357–67.

Prior, R.L. (2006) Phytochemicals. In: *Modern Nutrition in Health and Disease* (eds M.E. Shils, M. Shike & J. Olson). 10th edn. pp. 582–612. Lippincott, Williams and Wilkins, Philadelphia.

PWC 2009 Leveraging growth in the emerging functional foods industry: trends and market opportunities. PricewaterhouseCoopers, Delaware. www.pwc.com/us/en/transaction-services/publications/functional-foods.jhtml.

Rambaldi, A., Jacobs, B.P. & Gluud, C. (2007) Milk thistle for alcoholic and/or hepatitis B or C virus liver diseases. *Cochrane Database of Systematic Reviews*, Issue 4. Art. No.: CD003620. DOI: 10.1002/14651858.CD003620.pub3.

Rao, C.V., Desai, D., Simi, B., Kulkarni, N., Amin, S. *et al.* (1993) Inhibitory effect of caffeic acid esters on azoxymethane-induced biochemical changes and aberrant crypt loci formation in rat colon. *Cancer Research*, 53, 4182–8.

Rapala, J.M., Virtamo, J., Ripatti, S., Huttunen, J.K., Albanes, D. *et al.* (1997) Randomised trial of alpha-tocopherol and beta-carotene supplements on incidence of major coronary events in men with previous myocardial infarction. *Lancet*, 349, 1715–20.

Ray, J.G., Meier, C., Vermeulen, M.J., Boss, S., Wyatt, P.R. *et al.* (2002) Association of neural tube defects and folic acid food fortification in Canada. *Lancet*, 360, 2047–8.

Raz, R. & Gobis, L. (2009) Essential fatty acids and attention-deficit-hyperactivity disorder: A systematic review. *Developmental Medicine and Child Neurology*, 51, 580–92.

Rebouche, C.J. (2006) Carnitine. In: *Modern Nutrition in Health and Disease* (eds M.E. Shils, M.Shike & J. Olson) 10th edn. pp. 537–44. Lippincott, Williams and Wilkins, Philadelphia.

Record Trial Group (2005) Oral vitamin D_3 and calcium for secondary prevention of low-trauma fractures in elderly people (Randomised Evaluation of Calcium Or Vitamin S, RECORD): A randomised placebo-controlled trial. *The Lancet*, **365**, 1621–8.

Reddy, B.S. (1998) Prevention of colon cancer by pre- and probiotics: Evidence from laboratory studies. *British Journal of Nutrition*, **80**, S219–23.

Reginster, J.Y., Deroisy, R., Rovati, L.C., Lee, R.L., Lejeune, E. *et al.* (2001) Long-term effects of glucosamine sulphate on osteoarthritis progression: A randomised, placebo-controlled clinical trial. *The Lancet*, **357**, 251–6.

Reid, G., Burton, J. & Devillard, E. (2004) The rationale for probiotics in female urogenital healthcare. *Medscape General Medicine*, **6**(1), 49.

Rice, S. & Whitehead, S.A. (2006) Phyto-estrogens and breast cancer – promoters or protectors? *Endocrine-Related Cancer*, **13**, 995–1015.

Richardson, A.J. & Montgomery, P. (2005) The Oxford-Durham Study: A randomized controlled trial of dietary supplementation with fatty acids in children with developmental coordination disorder. *Pediatrics*, **115**, 1360–66.

Richmond, C. (2003) Obituary for David Horrobin. *British Medical Journal*, **326**, 885.

Richmond, V.L. (1986) Incorporation of methylsulfonylmethane sulphur into guinea pig serum proteins. *Life Sciences*, **39**, 263–8.

Riemersma, R.A., Wood, D.A., Macintyre, C.C.A., Elton, R.A., Gey, K.F. *et al.* (1991) Risk of angina pectoris and plasma concentrations of vitamins A, C, and E and carotene. *The Lancet*, **337**, 1–5.

Rimm, E.B., Stampfer, M.J., Ascheirio, A., Giovannucci, E.L., Colditz, G.A. *et al.* (1993) Vitamin E consumption and the risk of coronary heart disease in men. *New England Journal of Medicine*, **328**, 1450–55.

Roberfroid, M.B. (1998) Prebiotics and synbiotics: Concepts and nutritional properties. *British Journal of Nutrition*, **80**, S197–S202.

Roche, H.M., Noone, E., Nugent, A. & Gibney, M.J. (2001) Conjugated linoleic acid: A novel therapeutic nutrient? *Nutrition Research Reviews*, **14**, 173–87.

Ronca, G. & Conte, A. (1993) Metabolic fate of partially depolymerised shark chondroitin sulphate in man. *International Journal of Clinical Pharmacology Research*, **13**(Suppl.), 27–34.

Rosell, M., Wesley, A.M., Rydin, K., Klareskog, L. & Alfredsson, L. (2009) Dietary fish and fish oil and the risk of rheumatoid arthritis. *Epidemiology*, **20**, 896–901.

RTS (2005) *The European Market for Probiotics and Prebiotics*. RTS Resource Ltd, Wolverhampton. Available free online at www.ingredientsdirectory.com/reports/report2.pdf.

Rude, R.K. & Shils, M.E. (2006) Magnesium. In: *Modern Nutrition in Health and Disease* (eds M.E. Shils, M. Shike & J. Olson). 10th edn. pp. 23–47. Lippincott, Williams and Wilkins, Philadelphia.

Rumbold, A., Duley, L., Crowther, C.A. & Haslam, R.R. (2008) Antioxidants for preventing pre-eclampsia. *Cochrane Database of Systematic Reviews*, Issue 1. Art. No.: CD004227. DOI: 10.1002/14651858.CD004227.pub3.

Rutjes, A.W.S., Nüesch, E., Reichenbach, S. & Jüni, P. (2009) S-Adenosylmethionine for osteoarthritis of the knee or hip. *Cochrane Database of Systematic Reviews*, Issue 4. Art. No.: CD007321. DOI: 10.1002/14651858.CD007321.pub2.

Saavedra, J.M., Abi-Hanna, A., Moore, N. & Yolken, R.H. (2004) Long term consumption of infant formula containing live probiotic bacteria: Tolerance and safety. *American Journal of Clinical Nutrition*, **79**, 261–7.

Sacks, F.M., Willet, W.C., Smith, A., Brown, L.E., Rosner, B. *et al.* (1998) Effect on blood pressure of potassium, calcium and magnesium in women with low habitual intake. *Hypertension*, **31**, 131–8.

Salas-Salvado, J., Marquez-Sandoval, F. & Bullo, M. (2006) Conjugated linoleic acid intake in humans: A systematic review focusing on its effect on body composition, glucose, and lipid metabolism. *Critical Reviews in Food Science and Nutrition*, **46**, 479–88.

Sanders, T.A.B., Mistry, M. & Naismith, D.J. (1984) The influence of a maternal diet rich in linoleic acid on brain and retinal docosahexaenoic acid in the rat. *British Journal of Nutrition*, **51**, 57–66.

Sangkomkamhang, T., Sangkomkamhang, U.S. & Ngamjarus, C. (2010) Vitamin K for the prevention and treatment of osteoporosis in post-menopausal women (Protocol). *Cochrane Database of Systematic Reviews*, Issue 1. Art. No.: CD008329. DOI: 10.1002/14651858. CD008329.

Satia, J.A., Littman, A., Slatore, C.G., Galanko, J.A. & White, E. (2009) Associations of herbal and speciality supplements with lung and colorectal cancer risk in the VITamins and Lifestyle study. *Cancer Epidemiology, Biomarkers and Prevention*, **14**, 1419–28.

Schellenberg, R. (2001) Treatment for the premenstrual syndrome with agnus castus fruit extract: Prospective, randomised, placebo controlled study. *British Medical Journal*, **322**, 134–7.

Senok, A.C., Verstraelen, H., Temmerman, M. & Botta, G.A. (2009) Probiotics for the treatment of bacterial vaginosis. *Cochrane Database of Systematic Reviews*, Issue 4. Art. No.: CD006289. DOI: 10.1002/14651858.CD006289.pub2.

Shekelle, P., Morton, S. & Hardy, M. (2003) *Effect of Supplemental Antioxidants Vitamin C, Vitamin E, and Coenzyme Q$_{10}$ for the Prevention and Treatment of Cardiovascular Disease*. Evidence report/technology assessment No.83. Rockville MD: Agency for Health care Research and Quality. Available free online at www.ncbi.nlm.nih.gov/books/bv. fcgi?rid=hstat1a.chapter.16082.

Shepherd, J., Cobbe, S.M., Forde, I., Isles, J.C., Lorimer, A.R. *et al.* (1995) Prevention of coronary heart disease with pravastatin in men with hypercholesteremia. *New England Journal of Medicine*, **333**, 130–37.

Shikhman, A.R., Kuhn, K., Alaaeddine, N. & Lotz, M. (2001) N-Acetylglucosamine prevents IL-1β-mediated activation of human chondrocytes. *Journal of Immunology*, **166**, 5155–60.

Shils, M.E., Shike, M., Ross, A.C., Caballero, B. & Cousins, R.J. (2006) *Modern Nutrition in Health and Disease*. 10th edn. Lippincott, Williams and Wilkins, Philadelphia.

Silwinski, L., Folwarczna, J., Janiec, W., Grynkiewicz, G., Kuzyk, K. (2005) Differential effects of genistein, estradiol and raloxifene on rat osteoclasts in vitro. *Pharmacological Reports*, **57**, 352–9.

Singh, U. & Jiala, I. (2008) Alpha-lipoic acid supplementation and diabetes. *Nutrition Reviews*, **66**, 646–57.

Sircus, W. (1972) Carbenoxolone sodium. *Gut*, **13**, 816–24.

Smith, G.D., Song, F. & Sheldon, T.A. (1993) Cholesterol lowering and mortality: The importance of considering initial level of risk. *British Medical Journal*, **306**, 1367–73.

Smith, R. (2005) Investigating the previous studies of a fraudulent author. *British Medical Journal*, **331**, 288–91.

Smith, W.A., Fry, A.C., Tschume, L.C. & Bloomer, R.J. (2008) Effect of glycine propionyl-L-carnitine on aerobic and anaerobic exercise performance. *International Journal of Sport Nutrition and Exercise Metabolism*, **18**, 19–36.

Smolders, J. (2008) Vitamin D as an immune regulator in multiple sclerosis, a review. *Journal of Neuroimmunology*, **194**, 7–17.

Smolders, J., Damoiseaux, J., Menheere, P. & Hupperts, R. Vitamin D as an immune modulator in multiple sclerosis, a review. *Journal of Neuroimmunology*, **194**, 7–17.

Soh, S.E., Aw, M., Gerez, I., Chong, Y.S., Rauff, M. *et al.* (2009) Probiotic supplementation in the first 6 months of life in at risk Asian infants – effects on eczema and atopic sensitization at the age of 1 year. *Clinical and Experimental Allergy*, **39**, 571–8.

Soja, A.M. & Mortensen, S.A. (1997) Treatment of congestive heart failure with coenzyme Q10 illuminated by meta-analyses of clinical trials. *Clinical Aspects of Medicine*, 18(Suppl.), S159–68.

Sperber, S.J., Shah, L.P., Gilbert, R.D., Ritchey, T.W. & Monto, A.S. (2004) Echinacea purpurea for the prevention of experimental rhinovirus colds. *Clinical Infectious Disease*, **38**, 1367–71.

Srivastava, A, Mansel, R.E., Arvind, N., Prasad, K., Dhar, A. *et al.* (2007) Evidence-based management of Mastalgia: A meta-analysis of randomised trials. *Breast*, **16**, 503–12.

SSSS Group (Scandinavian Simvastatin Survival Study Group) (1994) Randomised trial of cholesterol lowering in 4444 patients with coronary heart disease: The Scandinavian Simvastatin Survival Study (4S). *The Lancet*, **344**, 1383–9.

Stammers, T., Sibbald, B. & Freeling, P. (1992) Efficacy of cod liver oil as an adjunct to non-steroidal anti-inflammatory drug treatment in the management of osteoarthritis in general practice. *Annals of Rheumatic Disease*, **51**, 128–9.

Stampfer, M.J., Hennekens, C.H., Manson, J.E., Colditz, G.A., Rosner, B. *et al.* (1993) Vitamin E consumption and the risk of coronary disease in women. *New England Journal of Medicine*, **328**, 1444–9.

Stephens, N.G., Parsons, A., Schofield, P.M., Kelly, F., Cheeseman, K. *et al.* (1996) Randomised controlled trial of vitamin E in patients with coronary disease: Cambridge Heart Antioxidant Study {CHAOS}. *The Lancet*, **347**, 781–6.

Stewart, J.J., Wood, M.J., Wood, C.D. & Mims, M.E. (1991) Effects of ginger on motion sickness susceptibility and gastric function. *Pharmacology*, **42**, 111–20.

Sutton, A.J., Duval, S.V., Tweedie, R.L., Abrams, K.R. & Jones, D.R. (2000) Empirical assessment of effect of publication bias on meta-analyses. *British Medical Journal*, **320**, 1574–7.

Szajewska, H. & Mrukowicz, J.Z. (2001) Probiotics in the treatment and prevention of acute infectious diarrhea in infants and children: A systematic review of published randomized, double-blind, placebo-controlled trials. *Journal of Pediatric Gastroenterology and Nutrition*, 33(Suppl. 2), S17–25.

Tacklind, J., MacDonald, R., Rutks, I. & Wilt, T.J. (2009) Serenoa repens for benign prostatic hyperplasia. *Cochrane Database of Systematic Reviews*, Issue 2. Art. No.: CD001423. DOI: 10.1002/14651858.CD001423.pub2.

Tanamaly, M.D., Tadros, F., Labeeb, S., Makld, H., Nessim, D. *et al.* (2004) Randomised double-blinded trial evaluating silymarin for chronic hepatitis C in an Egyptian village: Study description and 12-month results. *Digestive and Liver Diseases*, **36**, 752–9.

Taylor, G.R. & Williams, C.M. (1998) Effects of probiotics and prebiotics on blood lipids. *British Journal of Nutrition*, **80**, S225–30.

Taylor, J.A., Weber, W., Standish, L., Quinn, H., Goesling, J. *et al.* (2003) Efficacy and safety of Echinacea in treating upper respiratory tract infections in children. *Journal of the American Medical Association*, **290**, 2824–30.

Thal, L.J., Calvani, M., Amato, A. & Carta, A. (2000) A 1-year controlled trial of acetyl-l-carnitine in early-onset AD. *Neurology*, **55**, 805–10.

Thal, L.J., Carta, A., Clarke, W.R., Ferris, S.H., Friedland, R.P. *et al.* (1996) A 1-year multicenter placebo-controlled study of acetyl-L-carnitine in patients with Alzheimer's disease. *Neurology*, **47**, 705–11.

Thien, F.C., Leung, R., Baldo, B.A., Weiner, J.A., Plomley, R. *et al.* (1996) Asthma and anaphylaxis induced by royal jelly. *Clinical and Experimental Allergy*, **26**, 216–22.

Thomas, J.A. (2006) Oxidant defense in oxidative and nitrosative stress. In: *Modern Nutrition in Health and Disease* (eds M.E. Shils, M. Shike & J. Olson) 10th edn. pp. 685–94. Lippincott, Williams and Wilkins, Philadelphia.

Towheed, T., Maxwell, L., Anastassiades, T.P., Shea, B., Houpt, J. *et al.* (2005) Glucosamine therapy for treating osteoarthritis. *Cochrane Database of Systematic Reviews*, Issue 2. Art. No.: CD002946. DOI: 10.1002/14651858.CD002946.pub2.

Tung, J.M., Dolovich, L.R. & Lee, C.H. (2009) Prevention of Clostridium difficile infection with Saccharomyces boulardii: A systematic review. *Canadian Journal of Gastroenterology*, **23**, 817–21.

Turner, E.H., Mathews, A.M., Lindaratos, E. Tell, R.A. & Rosenthal, R. (2008) Selective publication of antidepressant trials and its influence on apparent efficacy, *New England Journal of Medicine*, **358**, 252–60.

Turnlund, J.R. (2006) Copper. In: *Modern Nutrition in Health and Disease* (eds M.E. Shils, M. Shike & J. Olson). 10th edn. pp. 286–99. Lippincott, Williams and Wilkins, Philadelphia.

USP (2010) Entry for saw palmetto, *United States Pharmacoepia*. www.usp.org/USPVerified/dietarySupplements/sawpalmetto.html.

Valenzuela, A. & Garrido, A. (1994) Biochemical bases of the pharmacological action of the flavonoid silymarin and of its structural isomer silibinin. *Biological Research*, **27**, 105–12.

Valtuena, S., Cashman, K., Robins, S.P., Cassidy, A., Kardinaal, A. *et al.* (2003) Investigating the role of phyto-oestrogens on bone health in postmenopausal women. *British Journal of Nutrition*, **89**(Suppl. 1), S87–99.

Van Etten, E., Decallonne, B. & Mathieu, C. (2002) 1,25-dihydroxycholecalciferol: endocrinology meets the immune system. *Proceedings of the Nutrition Society*, **61**, 375–80.

Van Gool, C.J., Zeegers, M.P. & Thils, C. (2004) Oral essential fatty acid supplementation in atopic dermatitis: A meta-analysis of placebo-controlled trials. *British Journal of Dermatology*, **150**, 728–40.

Vickers, A., Goyal, N., Harland, R. & Rees, R. (1998) Do certain countries produce only positive results? A systematic review of controlled trials. *Controlled Clinical Trials*, **19**, 159–66.

Viera, A.J. (2003) Management of carpal tunnel syndrome. *American Family Physician*, July 15. Available online at www.aafp.org/afp/20030715/265.html.

Vincent, A. & Fitzpatrick, L.A. (2000) Soy isoflavones: Are they useful in menopause? *Mayo Clinic Proceedings*, **75**, 1174–84.

Vittek, J. (1995) Effect of royal jelly on serum lipids in experimental and humans with atherosclerosis. *Experientia*, **51**, 927–35.

Vivekanathan, D.P., Penn, M.S., Sapp, S.K., Hsu, A. & Toppol, E.J. (2003) Use of antioxidant vitamins for the prevention of cardiovascular disease: Meta-analysis of randomised trials. *The Lancet*, **361**, 2017–23.

Vlaming, S., Biehler, A., Hennessy, E.M., Jamieson, C.P., Chattophadhyay, S. *et al.* (2001) Should the food intake of patients admitted to acute hospital services be routinely supplemented? A randomised placebo controlled trial. *Clinical Nutrition*, **20**, 517–26.

Vockley, J. & Renaud, D.L. (2006) Inherited metabolic diseases: Defects of β-oxidation. In: *Modern Nutrition in Health and Disease* (eds M.E. Shils, M. Shike & J. Olson). 10th edn. pp. 960–78. Lippincott, Williams and Wilkins, Philadelphia.

Vogel, G., Tuchweber, N. & Trost, W. (1984) Protection by silibinin against Amanita phalloides intoxication in beagles. *Toxicology and Applied Pharmacology*, 73, 355–62.

Vogler, B.K. & Ernst, E. (1999) Aloe vera: A systematic review of its clinical effectiveness. *British Journal of General Practice*, 49, 823–8.

Volpi, N. (2003) Oral absorption and bioavailability of ichthyic origin chondroitin sulphate in healthy male volunteers. *Osteoarthritis and Cartilage*, 11, 433–41.

Volpi, N. (2009) Quality of different chondroitin sulphate preparations in relation to their therapeutic activity. *Journal of Pharmacy and Pharmacology*, 61, 1271–80.

Wang, C., Chung, M., Lichtenstein, A., Balk, E., Kulpenick, B. *et al.* (2004) *Effects of Omega-3 Fatty Acids on Cardiovascular Disease*. Evidence Report/Technology Assessment No. 94. AHRQ Publication No. 04-E009–2. Rockville, MD: Agency for Healthcare Research and Quality. www.ncbi.nlm.nih.gov/books/bv.fcgi?rid=hstat1a.chapter.38290.

Wang, C., Harris, W.S., Chung, M., Lichtenstein, A., Balk, E.M. *et al.* (2006) n-3 Fatty acids from fish or fish oil supplements, but not alpha-linolenic acid, benefit cardiovascular disease outcomes in primary and secondary prevention studies: A systematic review. *American Journal of Clinical Nutrition*, 84, 5–17.

Wang, X.D., Liu, C., Bronson, R.T., Smith, D.E., Krinsky, N.I. *et al.* (1999) Retinoid signalling and activator protein-1 expression in ferrets given beta-carotene supplements and exposed to tobacco smoke. *Journal of the National Cancer Institute*, 91, 7–9.

Warri, A., Saarinen, N.M., Makela, S. & Hilakivi-Clarke, L. (2008) The role of genistein exposures in modifying breast cancer risk. *British Journal of Cancer*, 98, 1485–93.

Watanabe, F., Katsura, H., Takenaka, S., Fujita, T., Abe, K. *et al.* (1999) Pseudovitamin B_{12} is the predominant cobalamin of an algal health food, Spirulina tablets. *Journal of Agricultural and Food Chemistry*, 47, 4736–41.

WCRF/AICR (World Cancer Research Fund/American Institute for Cancer Research) (2007) *Food, Nutrition, Physical Activity, and the Prevention of Cancer: A Global Perspective*. Washington, DC: American Institute for Cancer Research.

Webb, G.P. (1992) Viewpoint II: Small animals as models for studies on human nutrition. In: *Nutrition and the Consumer* (ed. A.F. Walker & B.A. Rolls). pp. 279–97. London: Elsevier Applied Science.

Webb, G.P. (2001) Nutritional supplements: Benefits and risks. *Nursing and Residential Care*, 3, 477–81.

Webb, G.P. (2007) Nutritional supplements and conventional medicine: What should the physician know? *Proceedings of the Nutrition Society*, 66, 471–8.

Webb, G.P. (2008) *Nutrition: A Health Promotion Approach*. 3rd edn. London: Hodder Arnold.

Webb, G.P. (2009) Interpreting nutritional science: What have we learnt from the past? *British Nutrition Foundation Nutrition Bulletin*, 34, 309–15.

Werneke, U., Horn, O. & Taylor, D.M. (2004) How effective is St John's wort? The evidence revisited. *Journal of Clinical Psychiatry*, 65, 611–17.

Whiskey, E., Werneke, U. & Taylor, D. (2001) A systematic review and meta-analysis of Hypericum perforatum in depression: A comprehensive clinical review. *International Clinical Psychopharmacology*, 16, 239–52.

White, B. (2007) Ginger: An overview. *American Family Physician*, 75, 1689–91.

WHO (1970) *Fluorides and Human Health*. World Health Organization monographs series No 59. World Health Organization, Geneva.

Wickens, K., Black, P.N., Stanley, T.V., Mitchell, E., Fitzharris, P. *et al.* (2008) A differential effect of 2 probiotics in the prevention of eczema and atopy: A double-blind, randomized, placebo-controlled trial. *Journal of Allergy and Clinical Immunology*, 122, 788–94.

Williams, H.C. (2003) Evening primrose oil for atopic dermatitis. *British Medical Journal*, 327, 1358–9.

Wilson, J.H. (1994) Nutrition, physical activity and bone health in women. *Nutrition Research Reviews*, 7, 67–91.

Wilt, T.J., Ishani, A., Stark, G., MacDonald, R., Lau, J. *et al.* (1998) Saw palmetto extracts for treatment of benign prostatic hyperplasia: A systematic review. *Journal of the American Medical Association*, 280, 1604–9.

Wilt, T., Ishani, A., MacDonald, R., Stark, G., Mulrow, C. *et al.* (1999) Beta-sitosterols for benign prostatic hyperplasia. *Cochrane Database of Systematic Reviews*, Issue 3. Art. No.: CD001043. DOI: 10.1002/14651858.CD001043.

Wilt, T.J., Ishani, A., Stark, G., MacDonald, R., Lau, J. *et al.* (2000) Serenoa repens for benign prostatic hyperplasia. *Cochrane Database of Systematic Reviews*, Issue 3. Art. No. CD001423.

Wilt, T.J., Ishani, A. & MacDonald, R. (2002) Serenoa repens for benign prostatic hyperplasia. *Cochrane Database of Systematic Reviews*, Issue 3. Art. No. CD001423.

Winzenberg, T.M., Shaw, K.A., Fryer, J. & Jones, G. (2006) Calcium supplementation for improving bone mineral density in children. *Cochrane Database of Systematic Reviews*, Issue 2. Art. No.: CD005119. DOI: 10.1002/14651858.CD005119.pub2.

Wood, C.D., Manno, J.E., Wood, M.J., Manno, B.R. & Mims, M.E. (1988) Comparison of efficacy of ginger with various antimotion sickness drugs. *Clinical Research Practices and Drug Regulatory Affairs*, 6, 129–36.

Wyatt, K.M., Dimmock, P.W., Jones, P.W. & O'Brien, P.M.S. (1999) Efficacy of Vitamin B₆ in the treatment of premenstrual syndrome: systematic review. *British Medical Journal*, 318: 1375–81.

Yale, S.H. & Liu, K. (2004(*Echinacea purpurea* therapy for the treatment of the common cold: A randomized, double-blind, placebo-controlled trial. *Archives of Internal Medicine*, 164, 1237–41.

Yates, A.A. (2006) Dietary reference intakes: Rationale and applications. In: *Modern Nutrition in Health and Disease* (eds M.E. Shils, M. Shike & J. Olson). 10th edn. pp. 1655–72. Lippincott, Williams and Wilkins, Philadelphia.

Yeh, G.Y., Eisenberg, D.M., Kaptchuk, T.J. & Phillips, R.S. (2003) Systematic review of herbs and dietary supplements for glycaemic control in diabetes. *Diabetes Care*, 26, 1277–94.

Yuan, C.S., Wei, G., Dey, L., Karrison, T., Nahlik, L. *et al.* (2004) Brief communication: American ginseng reduces warfarin's effect in healthy patients: a randomized, controlled trial. *Annals of Internal Medicine*, 141, 23–7.

Yun, T.K. (2001) Panax ginseng – a non-organ-specific cancer preventative? *Lancet Oncology*, 2, 49–55.

Yun, T.K. & Choi, S.Y. (1998) Non-organ specific cancer prevention of ginseng: A prospective study in Korea. *International Journal of Epidemiology*, 27, 359–64. Free full text available at http://ije.oupjournals.org/cgi/reprint/27/3/359.

Zeisel, S.H. & Niculescu, M.D. (2006) Choline and phosphatidylcholine. In: *Modern Nutrition in Health and Disease* (eds M.E. Shils, M Shike & J Olson). 10th edn. pp. 525–36. Lippincott, Williams and Wilkins, Philadelphia.

Zhou, S. Chan, E, Pan, S.Q., Huang, M., Lee, E.J. (2004) Pharmacokinetic interactions of drugs with St John's wort. *Journal of Psychopharmacology*, 18, 262–76.

Ziegler, D., Reljanovic, M., Mehnert, H. & Gries, F.A. (1999) Alpha-lipoic acid in the treatment of diabetic neuropathy in Germany: Current evidence from clinical trials. *Experimental and Clinical Endocrinology and Diabetes*, 107, 421–30.

Ziegler, R.G. (1991) Vegetables, fruits and carotenoids and the risk of cancer. *American Journal of Clinical Nutrition*, 53, 251S–9S.

Zimmermann, M. & Delange, F. (2004) Iodine supplements of pregnant women in Europe: A review and recommendations. *European Journal of Clinical Nutrition*, 58, 979–84.

Zipitis, C.S. & Akobeng, A.K. (2008) Vitamin D supplementation in early childhood and risk of type 1 diabetes: A systematic review and meta-analysis. *Archives of Disease in Childhood*, 93, 512–17.

Index

Dietary Supplements and Functional Foods, 2nd Edition. Geoffrey P. Webb.
© 2011 Blackwell Publishing Ltd.